Artificial Intelligence for Bone Disorder

Scrivener Publishing
100 Cummings Center, Suite 541J
Beverly, MA 01915-6106

Publishers at Scrivener
Martin Scrivener (martin@scrivenerpublishing.com)
Phillip Carmical (pcarmical@scrivenerpublishing.com)

Artificial Intelligence for Bone Disorder

Diagnosis and Treatment

Rishabha Malviya
School of Pharmacy, Galgotias University, Greater Noida, India
Shivam Rajput
School of Pharmacy, Galgotias University, Greater Noida, India
and
Makarand Vaidya
Hindu Rao Hospital, New Delhi, India

Scrivener Publishing

WILEY

This edition first published 2024 by John Wiley & Sons, Inc., 111 River Street, Hoboken, NJ 07030, USA and Scrivener Publishing LLC, 100 Cummings Center, Suite 541J, Beverly, MA 01915, USA

For more information about Scrivener publications please visit www.scrivenerpublishing.com.

Wiley Global Headquarters
111 River Street, Hoboken, NJ 07030, USA

For details of our global editorial offices, customer services, and more information about Wiley products visit us at www.wiley.com.

Library of Congress Cataloging-in-Publication Data

ISBN 978-1-394-23088-4

Cover image: Pixabay.Com
Cover design by Russell Richardson

Set in size of 11pt and Minion Pro by Manila Typesetting Company, Makati, Philippines

Printed in the USA

10 9 8 7 6 5 4 3 2 1

Contents

Foreword

I am delighted to introduce the book "Artificial Intelligence for Bone Disorder: Diagnosis and Treatment," authored by Dr. Rishabha Malviya. This extensive collection of reports explores the relationship between artificial intelligence and bone problems, illuminating how AI can revolutionize orthopedics and radiology.

It is becoming increasingly apparent as we negotiate the changing landscape of healthcare that new technologies have enormous potential to revolutionize patient care. The integration of artificial intelligence, in particular, into the diagnosis and treatment of bone problems gives an intriguing prospect for improvements in healthcare. Artificial intelligence has emerged as a potent tool in many fields.

This book covers a wide range of issues. It thoroughly investigates how artificial intelligence can improve knowledge and management of bone fractures, tissue engineering for bone regeneration, deep supervised learning for fracture classification, treatment for osteoporosis, orthopedic care, treatment of spinal disorders, pediatric orthopedics, and diagnosis of bone cancer.

This book will be an essential tool for academicians, students, and healthcare professionals. The book offers a road map for utilizing the promise of artificial intelligence to enhance patient outcomes by digging into the complexities of AI algorithms, deep learning techniques, and their application to bone problems.

I appreciate Dr. Rishabha Malviya and all the authors who contributed to this important work with their commitment and knowledge. I am confident that "Artificial Intelligence for Bone Disorder: Diagnosis and Treatment" will inspire additional investigation and progress in the application of AI in bone healthcare, ultimately proving beneficial to patients and medical professionals worldwide.

I am assured that readers will find this book fascinating and informative information that encourages future research, collaborative efforts, and innovations in bone disorder diagnosis and treatment.

Dr. (Prof.) Seifedine Kadry
Professor
Noroff University College, Norway
FIET, SMIEEE, ACM

Preface

Healthcare is one of several sectors that Artificial Intelligence (AI) is revolutionizing. In recent years, AI has demonstrated incredible potential for transforming the diagnosis and management of a wide range of medical diseases. The field of bone problems is one area where AI has a lot of potential.

This book looks into the blending of AI and bone health care. It addresses the various uses of AI in the diagnosis and treatment of bone fractures, tissue engineering, orthopedic care, spinal problems, pediatric orthopedics, bone disease prediction, and imaging for bone cancer through a careful selection of chapters.

Thanks to a thorough analysis of the relationship between bone problems and artificial intelligence, the reader will gain unmatched insight into the most recent developments and prospects. This comprehensive volume proceeds from introductory chapters that provide a foundation in bone fracture detection and tissue engineering to an in-depth examination of the application of AI in particular domains like orthopedics, radiology, and pediatrics orthopedics.

The authors' combined efforts have produced an invaluable resource that connects the fields of AI and bone treatment. The book provides essential insights into the current state and future of AI in bone condition diagnosis and therapy, as well as a methodical examination of machine learning algorithms, deep learning approaches, and their real-world uses.

May this book spark your interest, inspire your creativity, and motivate readers to take advantage of artificial intelligence's promise to advance bone health care and ultimately help people worldwide.

The Authors
October 2023

1

Artificial Intelligence and Bone Fracture Detection: An Unexpected Alliance

Abstract
Bone fractures are the most frequent type of injury sustained in accidents. Clinicians mostly use radiographs and CT (computed tomography) scans to diagnose fractures, yet it is frequently impossible to make a correct diagnosis only from images. Also, a lack of doctors in areas where healthcare is scarce, a lack of specialized medical staff in overpopulated hospitals, or pressure caused by a high workload may all make it more likely that a fracture will be misdiagnosed or not heal well. "Artificial intelligence" (AI) is the process of programming computers to act like smart people with little or no human interaction. Using computer vision and AI techniques like deep learning and machine learning for image processing is becoming more and more important for recognizing bone fractures. This chapter begins by discussing bane fracture and its different kinds. Consequently, the function and uses of AI in bone fracture are described. This chapter also discusses various algorithms based on machine learning and deep learning and their importance in bone fracture detection.

Keywords: Artificial intelligence, bone fracture, deep learning, machine learning, radiology, algorithm, fracture detection

1.1 Introduction

The term "artificial intelligence" (AI) is used to describe the practice of utilizing computers to simulate intelligent behavior with little or no input from humans [1]. In addition, recent advances in AI, and notably machine learning and deep learning, have allowed machines to significantly improve their ability to encode and interpret imaging data [2]. In medical science, AI is used for a wide variety of tasks, including symptom identification and radiological im age processing. Machine learning is the iterative process that artificial intelligence utilizes to improve in response to the training technique, further enhancing the outputs for judgments and predictions.

Rishabha Malviya, Shivam Rajput and Makarand Vaidya. Artificial Intelligence for Bone Disorder: Diagnosis and Treatment, (1–24) © 2024 Scrivener Publishing LLC

The learning process involves various types of learning [3]. One type of machine learning, supervised learning, trained itself to anticipate future outcomes using a set of known data [4]. To categorize newly entered data, a trained model is then applied to the data using a classification technique [5]. The resulting groups are then used to make judgments. Unsupervised learning methods are another option that can be utilized to generate judgments in situations where trained models are not available [6]. Data analysis, computation, and application are all part of the learning process [7, 8]. Training in data collection is a common definition of learning. Like how training is a combination of numerous techniques, deep learning is based on supervised and unsupervised learning as well as the use of networks like artificial neural networks. Artificial intelligence is a branch of computer science that automates the process of combing through enormous datasets in search of recurring patterns and trends, frequently in datasets that are utterly unrelated to one another, like medical imaging for the detection of fractures. The application of machine learning and deep learning techniques has significant advantages in the disciplines of image processing, computer visualization, and medicine.

Layered artificial neural networks are the building blocks of deep learning, a subfield of machine learning. Each layer is composed of a predetermined number of units, each of which is a condensed representation of a neuron cell based on the anatomy of neurons seen in the human brain [9]. In specialized tasks, deep learning algorithms can match and occasionally even surpass human performance [10, 11]. Information technology has been revolutionized by deep learning, which has made it possible to quickly solve large-scale, data-driven challenges. The automated classification and detection of proximal humerus fractures using a deep learning algorithm is a prime example of artificial intelligence (also known as machine intelligence) in action, as it uses numerous layers of network systems to obtain features to enhance the quality of perception and accuracy. Deep learning is essential for the computation and processing needed by artificial intelligence. Deep learning uses neural networks, which are made up of input layers and hidden layers, to carry out the necessary computations and processing [12]. As a result, deep neural networks have emerged as a promising tool for improving the efficiency and precision of medical picture diagnosis. Deep learning has been gaining popularity over the past few years [13]. Recent studies have shown that deep learning can do difficult interpretation at the same level as human medical professionals [14, 15]. In the field of orthopedic traumatology, several studies have been carried out using deep learning in radiography to diagnose fractures [16]. However, research on the application of deep learning to CT imaging of fractures is few.

Any kind of bone break, from the tiniest hairline to the most severe severing, is considered a fracture. Fractures can be either closed or open, depending on the severity of the damage. The amount of force required to cause a fracture varies [17]. Both the patient's age and the affected bone region play a role in the degree of severity. Orthopedics is the medical specialty concerned with damaged bones, also known as fractures. Bone fractures can occur in any orientation after being broken by an outside force or stimulation, including but not limited to the vertical, horizontal, and oblique planes. Failure to diagnose a fracture in a clinical setting where specialist knowledge is lacking can have serious effects and reduce the likelihood of a positive result.

In most cases, an X-ray can detect and identify any form of fracture. Fracture confirmation via computed tomography (CT) or magnetic resonance imaging (MRI) can be performed later. X-rays are an electromagnetic radiation-based imaging technology used to provide images of structures beneath the skin. The patient is positioned properly for X-ray imaging of the affected area. Computer tomography, more commonly known as a "CT scan," is a medical imaging technique that employs a combination of a computer as well as an X-ray machine to produce cross-sectional images as well as three-dimensional reconstruction visuals to improve diagnostic capability and image clarity. To create images, magnetic resonance imaging, often known as MRI, makes use of the paired as well as unpaired magnetic fields of the proton nucleus of hydrogen atoms in water, which is prevalent throughout the body. Even if a fracture has not yet caused any noticeable symptoms, an MRI can help find it—for example, stress-related fractures as well as fractures that occur in situations where imaging procedures such as X-rays and CT scans are dangerous to perform during pregnancy. As a result of recent developments in machine learning, it is now possible to employ computers to assist with medical diagnosis, ushering in a veritable renaissance in the scientific community. It uses up-to-date, cutting-edge methods and tools to give a rapid diagnosis with increased precision. If a fracture is not detected on an X-ray, the patient could suffer serious consequences that hinder their rehabilitation.

1.2 Bone Fracture

There are various ways to categorize fractures. Examples of traumatic fractures include those sustained in motor vehicle accidents, physical altercations, train mishaps, slips and falls, and similar occurrences. Bones that have been compromised by cancer metastasis (bony metastasis) or osteoporosis (increased porosity of the bone) are more likely to suffer a pathological fracture. Implant-related fractures occur at mechanical weak points brought on by persistent pressure. Children and teenagers may only have a partial fracture line since their bones are still growing. These fractures, often known as "greenstick fractures," are incomplete due to the failure of one tension cortex. Children may experience a deformation of the bone without a clear fracture line. Numerous other factors, such as fracture pattern, fragment displacement, dislocation or subluxation of adjacent joints, quantity of pieces, etc., can be used in the classification process. The following Table 1.1 summarizes the common breakdowns and compares them across several dimensions.

Figure 1.1 depicts the various types of fractures that might occur. The first type of fracture is known as a stable and closed fracture, and it occurs when the bone fragments are ruled into a straight line and are just slightly out of place. The second type of fracture is known as an open or compound fracture, and it occurs when a bone breaks and protrudes completely through the skin. The bone may be visible in certain circumstances and hidden in others. Afterward, a transverse fracture occurs. An example of a transverse fracture is one in which the fracture line runs at an angle to the body's longitudinal axis. Next is oblique fractures, also called multiple fractures since they occur at different angles. Furthermore, a comminuted fracture occurs when the bone breaks into more than two pieces. Subsequently, a condition known as greenstick fracture occurs when bone fractures but do not fully separate. Kids may feel this way. Finally, spiral fractures occur when a break in the bone progresses in a spiral pattern.

However, only X-rays can correctly identify a fracture [18], even though a visual deformity, particularly a large one, may be discernible to the human eye. To provide a comprehensive description of a fracture, the following information must be provided: the name of the bone, the region of the bone, the pattern of the fracture line, the presence or absence of compression, the existence or absence of displacement of fracture fragments, the type and degree of displacement, the presence or absence of any pre-existing pathology as well as the existence or absence of any associated joint pathology, such as dislocation or subluxation. This information can be found in Table 1.1.

1.3 Deep Learning and Its Significance in Radiology

The term "deep learning" (DL) is utilized to designate a collection of approaches employed in the discipline of machine learning and the much

Table 1.1 Comparison of fractures with diagnosis.

Type of fractures	Symptoms	Diagnosis	Consequences if missed	Possibility of correction
Stable and closed	Pain, swelling, loss of transmitted movements, slight or no deformity	X-rays	Angulation, pain	Yes
Open and compound	Pain, bleeding, open wound, loss of transmitted movements, crepitus, deformity	X-rays	Malunion, infection, non-union, septic arthritis, osteomyelitis, Volkmann's ischemia, compartment syndrome	Less
Transverse	Pain, deformity, swelling, crepitus, loss of transmitted movements	X-rays	Angulation, persistent, stiffness, deformity, malunion, shortening, non-union	Less
Oblique	Pain, deformity, swelling, crepitus, loss of transmitted movements	X-rays	Angulation, stiffness, persistent deformity, malunion, non-union, shortening	Less
Comminuted	Gross swelling, total loss of transmitted movements, severe pain, crepitus, gross deformity	X-rays	Compartment syndrome, neurovascular injury, Volkmann's ischemia, subdeck's osteodystrophy malunion, nonunion	Maybe or may not
Greenstick	Pain, deformity, swelling, restricted mobility, angulation	X-rays	Angulation, stiffness persistent deformity, malunion	Yes
Spiral	Pain, deformity, swelling, loss of transmitted movements	X-rays	Deformity, angulation	Yes

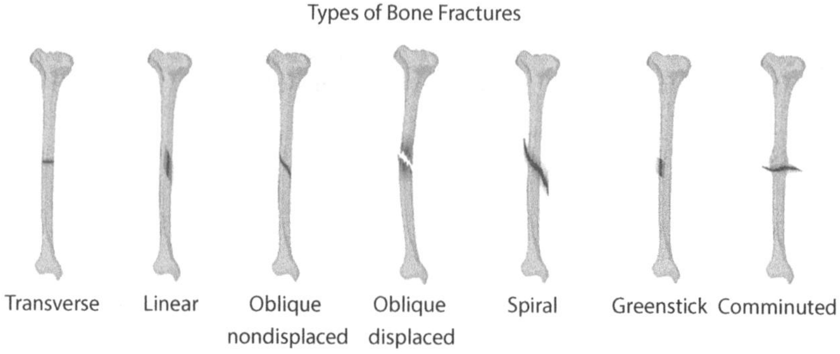

Figure 1.1 Different types of bone fracture.

broader subject of artificial intelligence. Both fields are subfields of the field of artificial intelligence. As a subfield of AI, deep learning is characterized by its reliance on simulated neural networks. The units, which are based on the architecture of the human brain, increase in number with each successive layer. The idea of deep learning revolutionized the field of information technology (IT) by providing large-scale answers to problems that had previously taken hours to resolve. The common goal of these algorithms is to comprehend the information at hand. For semantic image processing applications, deep learning has proven to be particularly effective [19].

Classification, segmentation, and noise reduction in medical images are just some of the many applications of DL approaches in use today. What is more, DL algorithms can learn from previous successes by using a technique known as transfer learning [20]. The significance of deep learning in radiology cannot be overstated. As a result, doctors will be able to give their patients better care and more accurate diagnosis. In the field of fracture diagnosis and localization on medical images such as radiographs and CT scans, deep learning achieves better results than humans under the current conditions [21].

1.4 Role of AI in Bone Fracture Detection and Its Application

As early as 1960, AI was being used to analyze X-ray pictures for medicinal purposes [22]. The data was initially converted to a numerical format for computation and analysis. Computer-aided detection was a later development in AI. Improvements in computational speed can be traced to the maturation of a system's ability to learn from past mistakes; this ability is known as machine learning. The advancement of AI systems in many fields is made possible through machine learning. AI models that undergo training and learning yield outcomes that are both more accurate and more efficient when applied to datasets [23, 24]. Artificial intelligence has proven very effective at sorting urgent situations from less urgent ones.

Bone fractures in X-rays can be identified by artificial intelligence systems that have been trained using machine learning methods. AI-enabled models can provide automatic diagnoses of bone fractures. When applied to X-ray pictures, a neural network that has been trained with appropriate data yields reliable findings. In addition, AI and, more specifically, deep learning, which includes neural networks, enhance the medical research area by allowing for enhanced visualization of imaging data. Bone fracture detection architecture development relies heavily on convolutional neural networks. It can produce results quickly and accurately.

Several studies have demonstrated that deep learning may be utilized to diagnose fractures [25] by undertaking a retrospective analysis to investigate the relevance of transfer learning using deep convolutional neural networks (CNNs), which had been pre-trained on photos that were not related to medicine, to the job of automating fracture recognition on plain wrist radiographs. The authors utilized the inception V3 convolutional neural network [26], which was trained for the IMageNet Large Visual Recognition Challenge on images other than radiography [27]. To complete the binary classification task, the top layer of the Inception V3 network was retrained with the help of a training dataset consisting of 1,389 radiographs annotated by humans. They were successful on the test dataset, with an area under the curve (AUC) of 0.95 (139 radiographs). This proved that the problem of fracture diagnosis on plain radiographs may be effectively applied to a CNN model pre-trained on non-medical pictures. Both the specificity and sensitivity were maximized at 0.90 and 0.88, respectively. Automated fracture analysis techniques like segmentation, edge recognition, and feature extraction have never been as accurate as they are now (prior studies only reported sensitivities and specificities in the 80%–85% range). There are still questions that need to be answered, even though this study proves the premise. At the end of the training phase, it was revealed that the accuracy of the training data and the accuracy of the validation data had a very minor but noticeable difference. Most likely, the problem was caused by excessive tailoring. There are a variety of approaches that can be taken to cut down on overfitting. It is possible to make the process of training more effective by eliminating the influence of attributes that are not important with automated segmentation of the most pertinent region of interest. One such strategy that could assist in lowering the incidence of overfitting is the application of cutting-edge augmentative approaches. In the realm of machine learning, another barrier that frequently arises is the size of the research sample [too small (1,000:10,000)]. The higher the size of the population that is being sampled, the more accurately it will reflect the overall population [28].

The researchers also employed plain AP (perfect anteroposterior) shoulder radiographs to investigate the effectiveness of deep learning in detecting and categorizing proximal humerus fractures. This was done by comparing the radiographs to a database of known fractures. The conclusions of the CNN network were contrasted with those of several specialists (general physicians, radiologists, and orthopedic surgeons). They used a pre-trained ResNet-152 model that was modified specifically for their proximal humerus fracture datasets, which included a total of 1,891 plain AP radiographs. The trained CNN had outstanding ability in distinguishing between normal and broken proximal humeri. On straightforward AP radiographs of the shoulder, the results for the classifying fracture type were also positive. The CNN performed better than primary care physicians and general orthopedic surgeons, and it was on par with shoulder specialists in terms of its effectiveness. This suggests that other fractures and orthopedic illnesses that can be accurately diagnosed with plain radiographs, such as those of the proximal humerus, could benefit from automated diagnosis and classification in the future [36].

The researchers carried out a study to test deep learning's capacity to automatically identify osteoporotic vertebral fractures (OVFs) on CT scans [29]. This evaluation was carried out as part of a retrospective study. The authors developed a machine learning system that relied solely on a deep neural network framework for all its functionality. Their OVF detection method consisted of two primary components: (1) a CNN-based feature extraction module and (2) an RNN (recurrent neural network) module that aggregated the retrieved features and produced the final diagnostic. Both modules were trained using the same data. A deep residual network, abbreviated as ResNet, was utilized to analyze the CT scans and extract the features [30]. For their training dataset, the researchers made use of 1,168 CT scans; for their validation set, they made use of 135 CT scans; and for their test dataset, they made use of 129 CT scans. On an independent test set, their system achieved levels of accuracy and F1 scores (mean of precision and recall) that were equivalent to those of expert radiologists. By eliminating the need for human intervention during OVF screening, this computerized detection system may help reduce false-negative errors in the diagnosis of asymptomatic, early-stage vertebral fractures.

1.4.1 Data Pre-Processing

The dataset can be pre-trained with non-medical pictures and then used for the task of automating fracture identification in plain radiographs. Preprocessing a dataset of broken photos can enhance data attributes and hide undesired aspects [31]. Pre-processing the data for a learning model takes a considerable amount of time. The goal here is to get the data ready for analysis and calculations. Overfitting is a potential issue during data retrieval and selection [32]. Overfitting occurs when the data absorbs irrelevant information, such as noise, during the learning process. The learning process itself takes considerable time, and the initial dataset acquisition is just the beginning. The next step is a labeling procedure that must be carefully supervised. This information is then separated into two groups: fractured and unbroken. The fracture's identification was verified by a surgeon with more than 3 years of experience. An orthopedic specialist's expertise is used to interpret a dataset of X-ray images obtained from a specialized hospital.

1.5 Primary Machine Learning-Based Algorithm in Bone Fracture Detection

Early fracture detection mechanisms relied on the neck-shaft angle (NSA) alone to function. As an example, if the NSA value is less than 116, a fracture is assumed to be present in the image. The mistake rate is close to 8% since the single feature is insufficient for identifying fractures. Therefore, researchers present a novel classification-based approach to detecting mild diseases by analyzing dragging characteristics in femur X-rays and performing the textural assessment of the bony trabecular pattern.

The process of feature extraction is crucial for using foundational machine learning methods for fracture identification. Gabor filters, Markov random field, and intensity gradient direction are techniques used for feature extraction from femur X-rays [33, 34]. Some researchers have exclusively used the Gabor filter for feature extraction while using classifiers for fracture identification [35]. Some scientists employ a gradient transformation using homotopic functions. Regression trees and SVM have several potential applications, including medical diagnosis and weather forecasting [36, 37]. It also expresses one take on the central theme and the supporting issues, disputes, challenges, etc., by analyzing the article's topic considering the overarching theme of the publication and comparing the results to previous or ongoing research or practice in the field.

1.5.1 Ensemble-Based Classification System

To enhance predictions, ensemble approaches combine multiple algorithms into a unified framework. Associating different kinds of learning models helps to refine the results. Since this is the case, ensemble methods are favored over alternative approaches. Ensemble-based classification systems are collections of classifiers that work together to provide a composite output [38]. Unlike the other techniques, which utilize the same learning method for all the datasets, the initial approach to the ensemble methodology is based on applying multiple learning methods on separate training sets. For accuracy, the classifier system combines the results of a small number of base classifiers [39].

To pick the best possible subset of classifiers, ensemble classifiers make use of selection procedures. There are two distinct ways that one can decide between two options: The most efficient classifier would be chosen to be used on the validation data in an entirely static setup. Both dynamic classifier selection and dynamic ensemble selection are valid applications of the dynamic methodology. Dynamic classifier selection uses a set of preselected classifiers as a foundation upon which to build an ensemble. The goal of dynamic ensemble selection is to find the most predictive ensemble combination [40]. Bagging and boosting are two examples of ensemble methods that have medical applications for fracture identification [41].

To better diagnose osteoporotic fractures, researchers have turned to ensemble-based learning techniques like bagging, boosting, and random subspaces [42]. Classifiers are developed from many models, each with its own unique set of properties. Bone fracture detection uses the ensemble method of 10-fold cross-validation [43]. In the research process, feature selection often comes first, followed by using a machine learning strategy. This method has the benefit of preventing additional, redundant bone testing.

1.5.2 Bagging

Bagging is a popular method that uses a single dataset to train many models. Some typical and recurring occurrences are the result of randomly selecting the initial functionality of a distinct dataset from the same dataset k time. Training several related datasets in parallel has many benefits, including reducing training time and enhancing the quality of results for tasks like decision trees that use many datasets. Joining the results of multiple classifiers where the majority value is the same increases precision. It relies solely on the arithmetic mean of results from the various basic classifiers. The bagging technique calculation formula is shown in Equation 1.1 as follows:

$$\text{Outcome}(O) = 1/n \sum_{i=1}^{n} Oi \tag{1.1}$$

Algorithm
Input:
D: dataset
C: number of classifiers
S: classification Scheme
Output:
Predicted output by Ensemble—a classifier model
Method:
1. For i to C do // create C models
2. Construct dataset Di from D
3. Apply Di with Ci and generate model
4. End;
5. Conjoint the outcomes in Ensemble S
6. Generate predicted value

Instead of randomly selecting from the training set, the authors advise using a method known as "wagging (weights aggregation)," which can be found in [44]. This tactic constantly rearranges the data collection, which makes it much simpler to identify any recurring trends or patterns. During the process of weighing, extra characteristics were assigned to each weight in the calculation. These characteristics included a random Gaussian distribution with a set standard deviation and a mean of zero for each weight. First, for testing, noise was introduced to the weights of the examples during each iteration of the technique. Next, a single classifier was induced when the operation was completed.

Bagging classification is the method that is utilized for fracture detection [45]. After labeling the X-rays and using filters to cut down on noise, the authors take a series of images using the X-ray machine. In addition to that, the bagging method is utilized as a classification strategy so that a basic classifier can be developed.

1.5.3 Boosting

Boosting is an alternative method that employs the same learning mechanism over numerous datasets to achieve its desired results. It is an example of an iterative approach. The accuracy of the classifier can be enhanced by applying weights to each instance, which is accomplished by the dynamic partitioning of training sets. After the fundamental classifiers have been developed and put to the ensemble, the first step is to reweigh each instance individually. The formation of a single prediction requires the combination of several weights derived from various base classifiers. The final prediction is the weighted average of all the predictions made by the individual base classifiers or the "conjoint."

The results from many base classifiers are averaged and weighted as shown in Equation 1.2 to produce the best results for boosting.

$$Outcome(O) = \sum_{i=1}^{n} w * Oi \tag{1.2}$$

The Adaptive Boosting (AdaBoost) algorithm is an example of a boosting ensemble technique. In this research, the researchers introduced MultiBoosting, an algorithmic approach to decision-making that is an extension of the AdaBoost method [46]. Greater precision in medical diagnosis may be achieved with the use of gradient boosting machines (GBM) [47]. It has been discovered that GBM produce reliable fracture predictions. Before feeding data into a GBM model, regression methods are used. For fracture prediction, a unique model is built with the R package.

1.5.4 Stacking

When multiple learning classifiers' results are combined into a single classifier, the resulting prediction exhibits less bias and variance error. These methods fall under the umbrella of ensemble learning. Stacking involves dividing a problem space into smaller pieces that may be handled by various kinds of learning algorithms. For each distinct problem partition, a unique learning model is constructed. The combined result is then used as a prediction.

1.5.5 Random Forest

At its core, it relies on the idea of categorizing attributes into different groups. It accomplishes this goal by applying separate feature subspaces to the same dataset used for training. The random forest can produce ensemble classifiers since it uses a huge number of trees. Classification using this method entails constructing several decision trees. The random forest method as well as the feature extraction procedure make it a breeze to perform an analysis of X-ray images [48]. The findings are based on tests that were carried out on a total of 145 X-ray scans. The method that has been suggested can be executed with the assistance of the feature extraction process, the random forest method, as well as the support vector machine method.

1.6 Deep Learning-Based Techniques for Fracture Detection

Fracture identification and characterization are two areas where deep learning could be useful in radiology, as evidenced by the instances (Figure 1.2). Overall, adding deep learning to current radiology procedures has the potential to increase the efficiency and precision of diagnostic tests while simultaneously reducing labor costs by relieving radiologists of some of their more tedious responsibilities. In addition, the algorithms used in deep learning are susceptible to problems such as inter- and intra-variance, both of which can be problematic for human-based diagnosis. Deep learning, when applied in the context of academic research, can identify and classify fractures on plain radiographs and CT scans at least as well as people can.

When using deep neural networks, accurate results can be achieved by merging the predictions generated by many training models [49]. They allow for greater data flexibility and scalability, and they offer new weight

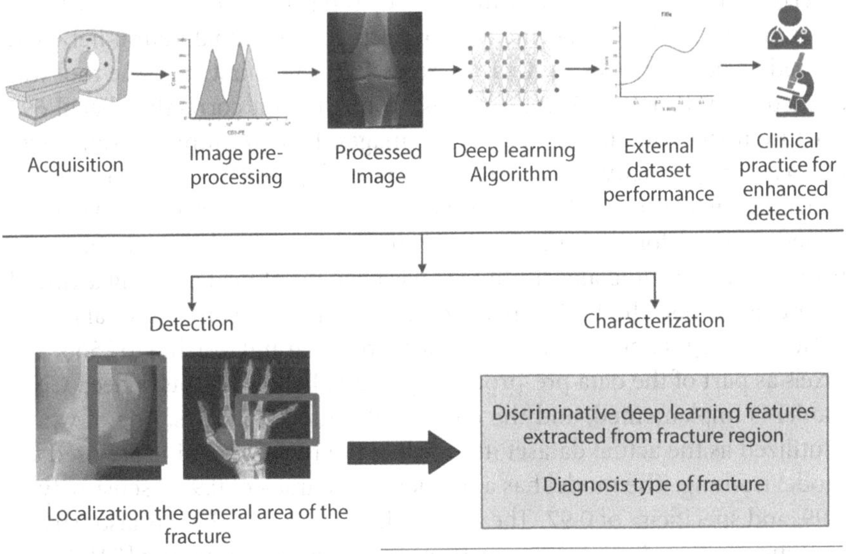

Figure 1.2 Deep learning-based work process for fracture detection.

sets with each iteration of deep learning, leading to unique predictions. The researchers also talk about a method called Adaptive Differential Parameter Optimization that uses artificial neural networks to identify bone fractures by the separation of fractured and unfractured lines [50]. The approach uses a probabilistic Hough transform for the data pre-processing and a neural network for the classification in order to differentiate between X-rays that contain fractures and those that do not have fractures. The area under the curve was 0.8149, while the overall rate of success was 74.4%.

A study was conducted to detect the wrist fracture using a convolutional neural network [28]. There are a total of 1,35,845 X-rays, each of which represents an image of a different portion of the body; however, only 34,990 were selected as they were of the wrist bone. From a total of 34,990 X-rays of the wrist, two test datasets were generated, with the first including 3,500 radiographs. There were 1,400 X-rays in the second dataset. There are two stages to the model's training process. It is first pre-trained, then honed and polished, to detect breaks in the wrist. The researchers generate an AUC curve with a sensitivity of 93.9% and a specificity of 94.5% and then compare these numbers across datasets to determine our performance. Specifically, the researchers use DenseNet, a specific type of neural network architecture, to analyze over 53,000 pelvic X-ray images [51]. Following the application of labeling, a 172-layer deep neural network is used, with each layer featuring 12 features/units. The model's receiver operating characteristic (ROC) curve boasts an accuracy range from 95% to over 99%.

Transfer learning, a specific type of deep convolutional neural network, is used to detect breaks in X-ray pictures [52]. As a first step, the tool was trained on a dataset of 11,112 photos, from which it correctly labeled 695 fracture images and 694 non-fracture images. By determining a sensitivity of 0.9 and a specificity of 0.88, an AUC value of approximately 0.954 may be generated, which is used in the performance evaluation process. An automated method for detecting and classifying proximal humerus fractures using a deep learning algorithm [53] has been developed utilizing artificial neural networks. The 1,891-image training dataset is a convolutional neural network. Images undergo manual square cropping and resizing to 256 × 256 pixels as part of the data pre-processing phase. Following this, a deep CNN model is implemented, and the data is split into 10 subsets, one of which is utilized as the actual dataset itself, while the remaining nine are used for model training. The model has a predictive accuracy of 0.996, sensitivity of 0.99, and specificity of 0.97. The area under the curve (AUC) is also 0.996.

Bone fracture diagnosis is greatly aided using deep learning [54]. Using a neural network of 1,024 neurons, X-rays of different bodily areas are classified as either fractured or unfractured in order to achieve this goal. The methodology was tested on 30 sample datasets and then applied to 70 datasets. Two of the most common types of pre-processing methods are the Haar wavelet transform and symmetric interferometric feature extraction. The procedure known as scale-invariant feature transform is a multi-stage process that comprises the extraction and orientation of features. This strategy makes use of deep learning in the form of a neural network, and it possesses accuracy of approximately 94%.

The researchers can now identify hip fractures in X-rays by employing a deep neural network [55]. The first is a dataset that has been pre-trained, and it consists of 25,505 limb X-rays (elbows, ankles, wrists, and feet). These datasets are used to train a deep convolutional neural network. In addition, 3,605 X-ray pictures make up the frontal pelvic dataset. In addition, the researchers have a dataset consisting of 100 pelvic X-rays taken for a separate evaluation. To begin, the dataset is preprocessed by having all photos resized to 512 × 512. Fracture identification is modeled using Densenet [56]. Both accuracy and AUC might vary widely depending on the data used. When first used, the pre-training stage achieves an accuracy of 99.5%. A direct application to hip fracture imaging, however, improved the accuracy to 90% and area under the curve to 0.98. In addition, the accuracy was determined after a questionnaire was given to four orthopedic surgeons and two radiologists, with a mean accuracy of 87.7% sensitivity and 98% specificity.

Deep learning algorithms can be broken down into two groups: single- and two-stage classifiers. Two-stage classifiers produce regions that could contain items. Then, a neural network assigns categories to these areas. One-stage detectors do both object localization and classification simultaneously, skipping the region proposal phase. Therefore, single-stage classifiers are quicker than multi-stage ones. When it comes to deep learning-based fracture detection algorithms, the Region-Based Convolutional Neural Network (R-CNN) and the You Only Look Once (YOLO) series are two of the more well-known options. The R-CNN series is less efficient in detecting changes than the YOLO series. Its performance in detecting fractures in real time falls short under realistic conditions.

1.6.1 R-CNN Series

The R-CNN is the pioneering deep learning-based object detection approach. One can use variations of R-CNN that are faster, such as Faster RCNN or Faster R-CNN. Since R-CNN requires around 47 s to analyze each test image, it is not feasible for use in real time. When using slow

R-CNN, the regions are only partially sent to CNN, but when using rapid R-CNN, the complete image is fed to the CNN so that it can generate a feature map. It is then common practice to square off the feature maps. Finally, the fully connected layer receives the converted regions of interest (ROIs) of a specified size from the ROI pooling layer [57]. If one wants faster results, then that individual can forget about selective search; it is a time-consuming, laborious process that will only slow down that person.

A convolutional neural network is used to analyze the input image and build a feature map when doing faster R-CNN, which is very similar to fast R-CNN. The different network is used to estimate region proposals rather than utilizing a selective search strategy on the feature map to find them. After a ROI pooling layer classifies the picture within the proposed zone and estimates the offset values for the bounding boxes, the proposed regions are shrunk [58].

1.6.2 YOLO Deep Learning Algorithm

Using a convolutional neural network, YOLO can detect objects with a single step. Its speed and efficiency have made it famous. There are several deep learning algorithms out there, but none of them can perform object detection in a single pass. There are a lot of deep learning methods out there, but none of them can do 100% accurate identification in just one go. Due to its ability to detect objects with just a single forward propagation *via* a neural network, YOLO outperforms any multi-step approach and is thus well suited to usage in real-time contexts. YOLO's central idea is to feed the network the entire image as input and then have it provide the location of the bounding box and the category to which it belongs as output [59].

The predictions and confidences for each of YOLO's five bounding boxes are based on the grid unit at the box's center and are derived from the image's features. In the YOLO basic frame, w and h were the projected width and height of the full image. You Only Look Once consists mostly of three parts as follows:

1. Backbone: a convolutional neural network that combines and generates a wide variety of visual features at multiple levels.
2. Neck: a collection of network layers that, before transferring the information to the prediction layer, combine and mix the attributes of the images being processed.

3. Head: the head can classify information, recognize bounding boxes, and anticipate the appearance of certain image components. The level of confidence reflects the precision with which the classification was made in light of the circumstances.

Within the YOLOv2 system, a newly developed training algorithm has been incorporated [60]. The k-means clustering method is utilized so that the bounding boxes can be grouped for the clustering process. As a result of the fact that enhancing the intersection over union is the primary objective of the process of developing the *a priori* box, the IOU value is used in the cluster analysis in the capacity of a distance indicator. It has a very significant improvement in accuracy and recall rate in comparison to YOLOv1. YOLOv3 makes use of both the more advanced basic classification network known as ResNet as well as the classifier known as Darknet53 [61]. A network topology that is analogous to an FPN is utilized in the process of simultaneously performing multiscale prediction. The percentage of false positives for backdrop detection has been significantly reduced, while there has been an increase in both accuracy and speed. YOLOv4 replaces the backbone network with CSPDarknet53 and employs spatial pyramid pooling (SPP) to enhance the receptive area, with PANet serving as the neck. This is done while maintaining the head that YOLOv3 provided. The structure of CSPNet makes it possible to obtain additional information on gradient combinations while simultaneously increasing processing performance. The many feature layers are wholly incorporated into the PANet topology, which considerably improves the faulty feature extraction [62].

1.6.3 YOLOv5

In the year 2020, Glenn and his team introduced the most recent version of the YOLO algorithms, which was called YOLOv5. The Darknet framework was utilized in the production of YOLO models. An organization by the name of Ultralystic adapts older versions of YOLO to the popular deep learning structure known as PyTorch, which is founded on the programming language Python. YOLOv5 had significant engineering improvements over the earlier versions of the software. Python, not C, is being used for the development of YOLOv5. Because YOLOv4 and YOLOv5 are written in two different languages and run on two different frameworks, it is challenging to evaluate how well the two versions perform in comparison to one another. Despite this, YOLOv5 has proven to be more effective than YOLOv4 in several scenarios and has earned a measure of credibility in the area of computer search [63].

The architecture of YOLOv5: YOLOv5 was different from the versions that came before it. PyTorch is utilized here in its place of Darknet. It utilizes CSPDarknet53 as its primary backbone. This backbone manages the recurring gradient information in big backbones, and the feature map contains gradient change. As a result, inference is carried out more quickly, accuracy is improved, and model size is reduced as a result of lower parameter values. It does this by utilizing a framework known as PANet, which speeds up the flow of information. PANet employs a brand new FPN that has a lot of levels. The model's transmission of lower-level features is improved as a result of this [64].

1.7 Conclusion

Overall, it is possible to conclude that bones play a crucial role in the structure of the human body. In the modern world, artificial intelligence is a cutting-edge idea in the study of medicine. There could be a surge in medical science as a result. The current chapter presents a thorough analysis of the use of artificial intelligence to detect bone fractures. Many reasons, such as an unhealthy lifestyle, the prevalence of traffic accidents, and other factors, have contributed to an increase in bone fractures during the past several years. Artificial intelligence must advance to be used in therapeutic settings such as bone fractures. More effort will lead to better performance, which will aid medical personnel in identifying the fracture.

References

1. Hamet, P. and Tremblay, J., Artificial intelligence in medicine. *Metabolism*, 69, S36–40, 2017 Apr 1.
2. Hosny, A., Parmar, C., Quackenbush, J., Schwartz, L.H., Aerts, H.J., Artificial intelligence in radiology. *Nat. Rev. Cancer*, 18, 8, 500–10, 2018 Aug.
3. Han, J., Pei, J., Tong, H., *Data mining: Concepts and techniques*, Morgan Kaufmann, Burlington, Massachusetts, United States, 2022 Jul 2.
4. Ilango, V., Subramanian, R., Vasudevan, V., A five step procedure for outlier analysis in data mining. *Eur. J. Sci. Res.*, 75, 3, 327–39, 2012.
5. Veni, C.K. and Rani, T.S., Ensemble based classification using small training sets: A novel approach, in: *2014 IEEE Symposium on Computational Intelligence in Ensemble Learning (CIEL)*, IEEE, pp. 1–8, 2014 Dec 9.

6. Mishra, D. and Soni, D., A comprehensive overview on data mining: Approaches and applications. *Int. J. Comput. Sci. Inf. Technol.*, 5, 6, 7814–6, 2014.
7. Koteeswaran, S., Visu, P., Janet, J., A review on clustering and outlier analysis techniques in datamining. *Am. J. Appl. Sci.*, 9, 2, 254, 2012.
8. Li, J., Roy, P., Khan, S.U., Wang, L., Bai, Y., Data mining using clouds: An experimental implementation of apriori over mapreduce, in: *12th International Conference on Scalable Computing and Communications (ScalCom)*, pp. 1–8, 2012 Dec.
9. McCulloch, W.S. and Pitts, W., A logical calculus of the ideas immanent in nervous activity. *Bull. Math. Biophys.*, 5, 115–33, 1943 Dec.
10. Mnih, V., Kavukcuoglu, K., Silver, D., Rusu, A.A., Veness, J., Bellemare, M.G., Graves, A., Riedmiller, M., Fidjeland, A.K., Ostrovski, G., Petersen, S., Human-level control through deep reinforcement learning. *Nature*, 518, 7540, 529–33, 2015 Feb.
11. Moravčík, M., Schmid, M., Burch, N., Lisý, V., Morrill, D., Bard, N., Davis, T., Waugh, K., Johanson, M., Bowling, M., Deepstack: Expert-level artificial intelligence in heads-up no-limit poker. *Science*, 356, 6337, 508–513, 2017 May 5.
12. Johari, N. and Singh, N., Bone fracture detection using edge detection technique, in: *Soft Computing: Theories and Applications: Proceedings of SoCTA 2016*, vol. 2, pp. 11–19, Springer Singapore, 2018.
13. Adams, M., Chen, W., Holcdorf, D., McCusker, M.W., Howe, P.D., Gaillard, F., Computer vs human: Deep learning versus perceptual training for the detection of neck of femur fractures. *J. Med. Imaging Radiat. Oncol.*, 63, 1, 27–32, 2019 Feb.
14. Lakhani, P. and Sundaram, B., Deep learning at chest radiography: Automated classification of pulmonary tuberculosis by using convolutional neural networks. *Radiology*, 284, 2, 574–582, 2017 Aug.
15. Ting, D.S., Cheung, C.Y., Lim, G., Tan, G.S., Quang, N.D., Gan, A., Hamzah, H., Garcia-Franco, R., San Yeo, I.Y., Lee, S.Y., Wong, E.Y., Development and validation of a deep learning system for diabetic retinopathy and related eye diseases using retinal images from multiethnic populations with diabetes. *JAMA*, 318, 22, 2211–2223, 2017 Dec 12.
16. Brett, A., Miller, C.G., Hayes, C.W., Krasnow, J., Ozanian, T., Abrams, K., Block, J.E., van Kuijk, C., Development of a clinical workflow tool to enhance the detection of vertebral fractures: Accuracy and precision evaluation. *Spine*, 34, 22, 2437–2443, 2009 Oct 15.
17. Maheshwari, J. and Mhaskar, V.A., *Essential orthopaedics: (including clinical methods)*, Jaypee Brothers Medical Publishers, New Delhi, India, 2019 Feb 28.
18. Meena, T. and Roy, S., Bone fracture detection using deep supervised learning from radiological images: A paradigm shift. *Diagnostics*, 12, 10, 2420, 2022 Oct 7.

19. Yasaka, K. and Abe, O., Deep learning and artificial intelligence in radiology: Current applications and future directions. *PLoS Med.*, 15, 11, e1002707, 2018 Nov 30.
20. Nakaura, T., Higaki, T., Awai, K., Ikeda, O., Yamashita, Y., A primer for understanding radiology articles about machine learning and deep learning. *Diagn. Interventional Imaging*, 101, 12, 765–70, 2020 Dec 1.
21. Montagnon, E., Cerny, M., Cadrin-Chênevert, A., Hamilton, V., Derennes, T., Ilinca, A., Vandenbroucke-Menu, F., Turcotte, S., Kadoury, S., Tang, A., Deep learning workflow in radiology: A primer. *Insights into Imaging*, 11, 1–5, 2020 Dec.
22. Lodwick, G.S., Keats, T.E., Dorst, J.P., The coding of roentgen images for computer analysis as applied to lung cancer. *Radiology*, 81, 2, 185–200, 1963 Aug.
23. Kalmet, P.H., Sanduleanu, S., Primakov, S., Wu, G., Jochems, A., Refaee, T., Ibrahim, A., Hulst, L.V., Lambin, P., Poeze, M., Deep learning in fracture detection: A narrative review. *Acta Orthop.*, 91, 2, 215–220, 2020 Mar 3.
24. Rainey, C., McConnell, J., Hughes, C., Bond, R., McFadden, S., Artificial intelligence for diagnosis of fractures on plain radiographs: A scoping review of current literature. *Intell.-Based Med.*, 5, 100033, 2021 Jan 1.
25. Urakawa, T., Tanaka, Y., Goto, S., Matsuzawa, H., Watanabe, K., Endo, N., Detecting intertrochanteric hip fractures with orthopedist-level accuracy using a deep convolutional neural network. *Skeletal Radiol.*, 48, 239–244, 2019 Feb.
26. Szegedy, C., Vanhoucke, V., Ioffe, S., Shlens, J., Wojna, Z., Rethinking the inception architecture for computer vision, in: *Proceedings of the IEEE Conference on Computer Vision and Pattern Recognition*, pp. 2818–2826, 2016.
27. Russakovsky, O., Deng, J., Su, H., Krause, J., Satheesh, S., Ma, S., Huang, Z., Karpathy, A., Khosla, A., Bernstein, M., Berg, A.C., Imagenet large scale visual recognition challenge. *Int. J. Comput. Vision*, 115, 211–252, 2015 Dec.
28. Lindsey, R., Daluiski, A., Chopra, S., Lachapelle, A., Mozer, M., Sicular, S., Hanel, D., Gardner, M., Gupta, A., Hotchkiss, R., Potter, H., Deep neural network improves fracture detection by clinicians. *Proc. Natl. Acad. Sci.*, 115, 45, 11591–11596, 2018 Nov 6.
29. Tomita, N., Cheung, Y.Y., Hassanpour, S., Deep neural networks for automatic detection of osteoporotic vertebral fractures on CT scans. *Comput. Biol. Med.*, 98, 8–15, 2018 Jul 1.
30. He, K., Zhang, X., Ren, S., Sun, J., Deep residual learning for image recognition, in: *Proceedings of the IEEE Conference on Computer Vision and Pattern Recognition*, pp. 770–778, 2016.
31. Khatik, I., A study of various bone fracture detection techniques. *Int. J. Eng. Comput. Sci.*, 6, 5, 21418–23, 2017 Jun.
32. Hodge, V. and Austin, J., A survey of outlier detection methodologies. *Artif. Intell. Rev.*, 22, 85–126, 2004 Oct.

33. Lim, S.E., Xing, Y., Chen, Y., Leow, W.K., Howe, T.S., Png, M.A., Detection of femur and radius fractures in X-ray images, in: *Proc. 2nd Int. Conf. on Advances in Medical Signal and Info. Proc*, vol. 65, 2004, Sep.
34. Lum, V.L., Leow, W.K., Chen, Y., Howe, T.S., Png, M.A., Combining classifiers for bone fracture detection in X-ray images, in: *IEEE International Conference on Image Processing 2005*, vol. 1, IEEE, pp. I–1149, 2005 Sep 14.
35. Yap, D.W., Chen, Y., Leow, W.K., Howe, T.S., Png, M.A., Detecting femur fractures by texture analysis of trabeculae, in: *Proceedings of the 17th International Conference on Pattern Recognition, ICPR 2004*, 2004 Aug 26, vol. 3, IEEE, pp. 730–733, 2004.
36. Wei, Z., Na, M., Huisheng, S., Hongqi, F., Feature extraction of X-ray fracture image and fracture classification, in: *2009 International Conference on Artificial Intelligence and Computational Intelligence*, vol. 2, IEEE, pp. 408–412, 2009 Nov 7.
37. Ordóñez, C., Matías, J.M., de Cos Juez, J.F., García, P.J., Machine learning techniques applied to the determination of osteoporosis incidence in post-menopausal women. *Math. Comput. Modell.*, 50, 5-6, 673–679, 2009 Sep 1.
38. Naz, M., Zafar, K., Khan, A., Ensemble based classification of sentiments using forest optimization algorithm. *Data*, 4, 2, 76, 2019 May 23.
39. Jurek, A., Bi, Y., Wu, S., Nugent, C., A survey of commonly used ensemble-based classification techniques. *Knowl. Eng. Rev.*, 29, 5, 551–581, 2014 Nov.
40. Abuassba, A.O., Zhang, D., Luo, X., Shaheryar, A., Ali, H., Improving classification performance through an advanced ensemble based heterogeneous extreme learning machines. *Comput. Intell. Neurosci.*, 2017, 663, 2017 May 4.
41. Chouhan, D.K. and Chouhan, N., Desaturating patient with long bone fractures: Diagnosis and management, in: *Acute Trauma Care in Developing Countries*, pp. 99–106, CRC Press, Boca Raton, Florida, 2023.
42. Kilic, N. and Hosgormez, E., Automatic estimation of osteoporotic fracture cases by using ensemble learning approaches. *J. Med. Syst.*, 40, 1–0, 2016 Mar.
43. Iliou, T., Anagnostopoulos, C.N., Anastassopoulos, G., Osteoporosis detection using machine learning techniques and feature selection. *Int. J. Artif. Intell. Tools*, 23, 05, 1450014, 2014 Oct 28.
44. Bauer, E. and Kohavi, R., An empirical comparison of voting classification algorithms: Bagging, boosting, and variants. *Mach. Learn.*, 36, 105–139, 1999 Jul.
45. Al-Ayyoub, M., Hmeidi, I., Rababah, H., Detecting hand bone fractures in X-ray images. *J. Multimed. Process. Technol.*, 4, 3, 155–168, 2013 Sep.
46. Webb, G.I., Multiboosting: A technique for combining boosting and wagging. *Mach. Learn.*, 40, 2, 159, 2000 Aug 1.
47. Atkinson, E.J., Therneau, T.M., Melton III, L.J., Camp, J.J., Achenbach, S.J., Amin, S., Khosla, S., Assessing fracture risk using gradient boosting machine (GBM) models. *J. Bone Miner. Res.*, 27, 6, 1397–404, 2012 Jun.

48. Cao, Y., Wang, H., Moradi, M., Prasanna, P., Syeda-Mahmood, T.F., Fracture detection in X-ray images through stacked random forests feature fusion, in: *2015 IEEE 12th International Symposium on Biomedical Imaging (ISBI)*, IEEE, pp. 801–805, 2015 Apr 16.
49. Thian, Y.L., Li, Y., Jagmohan, P., Sia, D., Chan, V.E., Tan, R.T., Convolutional neural networks for automated fracture detection and localization on wrist radiographs. *Radiol.: Artif. Intell.*, 1, 1, e180001, 2019 Jan 30.
50. Yang, A.Y., Cheng, L., Shimaponda-Nawa, M., Zhu, H.Y., Long-bone fracture detection using artificial neural networks based on line features of X-ray images, in: *2019 IEEE Symposium Series on Computational Intelligence (SSCI)*, IEEE, pp. 2595–2602, 2019 Dec 6.
51. Gale, W., Oakden-Rayner, L., Carneiro, G., Bradley, A.P., Palmer, L.J., Detecting hip fractures with radiologist-level performance using deep neural networks. *Computer Vision and Pattern Recognition (CVPR), arXiv preprint arXiv:1711.06504*, 3, 1–5, 2017 Nov 17.
52. Kim, D.H. and MacKinnon, T., Artificial intelligence in fracture detection: Transfer learning from deep convolutional neural networks. *Clin. Radiol.*, 73, 5, 439–45, 2018 May 1.
53. Chung, S.W., Han, S.S., Lee, J.W., Oh, K.S., Kim, N.R., Yoon, J.P., Kim, J.Y., Moon, S.H., Kwon, J., Lee, H.J., Noh, Y.M., Automated detection and classification of the proximal humerus fracture by using deep learning algorithm. *Acta Orthop.*, 89, 4, 468–73, 2018 Jul 4.
54. Dimililer, K., IBFDS: Intelligent bone fracture detection system. *Proc. Comput. Sci.*, 120, 260–7, 2017 Jan 1.
55. Cheng, C.T., Ho, T.Y., Lee, T.Y., Chang, C.C., Chou, C.C., Chen, C.C., Chung, I., Liao, C.H., Application of a deep learning algorithm for detection and visualization of hip fractures on plain pelvic radiographs. *Eur. Radiol.*, 29, 10, 5469–77, 2019 Oct.
56. Huang, G., Liu, Z., Maaten, L., Weinberger, K., Densely connected convolutional networks. *Comput. Vis. Pattern Recognit., arXiv preprint arXiv:1608.06993,* 1, 4700–4708, 2016.
57. Al-Zubaidi, F., Automated analysis of drill-core images using convolutional neural network, Doctoral dissertation, UNSW Sydney, Sydney Australia, 2022.
58. Lin, X., Yan, Z., Kuang, Z., Zhang, H., Deng, X., Yu, L., Fracture R-CNN: An anchor-efficient anti-interference framework for skull fracture detection in CT images. *Med. Phys.*, 49, 7179–7192, 2022 Nov 1.
59. Samothai, P., Sanguansat, P., Kheaksong, A., Srisomboon, K., Lee, W., The evaluation of bone fracture detection of YOLO series, in: *2022 37th International Technical Conference on Circuits/Systems, Computers and Communications (ITC-CSCC)*, IEEE, pp. 1054–1057, 2022 Jul 5.
60. Sha, G., Wu, J., Yu, B., Detection of spinal fracture lesions based on improved YOLOV2, in: *2020 IEEE International Conference on Artificial Intelligence and Computer Applications (ICAICA)*, IEEE, p p. 235–238, 2020 Jun 27.

61. Adarsh, P., Rathi, P., Kumar, M., YOLO v3-Tiny: Object detection and recognition using one stage improved model, in: *2020 6th International Conference on Advanced Computing and Communication Systems (ICACCS)*, IEEE, pp. 687–694, 2020 Mar 6.
62. Jeong, D., Road damage detection using YOLO with smartphone images, in: *2020 IEEE International Conference on Big Data (Big Data)*, IEEE, pp. 5559–5562, 2020 Dec 10.
63. Zhang, Q., Zhang, B., Chen, C., Li, L., Wang, X., Jiang, B., Zheng, T., A test method for finding early dynamic fracture of rock: Using DIC and YOLOv5. *Sensors*, 22, 17, 6320, 2022 Aug 23.
64. Mahendran, S.K. and Baboo, S.S., Automatic fracture detection using classifiers-a review. *Int. J. Comput. Sci. Issues (IJCSI)*, 8, 6, 340, 2011 Nov 1.

2

Integrating AI With Tissue Engineering: The Next Step in Bone Regeneration

Abstract
A branch of regenerative medicine called tissue engineering uses developments in biomaterial and stem cell research to support the body's natural healing processes. Three main elements that are required for tissue engineering are cells, growth agents, and a scaffold material. Metal, ceramic, or polymer scaffolds can be built to support bone regeneration. Many biomaterials have been tried with a wide variety of different cell types. An overview of contemporary approaches to bone regeneration is given in this chapter, with a focus on tissue engineering techniques that involve the fusion of diverse biomaterials with cells and growth hormones. Two of the many unanswered concerns in tissue engineering are the lack of an appropriate understanding of stem cells and the requirement for better biomaterial designs. Deep learning and artificial intelligence (AI) have the potential to improve the therapeutic outcomes and scientific understanding of regenerative medicine. This powerful technology will be even more effective at improving patient health outcomes with a better knowledge of how to apply AI to ongoing research and clinical practice.

Keywords: Bone regeneration, tissue engineering, bone biology, artificial intelligence, deep learning, bone structure, implant

2.1 Introduction

Even though it is encouraging that medical progress has led to a rise in life expectancy, this achievement also introduces a new set of hurdles, such as an increase in age-related diseases and the associated decrease in the value of life, as well as a significant rise in the costs to the economy and society [1, 2]. Osteoarthritis is a growing health concern worldwide [3, 4], affecting as many as 20% of the population and causing severe, chronic pain and disability in the joints and muscles.

Rishabha Malviya, Shivam Rajput and Makarand Vaidya. Artificial Intelligence for Bone Disorder: Diagnosis and Treatment, (25–58) © 2024 Scrivener Publishing LLC

Despite this, there is a possibility of unfavorable consequences, and the average lifespan of a prosthesis is less than 15 years due to strain and wear [5]. While joint replacement is a successful remedy for this multifactorial disease, it is not without its drawbacks. Poor outcomes are possible, and current prostheses typically only last between 10 and 15 years. Even those who have had knee replacement surgery and can no longer engage in physical activity such as sports or heavy lifting experience this. Research into bone regeneration has shifted away from the strategy of inserting bio-inert materials [6] in favor of using bioactive materials to harness the body's inherent curing processes to restore bone. While bio-inert materials were previously implanted, this signals a dramatic shift away from that practice. Despite decades of effort into creating bone tissue for organ transplantation, developing bio-fabricated bone that can be scaled up for clinical utilization remains a research objective [7]. The reasons for this include the complexity of fixing things like vascularization problems and tissue necrosis. However, recent advances in technology, especially artificial intelligence (AI), provide fresh resources and tailored approaches to tissue engineering for individual patients [8].

2.2 Anatomy and Biology of Bone

2.2.1 Bone Structure and Matrix

Bone is not a homogeneous tissue but a biomineralized structure in which living bone cells are arranged. Bone is formed when the matrix surrounding entangled cells becomes more rigid. The main components of bone are collagen fibers and tiny crystals of an inorganic bone mineral [9]. An estimated 30% of bone's biomineral medium is made up of organic components, while the remaining 70% is made up of inorganic ones [10]. Collagen makes up more than 90% of this organic component, while osteopontin (OPN), lipids, proteoglycan molecules, and other bone matrix proteins account for the remaining 10% [11]. Bone matrix proteins are essential for both the mechanical stability and tissue adhesion that the matrix provides. Hydroxyapatite (HA), the primary mineral in bone, crystallizes in a hexagonal crystal shape [12]. Crystalline HA, with the formula $Ca_{10}(PO_4)_6(OH)_2$, has been associated with surface binding and electrostatic interactions [13, 14]. Collagen HA crystals are created by assembling collagen triple helices in a parallel orientation [15].

2.2.2 Bone Cells

Besides the mineralized bone microenvironment, bone cells are critical to bone function. Bone is responsible for a variety of mechanical (protection, shape, mobility, and motility), synthetic (blood cell generation), and metabolic processes (mineral storage, fat storage, regulation of calcium and phosphate, and role in acid–base balance). In Figure 2.1, the four most significant cells (osteogenic, osteoblasts, osteocytes, and osteoclasts) that make up bone regeneration and structure are depicted as part of the basic multicellular unit (BMU) [16].

Bone marrow and other connective tissues include mesenchymal cells called osteoprogenitor cells, which give rise to osteoblasts. In the process of preparing the bone for development, they undergo differentiation and proliferation into osteoblasts, with the help of bone morphogenetic proteins (BMPs). Bone development and remodeling are both dependent on these cells [17]. They also produce a protein complex termed osteoid, which plays a part in bone matrix production, deposit, and mineralization. Upon reaching adulthood, osteoblasts either undergo apoptosis or develop into osteocytes as well as other bone-lining cells, creating a cuboidal cell layer inside the bone [18].

Most of the skeletal tissue is composed of cells called osteoblasts [19]. One may recognize them by the star-shaped outline characteristic of their structure. Osteocytes originate from mesenchymal stem cells (MSCs) that have differentiated into osteoblasts. Osteoblasts that have become encapsulated in the bone they helped create are no longer active. This group of cells is responsible for keeping the lines of communication open between osteocytes and osteoblasts. Their function in relaying information between distinct types of bone tissue is crucial. Osteocytes have been implicated in

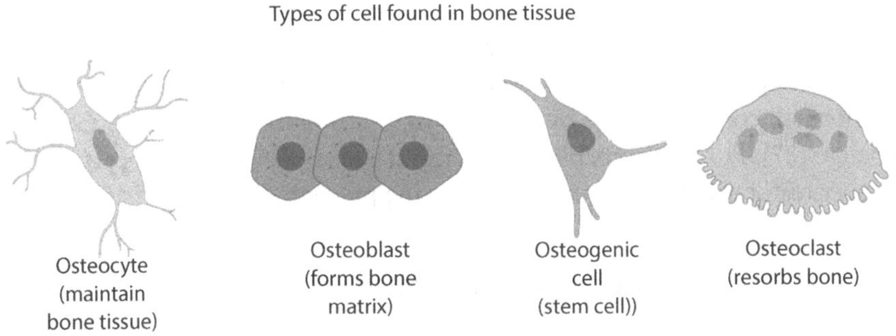

Figure 2.1 Types of cells that are found within bone tissue.

the regulation of calcium and phosphate homeostasis, and they respond to several different biochemical signaling pathways. Bone fragility and, potentially, osteoporosis come from abnormal osteocyte cell proliferation [20].

The surfaces of bones are populated by dormant osteoblasts, which give the bones their characteristic coating [21]. Lining cells are critically important in calcium homeostasis, osteoclastic differentiation, and the connection between bone resorption and bone production. They prevent osteoclasts from encountering the bone matrix by acting as a barrier [22].

Differentiated from the hematopoietic lineage, osteoclasts are multinucleated, massive cells. Their primary function is bone dissolution [23]. They secrete digestive acids and enzymes that break down bone tissue. Resorption describes this phenomenon. Injured bones can be remodeled with the aid of osteoclasts, which also clear out space for new blood vessels and nerves. Diseases like osteoporosis (characterized by elevated levels of osteoclast activity) and osteopetrosis (characterized by decreased levels of osteoclast activity) can be differentiated by their respective patterns of osteoclastic activity [24].

2.3 Bone Regeneration Mechanism

Bone fracture regeneration is a sophisticated, well-organized process that relies on a significant number of progenitor cells in addition to endothelial, inflammatory, and hematopoietic cells. Inflammation, bone formation, and remodeling are interconnected stages in the bone healing process [25]. Following a fracture, inflammation develops rapidly and persists for several days. When a bone breaks, blood rushes to the area, causing inflammation and clotting to form [26]. This provides the major structural framework for developing new bone. When inflamed blood clots are replaced with fibrous tissue and cartilage, bone formation can begin (recognized as a soft callus). Over several weeks following a fracture, X-rays will reveal the transition from soft callus to hard bone (identified as hard callus). The final stage of bone healing, called remodeling, might take several months. As the bone heals, it returns to its normal, compact shape by undergoing a formational and morphological change [27]. Furthermore, blood flow in the area benefits. After receiving the proper restorative treatment, weight-bearing promotes bone recovery.

2.3.1 Cellular Aspects of Bone Regeneration

Bio-scaffolds that have already been colonized by cells are crucial to the reparative process in tissue engineering. To create a bone construct, one can employ osteoblasts, induced pluripotent stem cells, embryonic stem cells, or mesenchymal stem cells. Osteoblasts, the autologous cells that can be recovered from bone biopsies, are rare and have little proliferation capability. Embryonic stem cells (ESCs) are pluripotent cells isolated from the inner mass of a blastocyst; they have many potential medical applications but have been met with controversy due to fears of immunologic incompatibility, teratoma formation, and ethical problems. The genetic editing of induced pluripotent stem cells (iPSCs) has prompted concerns regarding their clinical usage [28] despite their desirable qualities such as differentiation potential and autologous source. iPSCs were produced from somatic cells to overcome ESC problems. Finally, mesenchymal stromal cells are bone tissue regenerators. After an inflammatory reaction, normal bone repair involves mesenchymal and angiogenic activation [29]. MSCs are superior to iPSCs, ESCs, and osteoblasts for application in bone tissue engineering due to their ability to develop into bone-forming osteoblasts and chondrocytes *via* endochondral ossification [30]. Although MSCs were originally utilized in regenerative medicine due to their multipotency, new therapeutic approaches have evolved. Due to their "MSC tropism," these cells can be directed to certain wounds and home in on them in response to certain signals [31]. Because of their immunomodulatory and immunological escape properties, MSCs show the most potential as an allogenic cell therapy cell for addressing graft-versus-host disease and autoimmune disorders [32]. Bone and immune cells have a close relationship; therefore, this is important for bone healing. MSC express low levels of costimulatory CD40, CD40L, CD80, and CD86 as well as class II major histocompatibility complex (MHCII) [33]. Their immune regulation can be altered through paracrine signals including cytokines, chemokines, and extracellular vesicles as well as through direct cell-to-cell interactions [34]. Innate and adaptive immunity are possible. Recent research has focused on B and T cell modulation. Indoleamine 2,3-dioxygenase (IDO) induces apoptosis, suppressing B and T cell responses. Interactions between MSCs and NK (natural killer) cells, macrophages, monocytes, dendritic cells, and neutrophils can modulate the innate immune system. Living things are subject to environmental controls on their immunomodulatory activity. MSC responsiveness and secretome release are both affected by pro- and anti-inflammatory microenvironments [35]. Thus, various situations have been investigated to modify MSC secretory patterns to improve therapeutic efficacy. Hypoxia and priming with immunomodulatory substances precondition their immunological phenotype. First obtained from bone marrow, MSC is invasive to collect. Compared with bone marrow, adipose tissue is 500 times more productive in terms of MSC output [36].

They both can be traced back to a stem. The proliferation rate, longevity, and differentiation capacity of fetal (including placental), amnion, umbilical cord, and cord blood MSCs are superior to those of adult MSCs [37–40]. Immunomodulation is also affected by the source of MSCs. Although MSCs isolated from adipose tissue have greater immunomodulatory effects than those isolated from bone marrow, those isolated from umbilical cord blood have greater immunological escape and less risk of an allogenic immune response. Thus, the researcher's or clinician's application determines the MSC source modification [41].

Stem cells from mesenchymal origin (MSCs) have been employed in cell therapy and tissue engineering to restore bone [42]. Bone marrow transplantation and *in vitro*-cultured MSC are both used in MSC-based therapy [43]. Bone fractures, non-unions, anomalies of the jawbone, and osteonecrosis can all be effectively treated with MSC therapy, and studies suggest that it is safe. An updated search found 235 active and recruiting MSC clinical trials for various illnesses. MSCs are treating bone problems in 15 studies. MSC treatment has some drawbacks, including limited post-transplant survival and unknown dosage and administration [44]. MSC-based tissue engineering uses synthetic bone grafts to replenish MSCs *in situ.* Scaffolds that provide MSC to bone defects inhibit ectopic bone growth. Implantation of MSC on a cross-linked serum scaffold was shown to be effective in treating defects in the maxilla in pilot research [45]. Treatment of tibial, femoral, and humeral non-unions utilizing autologous, expanded MSCs as well as a bioceramic is feasible and safe in a multicentric, non-comparative experiment [46]. Preclinical research dominates nowadays. Several scaffold colonization techniques exist. Researchers showed how to simultaneously place cells and biomaterial on the scaffold. Encapsulated stromal cells in nanocomposite bio-inks generate three-dimensional constructions to aid bone regeneration and function [47]. Complex systems enable perfusion and interstitial flow and mimic native bone tissue structure [48]. The researchers successfully regenerated osteochondral tissue utilizing a three-layered stratified copolymeric scaffold colonized by MSCs and zone-specific growth factor administration—including MSCs, bone morphogenetic protein 7 (BMP7), and transforming growth factor (TGF) in the top layer, scaffolding and MSCs and TGF in the middle layer, and MSCs and BMP2 in the bottom layer of subchondral bone [49].

Mineralized stem cells aid in bone regeneration when implanted in metals, ceramics, polymers, and composites [50]. Using porous HA scaffolds modeled after the bone defect, Marcacci and colleagues seeded cells from the bone marrow stroma of four patients to treat substantial bone diaphysis defects. In the subsequent 5–7 months, the implant and bone joined, and the regrowth of bone lasted for another 7 years [51]. Integrating mesenchymal stem cells onto silica-coated calcium hydroxyapatite scaffolds improved the osteogenic potential of large critical-size bone lesions in rabbits. As a result, the presence of growth factors and scaffold–MSC constructions aided in the healing of bone [52]. Researchers showed that an MSC-colonized biphasic calcium phosphate (BCP) scaffold repaired a canine femoral head load-bearing bone lesion. BCP scaffolds with MSC increased bone formation and repair site strength and compressive modulus [53]. There are several types of research that have been processed that go into detail about how MSCs can be used with ceramics [54, 55]. Researchers showed that tibial non-unions with gaps smaller than 5 mm responded well to the injection of bone marrow aspirate concentrate (BMAC) with demineralized bone matrix [56]. Although both polyglycolic acid (PGA) and stem cells have demonstrated regenerative potential *in vivo* [58], faster degrading materials like polylactic glycolic acid (PLGA) are favored as they soften over time without affecting bone formation [57]. Implantation of a PLGA scaffold seeded with MSCs differentiated into cartilage-forming chondrocytes [59] and repaired critical-size and full-thickness femur fractures in rats. When human mesenchymal stem cells were implanted into chitosan/poly (butylene succinate) scaffolds in immunodeficient mice, the scaffolds' potential to generate osteoblasts was shown [60]. Both *in vivo* (in the animal) and *in vitro* (in the test tube), hyaluronate hydrogel implanted with mesenchymal stem cells derived from umbilical cord blood showed promise for the restoration of permanent articular cartilage in osteoarthritic knees [61]. Micro- and macroporous metal scaffolds are highly regulated and biocompatible. These morphologies improve serum protein adsorption, which promotes mesenchymal stem cell expansion [62]. Metals nevertheless tend to corrode [63]. Studies have shown that the addition of MSCs to the composite's biomaterial poly(3-hydroxybutyrate)/hydroxy alkanoates/alginate increases bone formation in a critical-size defect by a factor of 4 [64]. In a cranial defect model, researchers implanted MSCs isolated from an umbilical cord onto Geistlich Bio-Oss® collagen scaffolds, and 21 days later, the defect had healed [65]. In low concentrations, silver nanoparticles encapsulated in collagen have been shown to improve femoral fracture healing, mesenchymal stem cell proliferation, and bone formation (osteogenesis) [66, 67]. Indeed MSC and fibroblast (fibroblastic) chemotaxis to the fracture site, MSC proliferation, and TGF-/BMP signaling in MSCs can enhance fracture callus formation and early fracture gap closure [68]. The osteogenic potential of poly-lactic acid nanofibrous scaffolds is improved when nanoparticles encapsulated with copper, zinc, and imidazole metal–organic frameworks are attached to the scaffolds [69]. Several studies suggest that scaffold colonization with MSC may not necessarily promote bone healing contrasted to scaffold alone or scaffold with growth factors [70], even though these findings expand the disciplines of bone tissue engineering and regeneration. As a result, no product based on mesenchymal stem cells for bone repair has become the industry standard [71]. The widespread application of MSCs is hindered by problems with cell treatment [including standardization, quality control, good manufacturing practice (GMP) production, logistics, regulatory permission, tissue supplies, cost, etc.), tissue-engineered scaffolds, as well as the co-application of signals enhancing cell phenotypic and function *in vivo*. Using extracellular vesicles and MSC-released cytokines, secretome-based techniques have been employed to improve viable cell treatment and tissue transplantation. Despite promising research results, the translational application has struggled to standardize manufacturing and analytic procedures [72].

2.3.2 Tissue Engineering for Bone Regeneration

The production of red as well as white blood cells, the storage of minerals, and the ability to move and support the body are just some of the many ways in which healthy bone tissue is essential to human wellbeing [73]. Bone serves multiple functions and is made up of three distinct cell types (osteoblasts, osteocytes, and osteoclasts) that are respectively responsible for bone formation, mineralization, and resorption. Bone tissue is made up of the mineralized material of cortical bone and cancellous bone; however, there are many other types of tissue in bones, including bone marrow, blood vessels, cartilage, and nerves. The soft bone matrix is strengthened by the adherence of the inorganic mineral salt, calcium phosphate, in a chemical structure known as calcium hydroxyapatite, while normal bone cells repair, remodel, and rebuild. Bone regeneration is a difficult area of tissue engineering due to its mechanical, synthetic, and metabolic features, and there are many articles outlining recent advances in this field [74–76]. Figure 2.2 represents various bone regeneration strategies.

The goal of the tissue engineering approach to bone regeneration therapy is not merely to insert non-living scaffolds but, rather, to create new, cell-driven, functional tissues [77]. An alternate treatment for diseases needing bone regeneration is developed by fusing orthopedic surgery principles with those from biology, materials science, physics, and engineering [78]. In bone tissue engineering, growth hormones (for osteoinduction) and progenitor cells (for osteogenesis) are combined in biocompatible scaffolds, ideally in three-dimensional tissue-like constructions (for

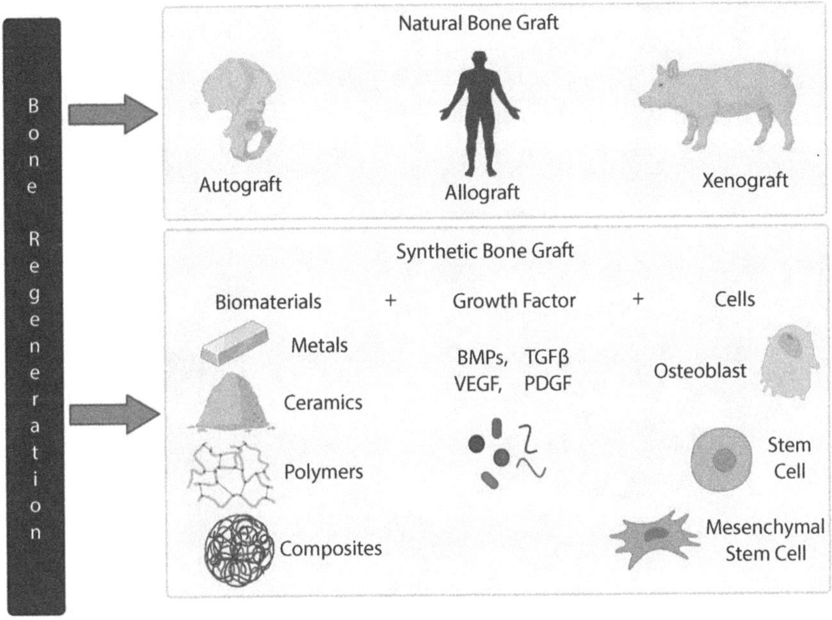

Figure 2.2 Regenerative bone tissue possibilities. Autograft, allograft, and xenograft are natural bone grafts. Metals (gray discs), ceramics (beige powder and gray microporous cylinder-shaped item), and polymers (green ribbon, green stiff cylinder-shaped hydrogel, light blue hydrogel mesh) can make synthetic bone grafts. BMPs, TGFβ, vascular endothelial growth factor (VEGF), and platelet-derived growth factor (PDGF) can be used to functionalize biomaterials (platelet-derived growth factor; light blue ribbon). Cells can colonize synthetic bone grafts.

osteoconduction and vascular ingrowth). Because of the high volume of grafting material required for treating significant bone lesions, composite grafts with reinforcements are the obvious choice. As an alternative to autologous bone transplant, composite grafts consisting of bone synthetic or bioabsorbable scaffolds planted with bone marrow aspirate or growth factors are already available [79]. Figure 2.3 describes the method of tissue engineering for bone regeneration.

Many animal studies and the initial pilot clinical studies using tissue-engineered structures for local bone regeneration have been conducted—credit goes to the many technological advancements made in the area of bone tissue engineering over the past few years, especially with the improved knowledge of bone healing at the molecular and cellular level. Culture-expanded, non-genetically modified MSCs have been used for bone repair in two research reporting on long bones and five studies

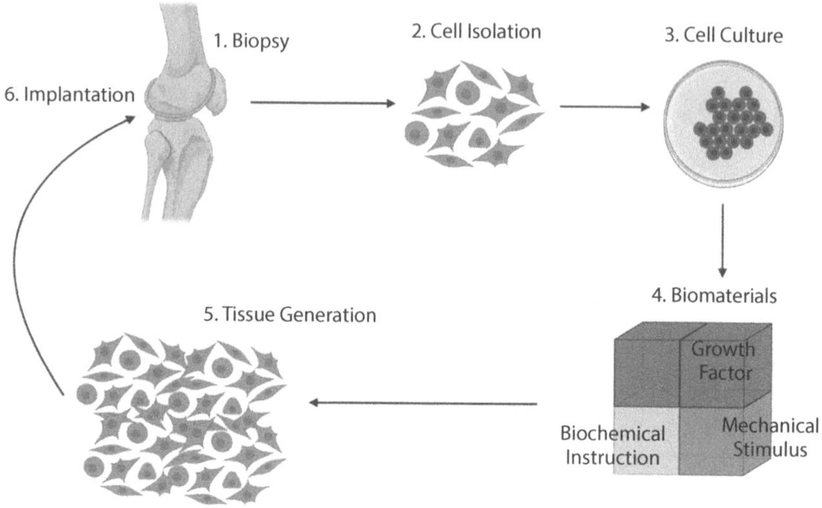

Figure 2.3 Tissue engineering and biomaterial paradigm for bone repair. After a tissue biopsy, the separated cells are put into a culture. Biomaterials are employed for tissue production and growth because of their multifaceted features, such as their biochemical and biophysical cell-instructive ones, which aid in both cell proliferation and the necessary differentiation. Tissue that has been artificially produced is implanted at the site of injury to promote healing and growth.

reporting on maxillofacial diseases [80]. The grafted MSCs showed signs of bone apposition; however, this was not enough to heal major defects. This is the case even if it is difficult to draw broad conclusions from so many different studies. To further reduce aseptic loosening in total joint arthroplasty, tissue engineering technique has been used to speed up fracture healing and improve bone–prosthesis interaction [81, 82].

Recent animal studies have shown that vascularized bioartificial bone grafts can be prefabricated *in vivo* using β-tricalcium phosphate (β-TCP) scaffolds stuffed with autogenous bone marrow for cell loading and transplanted into the latissimus dorsi muscle for possible applications at a later stage for segmental bone restructuring, demonstrating the concepts of bone transplantation with negligible donor site morbidity and no quantity restrictions [83].

There are still numerous questions about the effectiveness, safety, and cost of bone tissue engineering that need to be answered before it can be used routinely in clinical settings. Mutations or epigenetic alterations in cells that have been cultured and propagated *in vitro* may give tumorigenic potential. Nonetheless, tumor growth is unlikely, as shown by *in vitro* and *in vivo* testing [84]. Up to 11 years and 5 months after the implantation of autologous bone marrow-derived MSCs for cartilage repair, there had been no findings of tumor transformation among 41 patients (45 joints). Another key problem [85] is keeping cells alive and dense on three-dimensional biodegradable scaffolds. Because of this, various bioreactor technologies have been explored, and many more need to be created [86]. The degrading qualities of these materials should also protect the integrity of nearby tissues and the ongoing process of bone remodeling [87]. Constant research is being conducted to determine whether three-dimensional porous scaffolds can enhance cellular adhesion, proliferation, migration, and differentiation by modifying their nano-, micro-, and macro-scale architectures to achieve optimum surface porosity and chemistry.

2.3.3 Gene Therapy and Bone Regeneration

Gene therapy is an exciting new avenue for delivering growth factors in the domain of bone tissue engineering [88]. The target cell's genome is inserted with the desired genetic material, allowing for the sustained expression of bioactive substances within the cells themselves. Both viral (transfection) and non-viral (transduction) vectors can be used to move genes either in or out of a living organism, respectively. While being potentially easier because genetic material is administered directly into the host, the *in vivo* process has several safety issues. The indirect *ex vivo* technique involves removing cells from a living organism, such as a human, and then manipulating their deoxyribonucleic acid (DNA) in a laboratory. Despite the increased technical difficulty, this procedure is safer since it allows for assessing the cells for abnormal activity before reimplantation and selecting those with the highest gene expression [89].

While the use of gene therapy to administer growth factors for bone tissue regeneration has shown promise in animal studies [90, 91], many questions about its cost, effectiveness, and biological safety still need to be answered before it can be used on humans.

2.4 Understanding AI

Non-mathematicians are also able to use the tool thanks to its more generalized nature. Some several well-referenced publications and articles take a more mathematical or in-depth method to the topic [92]. The AIs that can predict the response of skeletal stem cells to topography and detect the depth of surfaces machined with lasers use deep learning. Despite its complex computing techniques and nonlinear mathematics, deep learning is a widely used machine learning architecture. As a result, this contributed to the "black box" description of AI. Common smartphone apps have a "magical black box" that can accurately label a picture of a cat using large image databases including ImageNet and Open Images [93]. Anyone can instantly alter their virtual look by sending in a photo of their face and receiving back a younger, more attractive version of themselves [94]. To some, it may appear like magic is required to make sense of data transformations (how the input has become the output), but this is not the case.

Artificial neural networks compute data transformation algorithms without comprehending the science or properties. They are universal approximators that can solve complex or time-consuming problems statistically [95]. Artificial neural networks resemble animal visual cortexes conceptually. Both have synapses connecting nodes (neurons). Data transformation as it propagates through neural networks makes them effective. Each node generates a new, weighted output by adding the previous weighted outputs of connected nodes. The dendrites of a neuron are responsible for relaying the electrical stimulation from those other neurons to the axon terminals. The synaptic weights among nodes in both natural and artificial neural networks increase with network sophistication. Backpropagation is an act of changing weights to better suit training instances in artificial neural networks, which automatically minimizes error [96]. Like brain plasticity in animals, stronger weightings strengthen connections that produce the right outputs and weaken those that do not.

Artificial neural networks comprising "hidden" nodes in between input and output layers are what deep neural networks (DNNs) are (Figure 2.4). These core, hidden layers adapt their performance with increasing depth. The first one processes the incoming data unmodified, while the second one uses the first one's modified data to do its abstract operations. Invisible layers are present at a higher degree of operation. With processing power, enough layers, and diverse input data, deep learning architecture can fine-tune synapses without the need for representation architecture or human–computer engineers. Using only backpropagation across all hidden layers, the network is taught for the first time without any science or prior knowledge of which attributes of the input data are important at each layer. Deep learning systems with fewer than 20 hidden layers can perform complex functions on their inputs that are sensitive to minute details (such as differentiating among distinct kinds of canine) but inadequate to large irrelevant variations like background, pose, lighting, and surrounding objects [97].

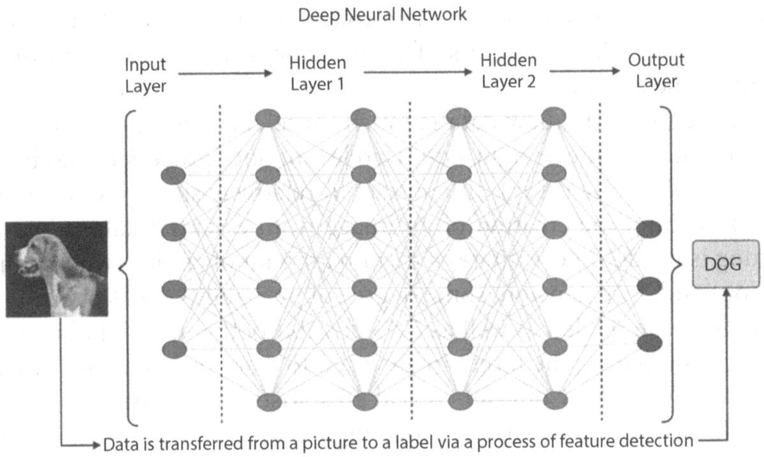

Figure 2.4 Deep neural network concept. The input layer, which has multiple nodes (circles), is connected to the first hidden layer, which weighs, sums, and transforms the data without human intervention before moving on to the next layer. The second hidden layer only receives input data from the first, enabling more abstract feature extraction. The output layer receives hidden layer data. Different networks can customize their hidden layers, nodes, and data transformation between layers.

So far, every single example of artificial intelligence has relied on convolutional neural networks (ConvNets or CNNs) that have long demonstrated superiority in imaging tasks [98, 99] within the medical field [100, 101]. Like the ventral route hierarchy in the visual cortex, which is critical for visual perception [102], this overall organization plays a role in visual perception. The convolutional and pooling layers of a ConvNet are inspired by visual neuroscience's archetypal simple and complex cells [103]. Extraction of image features is essential. The only way to see spatial details is to adjust the pixel position. However, the shape of a dog's ears is just as important as the color (measured in pixels) when it comes to determining the breed (spatial pixel arrangement). Without sacrificing any of the image's spatial context, the convolutional layer uses a weighted matrix to isolate relevant details. While the ConvNet learns (weights adjusted) to minimize loss, it may extract many features using a weight combination, such as one that concentrated on color, the other on edges, plus an additional blurring of unnecessary noise from the image. Not only is there a single goal to shoot for and an error metric to measure progress but features are also found and prioritized automatically. Hence, the pooling matrix reduces both the image size as well as the number of pixels that the network must process. This unifies characteristics that share a common semantic meaning and renders them robust against ambiguity (A brown dog is a brown dog regardless of its placement in a photograph or the quality of the lighting.).

However, creating new data is much more challenging. Whether the dog is on the left side or right side is irrelevant once processing has begun (there is a dog either way). In contrast to relatively straightforward feature extraction, the creation of an image from essential data (a picture of a dog is needed) necessitates a certain amount of choice (where to put the dog) and, by extension, some degree of probability (50% chance that it should be on the left as well as 50% possibility that it should be on the right) of comparing the target image used to train the ConvNet. Images produced by simple ConvNets reveal all statistically plausible outcomes throughout time rather than just one highly possible (the dog is on both sides and neither side simultaneously; a blurry mess rather than a clear picture of a dog on one side). This outcome minimizes loss but is useless because it is based on unrealistic input data. As a result, a second ConvNet is added into the design to fine-tune the loss function, leading to the crucial question of whether the generated ConvNet's output looks plausible. In today's modern world, blurry images are fake and unacceptable results. A conditionally generative adversarial network is made up of the generator and discriminator ConvNets, both of which are trained in a conditional generative adversarial network (cGAN). The generator tricks the discriminator into thinking that the images it produces are real.

Deep learning uses several network architectures, including the cGAN. A loss function, several hidden layers of more complex and hard-to-visualize data operations, and the ability to learn and improve without human interaction are hallmarks of today's most popular systems. Deep learning is very adaptable and becoming more affordable as computing advances lower graphics processing unit (GPU) and other hardware costs. It can be used for supervised learning, reinforcement learning, or other machine learning methods.

This review barely scratches the surface of AI, especially deep learning. In medicine and other fields, CNNs and cGANs are among many architectures that have influenced research and applications. The most important developments in deep learning and artificial intelligence over the past few decades have been narrowed down by several reputable research. The "deep learning" literature review by researchers provides a non-mathematical explanation of supervised, backpropagation, and unsupervised learning [97]. The mathematics of deep learning can be found in research conducted by researchers. The material presented here is appropriate for students at the beginning of their mathematical studies toward a degree.

Researchers explore cutting-edge theories like reinforcement learning and deep learning architectures that can take in a wide variety of data as well as successful applications like medical imaging and genomics. Data-driven medicine is explored by researchers, which also provides pictorial explanations of mathematical fundamentals [104]. It also discusses biomedical deep learning's triumphs and failures and how transparency and performance guarantees might improve applications.

2.5 Current AI Integration

Genomics (usually at the forefront of computer science integration), single-patient gene expression information, or national public health data converted into specific biomedical applications are driving the growth of deep learning in healthcare [105]. The deep learning have effect in medicine, biology, and healthcare [106]. Clinical imaging, electronic health records, genomics, smart health-tracking wearable devices, or even sensor-equipped smartphones are just some of the areas where deep learning is improving and inventing new techniques to connect data, patients, and medical professionals [107]. There is room for improvement in areas where doctors currently face challenges, such as determining whether novel variants in a patient's genome seem to be scientifically justified, whether plasma irregularities might be early-onset cancerous mutations, and also how cell characteristics are linked to tumor pathology [108, 109]. Minimal data processing and the capacity to extract features and characteristics without training in the life sciences are necessary for this. When it comes to medically evaluating, analyzing, and annotating huge amounts of data, the field of medical imaging is notoriously complex and perplexing [110, 111]. Abnormality detection, morphological identification, non-invasive cell counting, and stem cell behavior prediction are only some of the more complex tasks where deep learning is being employed [112–114].

Machine learning has contributed to the advancement of biomaterial science in several ways, such as the design of 3D scaffolds for cell control from geometrical fiber-based material matrices [115], the creation of blueprints for 3D bioprinting of tissue-specific microenvironments and patient-specific organs [116, 117], and the optimization of piezoelectric drop-on-demand printing [118]. Now, with the help of deep learning, biomaterials may be designed and manufactured with consideration for factors like patient and trauma type. Because topographical qualities influence cell motility, differentiation, proliferation, elongation, adhesion, and osteogenic gene expression, they are crucial biophysical parameters for cell-instructive biomaterials. Evidence suggests that utilizing deep learning on microtopographies can effectively detect cell sites in response to varying (unseen) surface patterning, resulting in statistically significant projection for adult skeletal stem cells using donors not employed during training [119]. Utilizing simpler machine learning models for morphology analysis, researchers have looked at how human bone marrow-derived mesenchymal stromal cells (HBMSCs) react to stimuli in their microenvironment. However, the stated results only included training accuracy, which makes it impossible to conduct a study and validation of actual usage [104]. Both research show promises for advancing the use of AI to tissue engineering issues if validation outcomes are in line with training accuracies. With a reliable deep learning-based model of stem cells, the time and money spent on laboratory experiments related to microtopography can be significantly reduced.

While dozens or even tens of thousands of images are typically thought to be necessary for deep learning to work well [120], these statistically meaningful predictions were made using only a batch of 200 photos. Randomly cropping, rotating, and inverting images are just a few examples of the data augmentation techniques that may be used to grow a small batch of photos into a huge, more valuable dataset containing thousands of images. The same issues that arise when amplifying trace DNA might arise when there is over-amplification of DNNs. A single, bad sample image would declare the whole training and testing process meaningless because the system would not be able to create enough data. If the training data is not well balanced, the network would not be able to discover the features it needs to handle the problem in the actual world. Training and testing on varied data are simplified by a big dataset, and accuracy is increased by preventing the network from over-training and over-fitting at the expense of generalizability and practicality. The training of a deep learning network might take many weeks; therefore, efficiency is of essence. It was demonstrated that deep learning may be used in areas with less data than genomics by training a model that accurately forecasted stem cell behavior without overfitting. Augmentation can expand training data without destabilizing training and improve results in smaller dataset-driving problems [121].

Research into stem cells has benefited from the application of artificial intelligence to better understand the potential to differentiate [122], recognize responses to microenvironmental cues [123], anticipate and examine immunosuppressive outcomes [125], detect pluripotent colony formation [124], and automate quality control [126]. Machine learning models projected 84% reliability upon 5 days of feature analysis and 90% accuracy after 7 days of testing in bioreactors [127] for cardiac myocytes produced from human pluripotent stem cells having therapeutic potential. Failures can be stopped and remedied, saving time and resources and revealing which features best predict cardiomyocyte content. This technique could not predict quality, functionality, or maturity. Even though their reliability was only 62.4%, the researchers in another study used machine intelligence to distinguish between good, semi-good, and dreadful colonies. Colonies that fell somewhere between "excellent" and "poor" were difficult for models to categorize. Either the model or the images were insufficient. With a quantitative approach, larger dataset, and more sophisticated network model, machine learning shows promise for quality control applications (83.8 percentage points of accuracy in finding good cultures).

After one high-quality stem cell colony has been cultivated, chronic graft-versus-host disease (GvHD) must be avoided because it is a major factor of morbidity and mortality after stem cell transplantation [128]. The relationship between chronic GvHD severity as well as National Institutes of Health (NIH) biomarkers is unknown, and clinical outcomes are still unpredictable to doctors but not to AI [129]. To reverse the process, machine learning was used to identify chronic GvHD phenotypes, and a clinical decision tree was the result. For risk assessment of patients with acute leukemia 100 days following stem cell transplantation [130], a decision tree model was developed using machine learning predictions. Advances in both theoretical and practical clinical knowledge are attributed to machine learning.

Research on animals is typically required as a bridge between cell culture models and human clinical trials. Animal testing is required to translate promising *in vitro* experiments into clinical applications of biomaterials, medicines, and methods in human medicine. *In vitro* data cannot predict *in vivo* results, so AI is a revolutionary technique for predicting results without animal testing [131]. The United Kingdom (UK) Home Office regulates animal research and requires extensive planning, training, competency evaluations, facility accreditation, and employee licensing. To save time, money, and animals, researchers should follow the prepared guidelines to swiftly amend the aspects to examine before beginning an experiment utilizing animals [132]. All the methodologies, data, and aspects examined during and before an *in vivo* study should be published to make it repeatable, buildable, and transparent [133], as recommended by the Arrive Guidelines. The National Coalition for the Replacement, Refinement, and Reduction of Animals in Research promotes the "3Rs" of animal experimentation: removing the need for animals altogether, improving animal welfare standards, and decreasing the number of animals used (National Centre for the Replacement, Refinement, and Reduction of Animals in Research).

Artificial intelligence is helping with the 3Rs of animal research. Nanomaterial toxicity modeling employs MPPD models, which allow for the prediction of micro- and nano-distribution in animal models [134]. Toxicology studies conducted using machine learning can complement *in vivo* studies [135]. Both computational neuroethology [136] and neurology studies employ deep learning to analyze how a subject's posture changes in response to external inputs. Recently, the discipline of behavior mapping was examined by researchers [137]. The current movement to limit animal exploitation in research provides a chance to enhance the 3Rs without compromising human therapeutic use.

2.6 Applying Deep Learning

2.6.1 Where Things Go Wrong

The application of deep learning is not without risk, and overfitting is just one of many potential issues that can develop. Knowing the goal of the network and the potential sources of bias in the training data is crucial. Both are important to keep in mind when applying deep learning because the consequences of misallocating resources or training a network with the wrong task or loss function will likely not be discovered until after a significant amount of time has been invested in collecting, processing, and training the data. Furthermore, even the right task can produce the wrong answer and an unusable network if the data is biased. The use of AI to automate the playing of several Nintendo Entertainment System (NES) games is a prime example of giving the wrong task to a network [138]. All these contests had one common goal: to be victorious. This can be construed in various ways, such as whether the network should be programmed to maximize the score, play time, level progression, or a mix of these and other factors. While the algorithm could play NES games like Super Mario Bros. when given the goal of winning, such play would be inhumanly exploitative of bugs, and hence the program failed at playing Tetris. It did not find out how to win by strategically placing blocks, but it did figure out how to pause the game right before it was done. This would cause the game to pause. A common tactic used by resentful older siblings is simply not playing the game, and this is what the algorithm had done.

Additionally crucial is the issue of possible data bias [139]. A network that can "augment clinical decision-making for dermatology professionals" [140] was reported to have been built in a 2017 Nature paper that received several thousand citations. In the research work, pictures of malignant tumors from a variety of patients were utilized to train and test the network. However, it is important to note that not all pictures feature a ruler. Researchers observed that, after publishing, the network became more accurate at predicting malignant tumors when a ruler was included in the image. This is not an illustration of a poorly trained network but, rather, one that was trained properly despite being given biased inputs. Images of malignant melanoma from the International Skin Imaging Collaboration (ISIC) Melanoma Project archive had a higher frequency of rulers [141]. The reason for this is that if a dermatologist has grounds for concern about a skin lesion, he or she is more likely to measure it with a ruler and document the results. More improvement may have been made in dermatology and oncology if the dataset had been more evenly split among benign and malignant lesion images and if the network had not selected the ruler feature as a crucial signal. Researchers working with AI need to exercise caution because the smallest error can severely compromise an entire dataset and network, lowering a widely cited cancer detection system to the accuracy of a basic ruler detector.

Reducing the gap between training and production environments is the most effective strategy for overcoming problems like erroneous task functions and biased datasets. Different categories [104] can be used to describe this discrepancy such as the following:

I. Target mismatch—The user is interested in knowing which biomaterials encourage differentiation, but the network has been trained to make predictions about proliferation.
II. Loss function mismatch—The squared error in estimating the total number of cells is the training loss function; however, all the bioengineer truly needs for the project to be regarded successful is for the colony to have a density that is higher than a particular threshold.
III. Mismatched data and biased selection—At any given time, donor cells could only be harvested from a single patient population.
IV. Nonstationary environments—The model does not include any changes to account for the change in cellular behavior that takes place as a result of expanding colony size.
V. Reactive and adversarial environments—As a direct result of using the model, the culture of the colony is altered; because of this, a second assumption concerning the rate of multiplication would not be correct.

VI. Confounding variables and causality—There is no correlation between the existence of a ruler and an increase in the likelihood that a lesion is malignant.

However, these challenges can be conquered by collaborative network design that incorporates data gathered from the end-user(s). If the activity at hand does not necessitate innovative data combinations or computer technology that is beyond conventional gaming or image processing computers, users can likewise employ AI in their study and train the network themselves utilizing publicly available deep learning architectures [142]. When the task at hand does not call for unusual data pairings or specific hardware, consumers can select this alternative. There will be less friction during implementation because the user will have a firm grasp of what to expect from the network and where its boundaries are.

2.6.2 How to Integrate AI

The first stage in implementing deep learning is deciding what the network will do. This must be a data-driven task that improves the field by saving time, resources, or knowledge. Data selection matters. There is a possibility that a network will be able to recognize COVID-19 cases using computed tomography (CT) scans of the lungs, which are more difficult to acquire [143]. Furthermore, chest X-rays are more readily available in other hospitals; hence, this could put the completion of the task and accessibility of the data at risk. Accessibility is crucial for generating a large, diverse training dataset and for real-world applications. After determining the data type and task, choose a network architecture. The response of adult skeletal stem cells to micro-patterned topographies can be predicted using deep learning, and placenta cells can be marked with nanoscale resolution [144]. The approximately 7,000-times-cited pix2pix architecture has found hundreds, if not thousands, of applications across several disciplines. As deep learning finds more and more uses in the biological sciences, many competing architectures produce results that differ slightly in precision and accuracy under the same conditions. Researchers in machine learning would do well to take advantage of the increasing number of available architectures, thanks to both Open Access publishing and a focus on practical applications [145]. The feasibility of a new application can be verified using alternative architectures and data formats.

Training the selected network architecture using data is a time-consuming but straightforward process. To optimize network performance, various hyperparameters must be modified. While the default settings provided by the network design builder will get good results, using your own judgment when selecting the optimizer and initiation functions that will be employed to convert data across the network will get you even better results. It is not uncommon for the optimization of a network's performance to require repeated tweaks to several hyperparameters, including the number of layers, the filters employed in each layer, the activation functions, and so on. When more layers and filters are added to a network, it takes longer to train and requires a larger GPU and more processing power. Training now permits alterations to the learning rate, unlike conventional hyperparameters. The network's error correction has a step size that determines how exactly data is transformed. If the network's steps are too large, it will either step over the optimal solution, leading it to fluctuate around it (which can be detected and rectified), or it will fail to locate it altogether (the network simply will not train successfully). If it is too tiny, the network risks settling for a suboptimal solution or wasting time (think of an adult attempting to travel a long distance while walking at the pace of a toddler). Figure 2.5 explains the relationship between clinicians and DNNs.

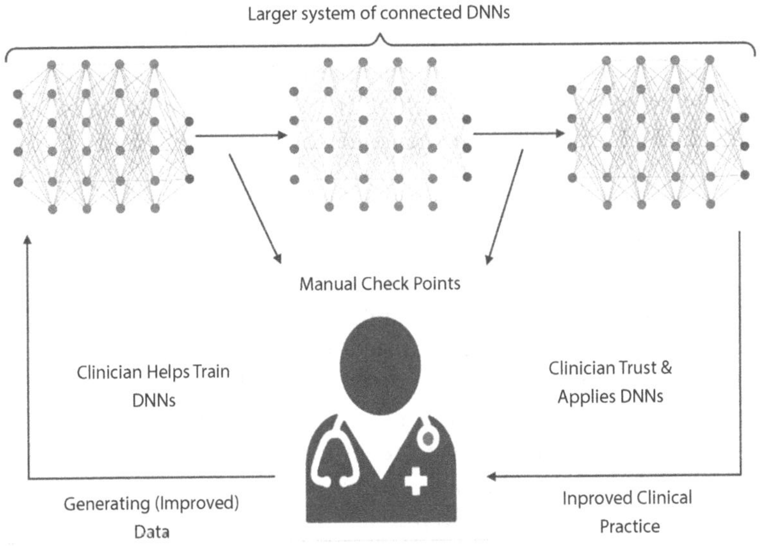

Figure 2.5 AI's future: clinician-centered. Clinicians continuously train connected DNNs with data. It creates several manual checkpoints to examine the DNN process, allowing for greater error correction and scientific knowledge. The clinician trusts the DNN system since they train and test it. DNN advancements make application and clinical practice easier. Improved data improves DNN training, which improves clinical practice in a positive feedback loop.

Testing is the most crucial aspect of the validation and accountability process because training does not always translate to real-world performance. Better test results can be expected when the testing data is consistent with the training data, but this is not indicative of generalizability. Overfitting can be detected through thorough testing, which should include data that was not used to train the network and, ideally, should include key features that were not included in the training data (to determine applicability). It is common practice to randomly select data from training datasets to use in testing, although this is not always the best approach. If a dataset contains many X-ray images of patients' lungs obtained by multiple doctors at three separate hospitals, then two of the hospitals should be utilized for training, preferably the ones with the least biased data (in terms of age, gender, race, etc., at adequate levels), and one for testing. To adequately train the network and for thorough testing of how effectively the AI may be deployed to varied situations, this would include variations in equipment, physicians, and patients from the training data. If the dataset is less varied, such as utilizing a single time-lapse experiment to train a network to predict cell behavior throughout time, pulling frames at random all through or from the center of the data will not challenge the network, which has seen similar information before and after the prediction point. More challenging would be to use data acquired at the end of a time-lapse experiment, after cell density, colony health, and illumination conditions are all likely to have altered. Without any training data, the network was still able to generate accurate predictions.

2.7 Conclusion

With the aging of the global population, tissue engineering's significance in regenerative medicine is only anticipated to increase. Although this science has advanced significantly over the past few decades, there are still numerous obstacles to overcome, including the design of biomaterials and a better understanding of stem cell behavior. Yet by incorporating AI into experimental research and clinical applications, many of the existing medical hurdles can be overcome, opening the door to patient- and trauma-specific treatments in the future. One day, artificial intelligence might be able to regrow bone.

References

1. Cooper, C., Mitchell, P., Kanis, J.A., Breaking the fragility fracture cycle. *Osteoporos. Int.*, 22, 2049–50, 2011 Jul.

2. Hiligsmann, M., Cooper, C., Arden, N., Boers, M., Branco, J.C., Brandi, M.L., Bruyère, O., Guillemin, F., Hochberg, M.C., Hunter, D.J., Kanis, J.A., Health economics in the field of osteoarthritis: An expert's consensus paper from the European Society for Clinical and Economic Aspects of Osteoporosis and Osteoarthritis (ESCEO), in: *Seminars in Arthritis and Rheumatism*, vol. 43, No. 3, WB Saunders, pp. 303–313, 2013 Dec 1.
3. Ackerman, I.N., Bohensky, M.A., De Steiger, R., Brand, C.A., Eskelinen, A., Fenstad, A.M., Furnes, O., Garellick, G., Graves, S.E., Haapakoski, J., Havelin, L.I., Substantial rise in the lifetime risk of primary total knee replacement surgery for osteoarthritis from 2003 to 2013: An international, population-level analysis. *Osteoarthr. Cartil.*, 25, 4, 455–61, 2017 Apr 1.
4. Inacio, M.C., Graves, S.E., Pratt, N.L., Roughead, E.E., Nemes, S., Increase in total joint arthroplasty projected from 2014 to 2046 in Australia: A conservative local model with international implications. *Clin. Orthop. Relat. Res.*, 475, 2130–7, 2017 Aug.
5. Rawal, B.R., Yadav, A., Pare, V., Life estimation of knee joint prosthesis by combined effect of fatigue and wear. *Proc. Technol.*, 23, 60–7, 2016 Jan 1.
6. Stevens, M.M., Biomaterials for bone tissue engineering. *Mater. Today*, 11, 5, 18–25, 2008 May 1.
7. Tang, D., Tare, R.S., Yang, L.Y., Williams, D.F., Ou, K.L., Oreffo, R.O., Biofabrication of bone tissue: Approaches, challenges and translation for bone regeneration. *Biomaterials*, 83, 363–82, 2016 Mar 1.
8. Armstrong, J.P. and Stevens, M.M., Emerging technologies for tissue engineering: From gene editing to personalized medicine. *Tissue Eng. Part A*, 25, 9-10, 688–92, 2019 May 1.
9. Uskoković, V., Janković-Cástvan, I., Wu, V.M., Bone mineral crystallinity governs the orchestration of ossification and resorption during bone remodeling. *ACS Biomater. Sci. Eng.*, 5, 7, 3483–98, 2019 Jun 11.
10. Wang, D., Jang, J., Kim, K., Kim, J., Park, C.B., "Tree to bone": Lignin/polycaprolactone nanofibers for hydroxyapatite biomineralization. *Biomacromolecules*, 20, 7, 2684–93, 2019 May 22.
11. Hu, C., Ashok, D., Nisbet, D.R., Gautam, V., Bioinspired surface modification of orthopedic implants for bone tissue engineering. *Biomaterials*, 219, 119366, 2019 Oct 1.
12. Qiu, Z.Y., Cui, Y., Wang, X.M., Natural bone tissue and its biomimetic, in: *Mineralized Collagen Bone Graft Substitutes*, pp. 1–22, Woodhead Publishing, Sawston, Cambridge, 2019 Jan 1.
13. Türk, S., Altınsoy, İ., Çelebi Efe, G., Ipek, M., Özacar, M., Bindal, C., Effect of solution and calcination time on sol-gel synthesis of hydroxyapatite. *J. Bionic Eng.*, 16, 311–8, 2019 Mar.
14. Samavedi, S., Whittington, A.R., Goldstein, A.S., Calcium phosphate ceramics in bone tissue engineering: A review of properties and their influence on cell behavior. *Acta Biomater.*, 9, 9, 8037–45, 2013 Sep 1.

15. Wang, Y., Azaïs, T., Robin, M., Vallée, A., Catania, C., Legriel, P., Pehau-Arnaudet, G., Babonneau, F., Giraud-Guille, M.M., Nassif, N., The predominant role of collagen in the nucleation, growth, structure and orientation of bone apatite. *Nat. Mater.*, 11, 8, 724–33, 2012 Aug.
16. Kular, J., Tickner, J., Chim, S.M., Xu, J., An overview of the regulation of bone remodelling at the cellular level. *Clin. Biochem.*, 45, 12, 863–73, 2012 Aug 1.
17. Standring, S., *Gray's anatomy*, 41st edn, Elsevier, Philadelphia, PA., 1584.
18. Sikavitsas, V.I., Temenoff, J.S., Mikos, A.G., Biomaterials and bone mechanotransduction. *Biomaterials*, 22, 19, 2581–93, 2001 Oct 1.
19. Noble, B.S. and Reeve, J., Osteocyte function, osteocyte death and bone fracture resistance. *Mol. Cell. Endocrinol.*, 159, 1–2, 7–13, 2000 Jan 25.
20. Teti, A., Bone development: Overview of bone cells and signaling. *Curr. Osteoporos. Rep.*, 9, 264–73, 2011 Dec.
21. Franz-Odendaal, T.A., Hall, B.K., Witten, P.E., Buried alive: How osteoblasts become osteocytes. *Dev. Dyn.: An Official Publication of the American Association of Anatomists*, 235, 1, 176–90, 2006 Jan.
22. Luginbuehl, V., Meinel, L., Merkle, H.P., Gander, B., Localized delivery of growth factors for bone repair. *Eur. J. Pharm. Biopharm.*, 58, 2, 197–208, 2004 Sep 1.
23. Boyle, W.J., Simonet, W.S., Lacey, D.L., Osteoclast differentiation and activation. *Nature*, 423, 6937, 337–42, 2003 May 15.
24. Kular, J., Tickner, J., Chim, S.M., Xu, J., An overview of the regulation of bone remodelling at the cellular level. *Clin. Biochem.*, 45, 12, 863–73, 2012 Aug 1.
25. Schindeler, A., McDonald, M.M., Bokko, P., Little, D.G., Bone remodeling during fracture repair: The cellular picture. *Semin. Cell Dev. Biol.*, 19, 5, 459–466, 2008 Oct 1. Academic Press.
26. Melo-Fonseca, F., Miranda, G., Domingues, H.S., Pinto, I.M., Gasik, M., Silva, F.S., Reengineering bone-implant interfaces for improved mechanotransduction and clinical outcomes. *Stem Cell Rev. Rep.*, 16, 1121–38, 2020 Dec.
27. Dimitriou, R., Tsiridis, E., Giannoudis, P.V., Current concepts of molecular aspects of bone healing. *Injury*, 36, 12, 1392–404, 2005 Dec 1.
28. Eslaminejad, M.B. and Faghihi, F., Mesenchymal stem cell-based bone engineering for bone regeneration, in: *Regenerative Medicine and Tissue Engineering-Cells and Biomaterials*, vol. 29, pp. 57–82, 2011 Aug.
29. Marzona, L. and Pavolini, B., Play and players in bone fracture healing match. *Clin. Cases Miner. Bone Metab.*, 6, 2, 159, 2009 May.
30. Knight, M.N. and Hankenson, K.D., Mesenchymal stem cells in bone regeneration. *Adv. Wound Care*, 2, 6, 306–16, 2013 Jul 1.
31. Kamdje, A.H., Kamga, P.T., Simo, R.T., Vecchio, L., Etet, P.F., Muller, J.M., Bassi, G., Lukong, E., Goel, R.K., Amvene, J.M., Krampera, M., Mesenchymal stromal cells' role in tumor microenvironment: Involvement of signaling pathways. *Cancer Biol. Med.*, 14, 2, 129, 2017 May.
32. Song, Y., Wu, H., Gao, Y., Li, J., Lin, K., Liu, B., Lei, X., Cheng, P., Zhang, S., Wang, Y., Sun, J., Zinc silicate/nano-hydroxyapatite/collagen scaffolds

promote angiogenesis and bone regeneration via the p38 MAPK pathway in activated monocytes. *ACS Appl. Mater. Interfaces*, 12, 14, 16058–75, 2020 Mar 17.
33. Chamberlain, G., Fox, J., Ashton, B., Middleton, J., Concise review: Mesenchymal stem cells: Their phenotype, differentiation capacity, immunological features, and potential for homing. *Stem Cells*, 25, 11, 2739–49, 2007 Nov.
34. Fierabracci, A., Del Fattore, A., Luciano, R., Muraca, M., Teti, A., Muraca, M., Recent advances in mesenchymal stem cell immunomodulation: The role of microvesicles. *Cell Transplant.*, 24, 2, 133–49, 2015 Feb.
35. Maffioli, E., Nonnis, S., Angioni, R., Santagata, F., Calì, B., Zanotti, L., Negri, A., Viola, A., Tedeschi, G., Proteomic analysis of the secretome of human bone marrow-derived mesenchymal stem cells primed by pro-inflammatory cytokines. *J. Proteomics*, 166, 115–26, 2017 Aug 23.
36. Fraser, J.K., Wulur, I., Alfonso, Z., Hedrick, M.H., Fat tissue: An underappreciated source of stem cells for biotechnology. *Trends Biotechnol.*, 24, 4, 150–4, 2006 Apr 1.
37. Hass, R., Kasper, C., Böhm, S., Jacobs, R., Different populations and sources of human mesenchymal stem cells (MSC): A comparison of adult and neonatal tissue-derived MSC. *Cell Commun. Signaling*, 9, 1, 1–4, 2011 Dec.
38. Cheng, H., Qiu, L., Ma, J., Zhang, H., Cheng, M., Li, W., Zhao, X., Liu, K., Replicative senescence of human bone marrow and umbilical cord derived mesenchymal stem cells and their differentiation to adipocytes and osteoblasts. *Mol. Biol. Rep.*, 38, 5161–8, 2011 Nov.
39. Fong, C.Y., Subramanian, A., Gauthaman, K., Venugopal, J., Biswas, A., Ramakrishna, S., Bongso, A., Human umbilical cord Wharton's jelly stem cells undergo enhanced chondrogenic differentiation when grown on nanofibrous scaffolds and in a sequential two-stage culture medium environment. *Stem Cell Rev. Rep.*, 8, 195–209, 2012 Mar.
40. Zhang, X., Hirai, M., Cantero, S., Ciubotariu, R., Dobrila, L., Hirsh, A., Igura, K., Satoh, H., Yokomi, I., Nishimura, T., Yamaguchi, S., Isolation and characterization of mesenchymal stem cells from human umbilical cord blood: Reevaluation of critical factors for successful isolation and high ability to proliferate and differentiate to chondrocytes as compared to mesenchymal stem cells from bone marrow and adipose tissue. *J. Cell. Biochem.*, 112, 4, 1206–18, 2011 Apr.
41. Marolt Presen, D., Traweger, A., Gimona, M., Redl, H., Mesenchymal stromal cell-based bone regeneration therapies: From cell transplantation and tissue engineering to therapeutic secretomes and extracellular vesicles. *Front. Bioeng. Biotechnol.*, 7, 352, 2019 Nov 27.
42. Yorukoglu, A.C., Kiter, A.H., Akkaya, S., Satiroglu-Tufan, N.L., Tufan, A.C., A concise review on the use of mesenchymal stem cells in cell sheet-based tissue engineering with special emphasis on bone tissue regeneration. *Stem Cells Int.*, 2017, 1–14, 2017 Oct.

43. Kon, E., Filardo, G., Roffi, A., Di Martino, A., Hamdan, M., De Pasqual, L., Merli, M.L., Marcacci, M., Bone regeneration with mesenchymal stem cells. *Clin. Cases Miner. Bone Metab.*, 9, 1, 24, 2012 Jan.
44. Shim, G., Lee, S., Han, J., Kim, G., Jin, H., Miao, W., Yi, T.G., Cho, Y.K., Song, S.U., Oh, Y.K., Pharmacokinetics and *in vivo* fate of intra-articularly transplanted human bone marrow-derived clonal mesenchymal stem cells. *Stem Cells Dev.*, 24, 9, 1124–32, 2015 May 1.
45. Redondo, L.M., García, V., Peral, B., Verrier, A., Becerra, J., Sánchez, A., Garcia-Sancho, J., Repair of maxillary cystic bone defects with mesenchymal stem cells seeded on a cross-linked serum scaffold. *J. Cranio-Maxillofac. Surg.*, 46, 2, 222–9, 2018 Feb 1.
46. Gómez-Barrena, E., Rosset, P., Gebhard, F., Hernigou, P., Baldini, N., Rouard, H., Sensebé, L., Gonzalo-Daganzo, R.M., Giordano, R., Padilla-Eguiluz, N., García-Rey, E., Feasibility and safety of treating non-unions in tibia, femur and humerus with autologous, expanded, bone marrow-derived mesenchymal stromal cells associated with biphasic calcium phosphate biomaterials in a multicentric, non-comparative trial. *Biomaterials*, 196, 100–8, 2019 Mar 1.
47. Cidonio, G., Glinka, M., Kim, Y.H., Kanczler, J.M., Lanham, S.A., Ahlfeld, T., Lode, A., Dawson, J.I., Gelinsky, M., Oreffo, R.O., Nanoclay-based 3D printed scaffolds promote vascular ingrowth *ex vivo* and generate bone mineral tissue *in vitro* and *in vivo*. *Biofabrication*, 12, 3, 035010, 2020 May 11.
48. Sladkova, M., Alawadhi, R., Jaragh Alhaddad, R., Esmael, A., Alansari, S., Saad, M., Mulla Yousef, J., Alqaoud, L., de Peppo, G.M., Segmental additive tissue engineering. *Sci. Rep.*, 8, 1, 1–1, 2018 Jul 18.
49. Qiao, Z., Lian, M., Han, Y., Sun, B., Zhang, X., Jiang, W., Li, H., Hao, Y., Dai, K., Bioinspired stratified electrowritten fiber-reinforced hydrogel constructs with layer-specific induction capacity for functional osteochondral regeneration. *Biomaterials*, 266, 120385, 2021 Jan 1.
50. Lozano, D., Gil-Albarova, J., Heras, C., Sánchez-Salcedo, S., Gómez-Palacio, V.E., Gómez-Blasco, A., Doadrio, J.C., Vallet-Regí, M., Salinas, A.J., ZnO-mesoporous glass scaffolds loaded with osteostatin and mesenchymal cells improve bone healing in a rabbit bone defect. *J. Mater. Sci.: Mater. Med.*, 31, 1–1, 2020 Nov.
51. Marcacci, M., Kon, E., Moukhachev, V., Lavroukov, A., Kutepov, S., Quarto, R., Mastrogiacomo, M., Cancedda, R., Stem cells associated with macroporous bioceramics for long bone repair: 6-to 7-year outcome of a pilot clinical study. *Tissue Eng.*, 13, 5, 947–55, 2007 May 1.
52. Maiti, S.K., Ninu, A.R., Sangeetha, P., Mathew, D.D., Tamilmahan, P., Kritaniya, D., Kumar, N., Hescheler, J., Mesenchymal stem cells-seeded bio-ceramic construct for bone regeneration in large critical-size bone defect in rabbit. *J. Stem Cells Regen. Med.*, 12, 2, 87, 2016.
53. Peng, J., Wen, C., Wang, A., Wang, Y., Xu, W., Zhao, B., Zhang, L., Lu, S., Qin, L., Guo, Q., Dong, L., Micro-CT-based bone ceramic scaffolding and its performance after seeding with mesenchymal stem cells for repair of

load-bearing bone defect in canine femoral head. *J. Biomed. Mater. Res. Part B: Appl. Biomater.*, 96, 2, 316–25, 2011 Feb.
54. Humbert, P., Brennan, M.Á., Davison, N., Rosset, P., Trichet, V., Blanchard, F., Layrolle, P., Immune modulation by transplanted calcium phosphate biomaterials and human mesenchymal stromal cells in bone regeneration. *Front. Immunol.*, 10, 663, 2019 Apr 2.
55. Mebarki, M., Coquelin, L., Layrolle, P., Battaglia, S., Tossou, M., Hernigou, P., Rouard, H., Chevallier, N., Enhanced human bone marrow mesenchymal stromal cell adhesion on scaffolds promotes cell survival and bone formation. *Acta Biomater.*, 59, 94–107, 2017 Sep 1.
56. Desai, P., Hasan, S.M., Zambrana, L., Hegde, V., Saleh, A., Cohn, M.R., Lane, J.M., Bone mesenchymal stem cells with growth factors successfully treat nonunions and delayed unions. *HSS J.*, 11, 2, 104–11, 2015 Jul.
57. Eppley, B.L. and Sadove, A.M., Effects of resorbable fixation on craniofacial skeletal growth: Modifications in plate size. *J. Craniofac. Surg.*, 5, 2, 110–4, 1994 May 1.
58. Taub, P.J., Yau, J., Spangler, M., Mason, J.M., Lucas, P.A., Bioengineering of calvaria with adult stem cells. *Plast. Reconstr. Surg.*, 123, 4, 1178–85, 2009 Apr 1.
59. Harada, N., Watanabe, Y., Sato, K., Abe, S., Yamanaka, K., Sakai, Y., Kaneko, T., Matsushita, T., Bone regeneration in a massive rat femur defect through endochondral ossification achieved with chondrogenically differentiated MSCs in a degradable scaffold. *Biomaterials*, 35, 27, 7800–10, 2014 Sep 1.
60. Costa-Pinto, A.R., Correlo, V.M., Sol, P.C., Bhattacharya, M., Srouji, S., Livne, E., Reis, R.L., Neves, N.M., Chitosan-poly (butylene succinate) scaffolds and human bone marrow stromal cells induce bone repair in a mouse calvaria model. *J. Tissue Eng. Regen. Med.*, 6, 1, 21–8, 2012 Jan.
61. Park, Y.B., Ha, C.W., Lee, C.H., Yoon, Y.C., Park, Y.G., Cartilage regeneration in osteoarthritic patients by a composite of allogeneic umbilical cord blood-derived mesenchymal stem cells and hyaluronate hydrogel: Results from a clinical trial for safety and proof-of-concept with 7 years of extended follow-up. *Stem Cells Transl. Med.*, 6, 2, 613–21, 2017 Feb.
62. Chen, H., Wang, C., Zhu, X., Zhang, K., Fan, Y., Zhang, X., Fabrication of porous titanium scaffolds by stack sintering of microporous titanium spheres produced with centrifugal granulation technology. *Mater. Sci. Eng.: C*, 43, 182–8, 2014 Oct 1.
63. Chou, D.T., Wells, D., Hong, D., Lee, B., Kuhn, H., Kumta, P.N., Novel processing of iron–manganese alloy-based biomaterials by inkjet 3-D printing. *Acta Biomater.*, 9, 10, 8593–603, 2013 Nov 1.
64. Volkov, A.V., Muraev, A.A., Zharkova, I.I., Voinova, V.V., Akoulina, E.A., Zhuikov, V.A., Khaydapova, D.D., Chesnokova, D.V., Menshikh, K.A., Dudun, A.A., Makhina, T.K., Poly (3-hydroxybutyrate)/hydroxyapatite/alginate scaffolds seeded with mesenchymal stem cells enhance the regeneration of critical-sized bone defect. *Mater. Sci. Eng.: C*, 114, 110991, 2020 Sep 1.

65. Kosinski, M., Figiel-Dabrowska, A., Lech, W., Wieprzowski, L., Strzalkowski, R., Strzemecki, D., Cheda, L., Lenart, J., Domanska-Janik, K., Sarnowska, A., Bone defect repair using a bone substitute supported by mesenchymal stem cells derived from the umbilical cord. *Stem Cells Int.*, 2020, 1–15, 2020 Mar 18.
66. Sherry, B., Smith, A.L., Kronmal, R.A., Anemia during Haemophilus influenzae type b meningitis: Lack of an effect of chloramphenicol, in: *Developmental Pharmacology and Therapeutics*, vol. 12, pp. 188–99, 1989.
67. Zhang, X.F., Shen, W., Gurunathan, S., Silver nanoparticle-mediated cellular responses in various cell lines: An *in vitro* model. *Int. J. Mol. Sci.*, 17, 10, 1603, 2016 Sep 22.
68. Zhang, R., Lee, P., Lui, V.C., Chen, Y., Liu, X., Lok, C.N., To, M., Yeung, K.W., Wong, K.K., Silver nanoparticles promote osteogenesis of mesenchymal stem cells and improve bone fracture healing in osteogenesis mechanism mouse model. *Nanomed.: Nanotechnol. Biol. Med.*, 11, 8, 1949–59, 2015 Nov 1.
69. Telgerd, M.D., Sadeghinia, M., Birhanu, G., Daryasari, M.P., Zandi-Karimi, A., Sadeghinia, A., Akbarijavar, H., Karami, M.H., Seyedjafari, E., Enhanced osteogenic differentiation of mesenchymal stem cells on metal–organic framework based on copper, zinc, and imidazole coated poly-l-lactic acid nanofiber scaffolds. *J. Biomed. Mater. Res. Part A*, 107, 8, 1841–8, 2019 Aug.
70. De Kok, I.J., Jere, D., Padilla, R.J., Cooper, L.F., Evaluation of a collagen scaffold for cell-based bone repair. *Oral. Craniofac. Tissue Eng.*, 2, 3, 190–197, 2012 Sep 1.
71. Eslaminejad, M.B., Mirzadeh, H., Mohamadi, Y., Nickmahzar, A., Bone differentiation of marrow-derived mesenchymal stem cells using β-tricalcium phosphate–alginate–gelatin hybrid scaffolds. *J. Tissue Eng. Regener. Med.*, 1, 6, 417–24, 2007 Nov.
72. Marolt Presen, D., Traweger, A., Gimona, M., Redl, H., Mesenchymal stromal cell-based bone regeneration therapies: From cell transplantation and tissue engineering to therapeutic secretomes and extracellular vesicles. *Front. Bioeng. Biotechnol.*, 7, 352, 2019 Nov 27.
73. Clarke, B., Normal bone anatomy and physiology. *Clin. J. Am. Soc. Nephrol.*, 3, Supplement 3, S131–9, 2008 Nov 1.
74. Grayson, W.L., Bunnell, B.A., Martin, E., Frazier, T., Hung, B.P., Gimble, J.M., Stromal cells and stem cells in clinical bone regeneration. *Nat. Rev. Endocrinol.*, 11, 3, 140–50, 2015 Mar.
75. Gaharwar, A.K., Singh, I., Khademhosseini, A., Engineered biomaterials for *in situ* tissue regeneration. *Nat. Rev. Mater.*, 5, 9, 686–705, 2020 Sep.
76. Montoya, C., Du, Y., Gianforcaro, A.L., Orrego, S., Yang, M., Lelkes, P.I., On the road to smart biomaterials for bone research: Definitions, concepts, advances, and outlook. *Bone Res.*, 9, 1, 12, 2021 Feb 11.
77. Salgado, A.J., Coutinho, O.P., Reis, R.L., Bone tissue engineering: State of the art and future trends. *Macromol. Biosci.*, 4, 8, 743–65, 2004 Aug 9.

78. Rose, F.R. and Oreffo, R.O., Bone tissue engineering: Hope vs hype. *Biochem. Biophys. Res. Commun.*, 292, 1, 1–7, 2002 Mar 22.
79. Giannoudis, P.V., Dinopoulos, H., Tsiridis, E., Bone substitutes: An update. *Injury*, 36, 3, S20–7, 2005 Nov 1.
80. Chatterjea, A., Meijer, G., Van Blitterswijk, C., De Boer, J., Clinical application of human mesenchymal stromal cells for bone tissue engineering. *Stem Cells Int.*, 2010, 1–13, 2010 Nov 11.
81. Kim, S.J., Shin, Y.W., Yang, K.H., Kim, S.B., Yoo, M.J., Han, S.K., Im, S.A., Won, Y.D., Sung, Y.B., Jeon, T.S., Chang, C.H., A multi-center, randomized, clinical study to compare the effect and safety of autologous cultured osteoblast (Ossron™) injection to treat fractures. *BMC Musculoskelet. Disord.*, 10, 1, 1–9, 2009 Dec.
82. Ohgushi, H., Kotobuki, N., Funaoka, H., Machida, H., Hirose, M., Tanaka, Y., Takakura, Y., Tissue engineered ceramic artificial joint—*Ex vivo* osteogenic differentiation of patient mesenchymal cells on total ankle joints for treatment of osteoarthritis. *Biomaterials*, 26, 22, 4654–4661, 2005 Aug 1.
83. Kokemueller, H., Spalthoff, S., Nolff, M., Tavassol, F., Essig, H., Stuehmer, C., Bormann, K.H., Rücker, M., Gellrich, N.C., Prefabrication of vascularized bioartificial bone grafts *in vivo* for segmental mandibular reconstruction: Experimental pilot study in sheep and first clinical application. *Int. J. Oral. Maxillofac. Surg.*, 39, 4, 379–387, 2010 Apr 1.
84. Tarte, K., Gaillard, J., Lataillade, J.J., Fouillard, L., Becker, M., Mossafa, H., Tchirkov, A., Rouard, H., Henry, C., Splingard, M., Dulong, J., Clinical-grade production of human mesenchymal stromal cells: Occurrence of aneuploidy without transformation. *Blood, J. Am. Soc. Hematol.*, 115, 8, 1549–1553, 2010 Feb 25.
85. Weinand, C., Xu, J.W., Peretti, G.M., Bonassar, L.J., Gill, T.J., Conditions affecting cell seeding onto three-dimensional scaffolds for cellular-based biodegradable implants. *J. Biomed. Mater. Res. Part B: Appl. Biomater.*, 91, 1, 80–7, 2009 Oct.
86. Yoshioka, T., Mishima, H., Ohyabu, Y., Sakai, S., Akaogi, H., Ishii, T., Kojima, H., Tanaka, J., Ochiai, N., Uemura, T., Repair of large osteochondral defects with allogeneic cartilaginous aggregates formed from bone marrow-derived cells using RWV bioreactor. *J. Orthop. Res.*, 25, 10, 1291–1298, 2007 Oct.
87. Patterson, T.E., Kumagai, K., Griffith, L., Muschler, G.F., Cellular strategies for enhancement of fracture repair. *JBJS*, 90, Supplement_1, 111–119, 2008 Feb 1.
88. Caplan, A.I., Mesenchymal stem cells and gene therapy. *Clin. Orthop. Relat. Res. (1976-2007)*, 379, S67–70, 2000 Oct 1.
89. Chen, Y., Orthopedic applications of gene therapy. *J. Orthop. Sci.*, 6, 2, 199–207, 2001 Apr 1.

90. Calori, G.M., Donati, D., Di Bella, C., Tagliabue, L., Bone morphogenetic proteins and tissue engineering: Future directions. *Injury*, 40, S67–76, 2009 Dec 1.
91. Tang, Y., Tang, W., Lin, Y., Long, J., Wang, H., Liu, L., Tian, W., Combination of bone tissue engineering and BMP-2 gene transfection promotes bone healing in osteoporotic rats. *Cell Biol. Int.*, 32, 9, 1150–1157, 2008 Sep.
92. Mackay, B.S., Marshall, K., Grant-Jacob, J.A., Kanczler, J., Eason, R.W., Oreffo, R.O., Mills, B., The future of bone regeneration: Integrating AI into tissue engineering. *Biomed. Phys. Eng. Express*, 7, 5, 052002, 2021 Jul 30.
93. Sharma, A., Mishra, A., Bansal, A., Bansal, A., Bone fractured detection using machine learning and digital geometry, in: *Mobile Radio Communications and 5G Networks: Proceedings of MRCN 2020*, pp. 369–376, Springer Singapore, 2021.
94. Parkin, S., The rise of the deepfake and the threat to democracy, The Guardian, 2019 Jun; 22.
95. Hornik, K., Stinchcombe, M., White, H., Multilayer feedforward networks are universal approximators. *Neural Networks*, 2, 5, 359–366, 1989 Jan 1.
96. Rumelhart, D.E., Hinton, G.E., Williams, R.J., Learning representations by back-propagating errors. *Nature*, 323, 6088, 533–6, 1986 Oct 9.
97. LeCun, Y., Bengio, Y., Hinton, G., Deep learning. *Nature*, 521, 7553, 436–444, 2015 May 28.
98. Donahue, J., Anne Hendricks, L., Guadarrama, S., Rohrbach, M., Venugopalan, S., Saenko, K., Darrell, T., Long-term recurrent convolutional networks for visual recognition and description. *Proc. IEEE Conf. Comput. Vis. Pattern Recognit.*, 2625–2634, 2015.
99. Dong, C., Loy, C.C., He, K., Tang, X., Image super-resolution using deep convolutional networks. *IEEE Trans. Pattern Anal. Mach. Intell.*, 38, 2, 295–307, 2015 Jun 1.
100. Liang, L., Liu, M., Sun, W., A deep learning approach to estimate chemically-treated collagenous tissue nonlinear anisotropic stress-strain responses from microscopy images. *Acta Biomater.*, 63, 227–235, 2017 Nov 1.
101. Dzobo, K., Adotey, S., Thomford, N.E., Dzobo, W., Integrating artificial and human intelligence: A partnership for responsible innovation in biomedical engineering and medicine. *Omics: J. Integr. Biol.*, 24, 5, 247–263, 2020 May 1.
102. Felleman, D.J. and Van Essen, D.C., Distributed hierarchical processing in the primate cerebral cortex. *Cereb. Cortex (New York, NY: 1991)*, 1, 1, 1–47, 1991 Jan 1.
103. Hubel, D.H. and Wiesel, T.N., Receptive fields of single neurones in the cat's striate cortex. Republication of *J. Physiol.*, 148, 574–591, 1959, *J. Physiol.*, 587, Pt 12, 2721–32, 2009 Jun 15.
104. Wainberg, M., Merico, D., Delong, A., Frey, B.J., Deep learning in biomedicine. *Nat. Biotechnol.*, 36, 9, 829–838, 2018 Oct.
105. Ching, T., Himmelstein, D.S., Beaulieu-Jones, B.K., Kalinin, A.A., Do, B.T., Way, G.P., Ferrero, E., Agapow, P.M., Zietz, M., Hoffman, M.M., Xie, W.,

Opportunities and obstacles for deep learning in biology and medicine. *J. R. Soc. Interface*, 15, 141, 20170387, 2018 Apr 30.
106. Moen, E., Bannon, D., Kudo, T., Graf, W., Covert, M., Van Valen, D., Deep learning for cellular image analysis. *Nat. Methods*, 16, 12, 1233–1246, 2019 Dec.
107. Miotto, R., Wang, F., Wang, S., Jiang, X., Dudley, J.T., Deep learning for healthcare: Review, opportunities and challenges. *Briefings Bioinf.*, 19, 6, 1236–1246, 2018 Nov.
108. Forshew, T., Murtaza, M., Parkinson, C., Gale, D., Tsui, D.W., Kaper, F., Dawson, S.J., Piskorz, A.M., Jimenez-Linan, M., Bentley, D., Hadfield, J., Noninvasive identification and monitoring of cancer mutations by targeted deep sequencing of plasma DNA. *Sci. Transl. Med.*, 4, 136, 136ra68, 2012 May 30.
109. Malta, T.M., Sokolov, A., Gentles, A.J., Burzykowski, T., Poisson, L., Weinstein, J.N., Kamińska, B., Huelsken, J., Omberg, L., Gevaert, O., Colaprico, A., Machine learning identifies stemness features associated with oncogenic dedifferentiation. *Cell*, 173, 2, 338–354, 2018 Apr 5.
110. Cao, C., Liu, F., Tan, H., Song, D., Shu, W., Li, W., Zhou, Y., Bo, X., Xie, Z., Deep learning and its applications in biomedicine. *Genom. Proteom. Bioinform.*, 16, 1, 17–32, 2018.
111. MacKay, B., Blundell, S., Etter, O., Xie, Y., McDonnell, M., Tom, D., Praeger, M., Grant-Jacob, J., Eason, R.W., Lewis, R., Mills, B., Automated 3D labelling of fibroblasts and endothelial cells in SEM-imaged placenta using deep learning. *Bioimaging*, 2, 46–53, 2022.
112. Lerouge, J., Hérault, R., Chatelain, C., Jardin, F., Modzelewski, R., IODA: An input/output deep architecture for image labeling. *Pattern Recognit.*, 48, 9, 2847–2858, 2015 Sep 1.
113. Liao, S., Gao, Y., Oto, A., Shen, D., Representation learning: A unified deep learning framework for automatic prostate MR segmentation, in: *Medical Image Computing and Computer-Assisted Intervention–MICCAI 2013: 16th International Conference, Proceedings, Part II*, Nagoya, Japan, 16, pp. 254–261, Springer Berlin Heidelberg, 2013.
114. Jacobsen, G., Xu, T., Popov, S., Li, J., Friberg, A.T., Zhang, Y., Phase noise influence in coherent optical OFDM systems with RF pilot tone: Digital IFFT multiplexing and FFT demodulation. arXiv preprint arXiv:1607.04899, *J. Opt. Commun.*, 33, 217–226, 2016 Jul 17.
115. Tourlomousis, F., Jia, C., Karydis, T., Mershin, A., Wang, H., Kalyon, D.M., Chang, R.C., Machine learning metrology of cell confinement in melt electrowritten three-dimensional biomaterial substrates. *Microsyst. Nanoeng.*, 5, 1, 15, 2019 Mar 25.
116. Kim, J., McKee, J.A., Fontenot, J.J., Jung, J.P., Engineering tissue fabrication with machine intelligence: Generating a blueprint for regeneration. *Front. Bioeng. Biotechnol.*, 7, 443, 2020 Jan 10.
117. Ng, W.L., Chan, A., Ong, Y.S., Chua, C.K., Deep learning for fabrication and maturation of 3D bioprinted tissues and organs. *Virtual Phys. Prototyping*, 15, 3, 340–358, 2020 Jul 2.

118. Shi, J., Song, J., Song, B., Lu, W.F., Multi-objective optimization design through machine learning for drop-on-demand bioprinting. *Engineering*, 5, 3, 586–593, 2019 Jun 1.
119. Mackay, B.S., Praeger, M., Grant-Jacob, J.A., Kanczler, J., Eason, R.W., Oreffo, R.O., Mills, B., Modeling adult skeletal stem cell response to laser-machined topographies through deep learning. *Tissue Cell*, 67, 101442, 2020 Dec 1.
120. Kassani, S.H. and Kassani, P.H., A comparative study of deep learning architectures on melanoma detection. *Tissue Cell*, 58, 76–83, 2019 Jun 1.
121. Karras, T., Aittala, M., Hellsten, J., Laine, S., Lehtinen, J., Aila, T., Training generative adversarial networks with limited data. *Adv. Neural Inf. Process. Syst.*, 33, 12104–12114, 2020.
122. Matsuoka, F., Takeuchi, I., Agata, H., Kagami, H., Shiono, H., Kiyota, Y., Honda, H., Kato, R., Morphology-based prediction of osteogenic differentiation potential of human mesenchymal stem cells. *PLoS One*, 8, 2, e55082, 2013 Feb 21.
123. Chen, D., Sarkar, S., Candia, J., Florczyk, S.J., Bodhak, S., Driscoll, M.K., Simon Jr., C.G., Dunkers, J.P., Losert, W., Machine learning based methodology to identify cell shape phenotypes associated with microenvironmental cues. *Biomaterials*, 104, 104–118, 2016 Oct 1.
124. Fan, K., Zhang, S., Zhang, Y., Lu, J., Holcombe, M., Zhang, X., A machine learning assisted, label-free, non-invasive approach for somatic reprogramming in induced pluripotent stem cell colony formation detection and prediction. *Sci. Rep.*, 7, 1, 13496, 2017 Oct 18.
125. Marklein, R.A., Klinker, M.W., Drake, K.A., Polikowsky, H.G., Lessey-Morillon, E.C., Bauer, S.R., Morphological profiling using machine learning reveals emergent subpopulations of interferon-γ–stimulated mesenchymal stromal cells that predict immunosuppression. *Cytotherapy*, 21, 1, 17–31, 2019 Jan 1.
126. Joutsijoki, H., Haponen, M., Rasku, J., Aalto-Setälä, K., Juhola, M., Machine learning approach to automated quality identification of human induced pluripotent stem cell colony images. *Comput. Math. Methods Med.*, 2016, 1–16, 2016 Jul 14.
127. Williams, B., Löbel, W., Finklea, F., Halloin, C., Ritzenhoff, K., Manstein, F., Mohammadi, S., Hashemi, M., Zweigerdt, R., Lipke, E., Cremaschi, S., Prediction of human induced pluripotent stem cell cardiac differentiation outcome by multifactorial process modeling. *Front. Bioeng. Biotechnol.*, 8, 851, 2020 Jul 23.
128. Arora, M., Cutler, C.S., Jagasia, M.H., Pidala, J., Chai, X., Martin, P.J., Flowers, M.E., Inamoto, Y., Chen, G.L., Wood, W.A., Khera, N., Late acute and chronic graft-versus-host disease after allogeneic hematopoietic cell transplantation. *Biol. Blood Marrow Transplant.*, 22, 3, 449–455, 2016 Mar 1.
129. Gandelman, J.S., Byrne, M.T., Mistry, A.M., Polikowsky, H.G., Diggins, K.E., Chen, H., Lee, S.J., Arora, M., Cutler, C., Flowers, M., Pidala, J., Machine learning reveals chronic graft-versus-host disease phenotypes and

stratifies survival after stem cell transplant for hematologic malignancies. *Haematologica*, 104, 1, 189, 2019 Jan.

130. Shouval, R., Labopin, M., Bondi, O., Mishan Shamay, H., Shimoni, A., Ciceri, F., Esteve Reyner, J., Giebel, S., Gorin, N.C., Schmid, C., Polge, E., Prediction of allogeneic hematopoietic stem-cell transplantation mortality 100 days after transplantation using a machine learning algorithm: A European group for blood and marrow transplantation acute leukemia working party retrospective data mining study. *J. Clin. Oncol.*, 33, 28, 3144–3151, 2015 Oct 1.
131. Hulsart-Billström, G., Dawson, J.I., Hofmann, S., Müller, R., Stoddart, M.J., Alini, M., Redl, H., El Haj, A., Brown, R., Salih, V., Hilborn, J., A surprisingly poor correlation between *in vitro* and *in vivo* testing of biomaterials for bone regeneration: Results of a multicentre analysis. *Eur. Cells Mater.*, 31, 312–322, 2016.
132. Smith, A.J., Clutton, R.E., Lilley, E., Hansen, K.E., Brattelid, T., PREPARE: Guidelines for planning animal research and testing. *Lab. Anim.*, 52, 2, 135–141, 2018 Apr.
133. Kilkenny, C., Browne, W.J., Cuthill, I.C., Emerson, M., Altman, D.G., Improving bioscience research reporting: The arrive guidelines for reporting animal research. *Animals*, 4, 1, 35–44, 2014 Feb 3.
134. Singh, A.V., Ansari, M.H., Rosenkranz, D., Maharjan, R.S., Kriegel, F.L., Gandhi, K., Kanase, A., Singh, R., Laux, P., Luch, A., Artificial intelligence and machine learning in computational nanotoxicology: Unlocking and empowering nanomedicine. *Adv. Healthcare Mater.*, 9, 17, 1901862, 2020 Sep.
135. Guan, D., Fan, K., Spence, I., Matthews, S., Combining machine learning models of *in vitro* and *in vivo* bioassays improves rat carcinogenicity prediction. *Regul. Toxicol. Pharm.*, 94, 8–15, 2018 Apr 1.
136. Mathis, M.W. and Mathis, A., Deep learning tools for the measurement of animal behavior in neuroscience. *Curr. Opin. Neurobiol.*, 60, 1–1, 2020 Feb 1.
137. Pereira, T.D., Shaevitz, J.W., Murthy, M., Quantifying behavior to understand the brain. *Nat. Neurosci.*, 23, 12, 1537–49, 2020 Dec.
138. M., T.,VII, The first level of super Mario bros. is easy with lexicographic.
139. Cirillo, D., Catuara-Solarz, S., Morey, C., Guney, E., Subirats, L., Mellino, S., Gigante, A., Valencia, A., Rementeria, M.J., Chadha, A.S., Mavridis, N., Sex and gender differences and biases in artificial intelligence for biomedicine and healthcare. *NPJ Digital Med.*, 3, 1, 81, 2020 Jun 1.
140. Esteva, A., Kuprel, B., Novoa, R.A., Ko, J., Swetter, S.M., Blau, H.M., Thrun, S., Dermatologist-level classification of skin cancer with deep neural networks. *Nature*, 542, 7639, 115–8, 2017 Feb.
141. Mackay, B.S., Marshall, K., Grant-Jacob, J.A., Kanczler, J., Eason, R.W., Oreffo, R.O., Mills, B., The future of bone regeneration: Integrating AI into tissue engineering. *Biomed. Phys. Eng. Express*, 7, 5, 052002, 2021 Jul 30.

142. Isola, P., Zhu, J.Y., Zhou, T., Efros, A.A., Image-to-image translation with conditional adversarial networks, in: *Proceedings of the IEEE Conference on Computer Vision and Pattern Recognition*, pp. 1125–1134, 2017.
143. MaJ, Z. and XiaoM, G., A deep learning algorithm using CT images to screen for corona virus disease (COVID-19). *medRxiv*, 31, 6096–6104, 2020.
144. Kusumoto, D. and Yuasa, S., The application of convolutional neural network to stem cell biology. *Inflamm. Regen.*, 39, 1, 1–7, 2019 Dec.
145. Sonnenburg, S., Braun, M.L., Ong, C.S., Bengio, S., Bottou, L., Holmes, G., LeCunn, Y., Muller, K.R., Pereira, F., Rasmussen, C.E., Ratsch, G., The need for open source software in machine learning. *J. Mach. Learn. Res.*, 8, 2443–2466, 2007.

3

Deep Supervised Learning on Radiological Images to Classify Bone Fractures: A Novel Approach

Abstract
Several researchers in recent years have proposed several ways to classify bone fractures. Despite this, there is no well-defined system for categorizing the many fractures that might occur in a human body. The use of X-rays to identify bone fractures is just one such application, yet this can also occur with smaller fissures. This highlights the need to quickly diagnose a patient with a fracture and start treatment. Because of this, it is crucial to design efficient and intelligent systems. Still it is a regular emergency when a fracture is not properly diagnosed. Patients' access to care and treatment is limited and often delayed as a result. The potential use of deep learning (DL) and other forms of artificial intelligence to aid radiologists in the identification of bone fractures is now receiving a great deal of attention. The analysis of medical images is a promising area for the use of DL. In this chapter, we investigate how deep supervised learning can be used to analyze X-ray pictures and categorize the many types of bone fractures.

Keywords: Deep supervised learning, radiological images, bone fracture, bone classification, X-ray, deep learning

3.1 Introduction

There has been widespread application of image processing methods across the medical sector. Applications of wavelet transform in medical image processing are discussed by researchers [1]. The ability to store more photos in the same amount of disc or memory space makes this application crucial in the medical industry. To get the best and most precise findings, researchers employed image processing techniques supported by artificial intelligence technologies like back-propagation neural networks [2].

Rishabha Malviya, Shivam Rajput and Makarand Vaidya. Artificial Intelligence for Bone Disorder: Diagnosis and Treatment, (59–78) © 2024 Scrivener Publishing LLC

Automatic illness identification, categorization, segmentation, and quantification are just some of the numerous uses of AI in radiology, such as Intelligent Bone Fracture Detection System (Figure 3.1). Studies have revealed that the form of artificial intelligence known as deep learning (DL) is more accurate than human doctors when it comes to diagnosing ailments based on medical pictures [3]. The key areas of study for DL in medical imaging include X-ray, computed tomography (CT), and bone magnetic resonance imaging (MRI). Because the sheer volume of data presents a challenge for doctors and other medical professionals, researchers need DL algorithms that are both more advanced and more suited to the data that is specific to bone imaging. The ever-growing quantity of literature that is dedicated to the study of artificial intelligence systems in radiography reflects the growing interest in developing such systems in this field. About a decade ago, there were seldom more than a hundred articles published annually in radiology that dealt with AI. Subsequently, researchers saw a meteoric rise in the number of annual publications, from a thousand to 2,000. DL is applied during the picture capture and reshaping process to improve acquisition speed, image quality, and cost. It also can translate across different modalities, register pictures, and remove noise from them. Computer-aided diagnosis, segmentation, and anomaly detection are just a few of the medical image processing applications that are benefiting from the proliferation of DL systems.

Annotation and data labeling are two additional actions that are crucial. However, due to diverse experiences and different environments, there are considerable inter-user and intra-user labeling changes as well as distinct resolution and procedure variations [4]. In some cases, this might cause labeling errors due to noise, so there is still a lot of work to be done in DL when it comes to standardizing picture labeling.

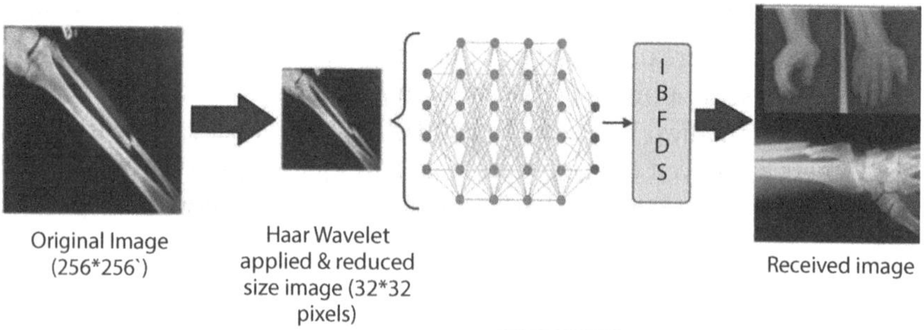

Figure 3.1 Diagrammatic representation of intelligent bone fracture detection system.

In the field of radiology, a technique known as computational radiology [5] is one that makes use of artificial intelligence (AI) tools, most notably DL research, to assist medical professionals by automating image processing and analytics. This technique can even be used in co-clinical studies. Computerized tools, which are also known as decision support systems, can be developed for a wide variety of purposes. Some of these purposes include, but are not limited to, the detection of clinical findings, the identification of the illness extent, the classification of clinical conclusions (for example, into malignant and benign tissue) as well as a great number of other purposes. Due to time constraints as well as a lack of capabilities for visualization and quantification, these are often included in modern radiological reports. In the field of bone radiology, various examples of DL are depicted in Figure 3.2.

The goal of the researchers was to examine the best ways to compress and modulate data for the secure digital transmission of the human voice. The major goal was to improve data transfer rates, reduce bit error rates, and reduce bandwidth use. Researchers who have developed a method for sending data through a voice channel are compared against the suggested method to gauge its efficacy [6]. To further describe the structure of particle assemblies from two-dimensional pictures, a rotational Haar wavelet transform (RHWT) technique is developed. Maximum energy ratio provides information about the fabric's orientation and strength [7].

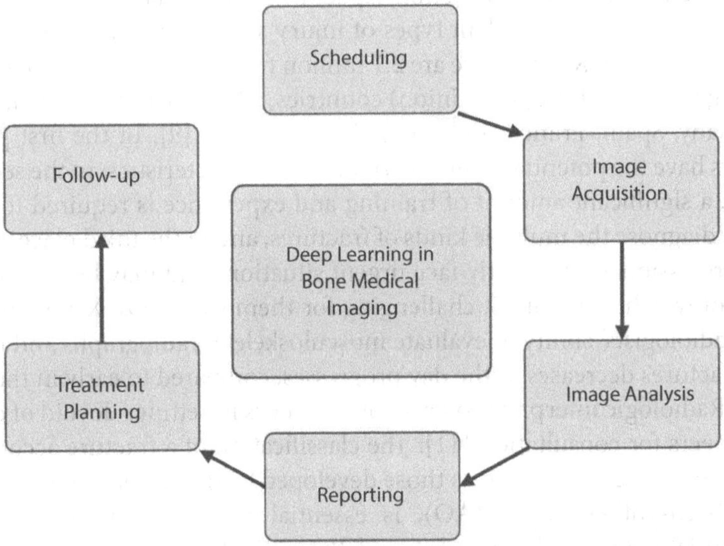

Figure 3.2 Diagrammatic representation of machine learning in the field of radiology.

There is no universally agreed-upon number of elements that constitute a "feature" depiction of any given film. Separating and cataloging these components can be accomplished using several approaches and procedures. Highlights from a filtered picture provide a layout of the parts, as described by researchers. Images are often transformed into a large collection of neighborhood vectors using the well-praised scale-invariant feature transform (SIFT) technique, which is then highlighted using the researchers [8]. These vectors are considered invariant under transformations such as scaling, pivoting, or reinterpreting the pictures. SIFT indicates a high component number for primate vision. A method of separation is utilized to get these constituents.

3.2 Common Bone Disorder

Radiologists and orthopedic surgeons examine MRI, X-rays, or CT scans of the affected portion to identify any abnormalities. Significant progress in DL in recent years has allowed for the deployment and evaluation of deep learning models in the healthcare sector. As a field, orthopedics have several challenges, one of the most significant being musculoskeletal. Arthritis, bursitis, tendinitis, and many more disorders all affect the musculoskeletal system. They induce excruciating pain immediately but worsen over time, sometimes to the point where they become disabling. Consequently, DL's early detection capabilities are crucial.

One of the most prevalent types of injury seen nowadays is bone fracture as a result of X-ray. There are 2.7 million fractures that occur each year among the EU 6 (European Union) countries, which include Sweden, Italy, Germany, Spain, France, and the United Kingdom [9]. In the first place, X-rays have the potential to hide certain bone characteristics; in the second place, a significant amount of training and experience is required to correctly diagnose the multiple kinds of fractures, and in the third place, medical professionals frequently face urgent situations and may be exhausted, both of which can make it challenging for them to analyze X-ray images. The radiologists' ability to evaluate musculoskeletal radiographs and identify fractures decreases as the day progresses, compared to early in the day [10]. Radiologic interpretation also often occurs in settings devoid of qualified peers for consultation [11]. The classification of a fracture according to recognized criteria, such as those developed by the Arbeitsgemeinschaft für Osteosynthesefragen (AO), is essential for establishing the most appropriate course of treatment and the patient's prognosis. An aiding computer-aided design (CAD) system in such a setting might potentially have a significant effect on patient outcomes.

3.3 Deep Supervised Learning's Importance in Orthopedics and Radiology

In radiology, the implementation of deep learning methods, in contrast to more conventional methods, provides the chance to increase the accuracy and speed of medical diagnostics as well as to minimize the load of work on radiologists by having time-consuming processes conducted by the computer rather than by the radiologists themselves, yet there are substantial issues related to both inter- and intra-observer inconsistency, which can hurt the performance of deep learning systems. In the realm of academic research, DL is performing exceptionally well; actually, it has even eclipsed the efficiency of humans when it comes to detecting and classifying fractures based on radiographic images. Researchers have shown a substantial level of interest in deep learning over the previous several years. Recent research has demonstrated that deep learning is competent for completing sophisticated evaluations at the same level as those conducted by professionals in the medical field [12]. Several studies [13] in the field of orthopedic traumatology have applied deep learning to radiographs to detect and classify fractures. This was done to improve the accuracy of fracture diagnosis. On the other hand, the use of deep learning in the diagnosis of fractures on CT images has received a comparatively low amount of attention [14]. Although it has been for a long time, this is still the case. Estimating the parameters for fracture detection using DL has a very good chance of being successful. These parameters include normal distal radius angles, radial height, radial inclination, palmar tilts, and other features with a similar profile.

3.4 Perspective From the Past

The breakthrough of DL techniques was made possible as a direct result of convolutional neural network's (CNN) dominance over the ImageNet data set. This dominance was demonstrated in a large-scale picture categorization task in 2012 [15], which took place after CNN had already established its mastery over the data set. At that period, DL was the most well-known machine learning approach, which sparked a dispute in the community of medical imaging specialists regarding whether DL could be utilized in medical imaging. DL was the most well-known machine learning technique during that period. The concerns, which are referred to collectively as the data challenge, functioned as the jumping-off point for the conversation. The most critical of these problems was a lack of properly labeled data, and it was this shortcoming that served as the starting point.

Methods were created in 2015–2016 that made use of "transfer learning" (TL), which is also named "learning from nonmedical features", to utilize the experience that was gained from trying to resolve a reference problem to solve a different but related target problem. These methods were developed in 2015. Imaging of the bone was accomplished using these methods. The application of the DL approach in the field of medical imaging is made possible by a great number of different methods. Applying a deep network that had been perfect as well as trained on ImageNet to a problem statement relevant to medical imaging accelerated the training convergence and boosted the accuracy. This was demonstrated by a few distinct research [16]. The creation of synthetic data augmentation was an alternative strategy that was made available throughout the years 2017 and 2018 to analyze restricted data sets. At this point, classical augmentation is a necessary component of the training process for every network. This is the case regardless of the type of network. However, the key obstacles that had to be resolved were whether it would be feasible to synthesize medical information making use of approaches such as generative modeling as well as if the synthesized information would serve as valid medical models and, in actuality, enhance the implementation of the medically assigned task. In the study [17], synthetic image augmentation with the generative adversarial network (GAN) was utilized to construct lesion image samples that have not been detected as synthetic by trained radiologists while simultaneously enhancing CNN performance in diagnosing liver lesions. This was accomplished without compromising the integrity of the original synthetic images. This was performed without causing any damage to the quality of the original photographs. Vibrational encoders, GANs as well as variants upon those two types of encoders have all been the subject of recent research, and their advancement has advanced as a result of this research. The U-Net architecture [18] is among the most major contributions that have emerged from the medical imaging field in recent years. Its focus is on the extraction of data about bone disease from images, making it one of the most important advances in this area.

3.5 Essential Deep Learning Methods for Bone Imaging

There are important repercussions for clinical practice that may be drawn from the ability to reconstruct high-quality images with very few doses of contrast medium and/or relatively fast acquisition times. Image enhancement in clinical practice involves adjusting the intensities of individual pixels to generate a product that is more suitable for presentation or additional research. Some of the approaches that may be used to improve the picture are magnetic resonance (MR) bias field correction, super-resolution, denoising, and image harmonization. In recent times, there has been a lot of focus placed on modalities such as translation and synthesis, which might be interpreted as processes that improve images. Target lesion segmentations, clinical measurements, therapeutic planning, and surgical preparation can all be assisted by deep learning. Utilizing image segmentation accomplished by label transition, DL-based registration is a technique that sees extensive application in multimodal fusion, population analysis, and longitudinal research. Other machine learning and pre-processing methods include the recognition of targets and landmarks, the identification of views or pictures, and the development of automatic reports [19].

The model capacity and generalization capabilities of deep learning models are significantly better than those of simple neural network models. Deep learning approaches that have been trained on enormous data sets produce remarkable outcomes for a single job. These results far transcend those produced by regular algorithms and abilities.

3.5.1 Network Structure

Visual Geometry Group Network (VGGNet) [20], residual neural network (ResNet) [21], and Inception Net [22] are all examples of a movement in research that began with AlexNet (the convolutional neural network that is eight-layer-deep) that seeks to develop deeper networks which apply them in defect visualization in bone. This trend was first exhibited by AlexNet. AlexNet was the catalyst for the beginning of this movement. Both DenseNet (densely connected convolutional networks) [23] and U-Net (convolutional networks for biomedical image segmentation) provide evidence that the utilization of skip connections makes it simpler to build a deep network which is even more complex. To keep up with the segmentation, the U-net was built, and additional networks were developed to undertake photo categorization. Deeper supervision results in even greater improvements to one's capacity for discrimination [24]. In bone imaging, the method of adversarial learning is used widely for a variety of purposes, including the segmentation of images, the restoration of medical images, and the improvement of picture quality. Whether accumulating bone imaging data or making a systematic choice, the attention mechanism allows the automatic identification of "where" and "what" to concentrate on by detecting "where" and "what" to pay attention to. While trying to figure out "where" and "what" to pay attention to, this is valuable information to have. Two different techniques may be employed to influence channel attention. These are squeeze and excitement. Three pieces of study combine attention with either the GAN or the U-Net [25]. Two of these research studies integrate attention with the GAN. The generator and the discriminator are the two components that make up a GAN, which is an adversarial network. A generator is responsible for discovering the significant qualities, and after it has done so, it constructs feature maps by mapping those traits to a latent space. The discriminator will finally be able to discern between the feature maps that were generated by the generator and the true distribution of data that it has learned. Attention gates are incorporated into the pipeline so that significant feature vectors may be represented effectively without adding to the overall level of complexity of the calculation. An image encoder receives the newly learned features, which take the form of a scattering of raw vectors, and uses them to create the encoded picture. Afterward, it is sent to an output layer where the appropriate output can be made.

3.5.2 Haar Wavelet Transforms

Mathematically, wavelets may be used to break down a function into smaller and smaller pieces. Compressing images with wavelet transforms results in higher compression ratios and peak signal-to-noise ratio values, as stated by researchers [26]. Traditional approaches to image processing and analysis utilize continuous or discrete image transformations. Transforming images is often used in many fields, including picture filtering, data description, etc. Wavelet theorems have been at the heart of widely used techniques for image processing, denoising, and compression for well over two decades. The Haar functions are the simplest wavelets; hence, they find widespread application in many discrete picture transformation and processing techniques.

It takes a lot of space to save digital photos, and it can be a lengthy process to download an image from the internet. Researchers use the

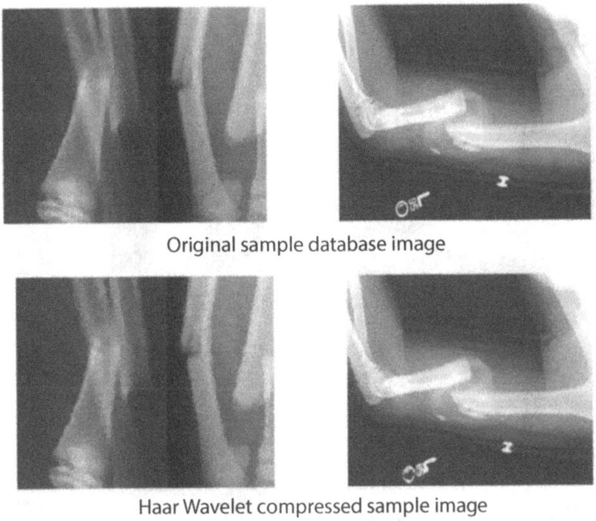

Figure 3.3 Diagrammatic representation of Haar wavelet image compression.

Haar wavelet transform to reduce the storage requirements of digital images [27]. To process data, the Haar wavelet performs addition and subtraction between neighboring components, first along the horizontal axis and then along the vertical axis [28]—for example, in a prior research, Haar image compression has been used for adaptive data concealing, where the original picture is divided into 8 × 8 sub-blocks and then reconstructed with acceptable quality after compression. Figure 3.3 displays examples of the application of the Haar wavelet transform on photos taken from the original image database, which contains unprocessed photographs.

3.5.3 Scale-Invariant Feature Transform Algorithm

Another method for feature extraction is the SIFT, as demonstrated by the researcher. The approach relies on the statistics of the orientations of picture intensity gradients. The image structures of each point of interest acquire these intensities (Figure 3.4). The descriptor is employed in a matching process between photos with similar interest locations. The SIFT, in its simplest form, is a technique used in computer vision for locating and illustrating details inside images. On the other hand, researchers discovered that the SIFT method may extract feature points with strong invariance that are resilient to a wide range of challenges [29]. Together

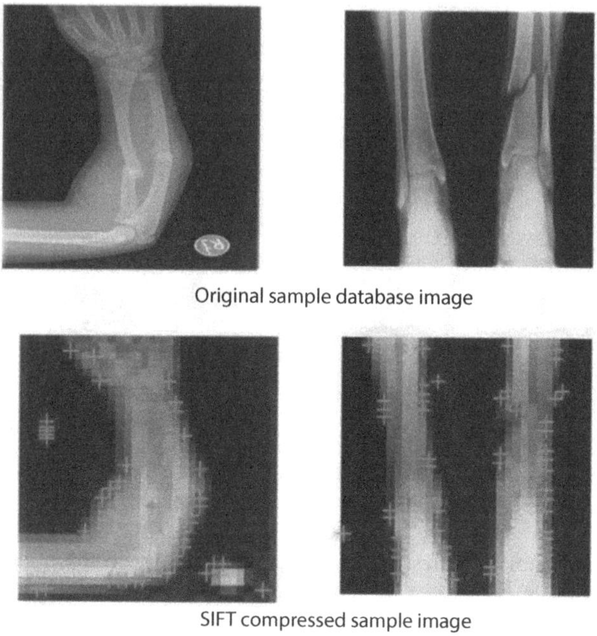

Figure 3.4 Some examples of photos processed using standard for image feature extraction (SIFT). The images' features, retrieved with the SIFT technique, are then utilized to train the back-propagation network. Following training and convergence, the neural network is put to the test using testing images that have undergone a feature extraction phase using the SIFT.

with smart classifiers like neural networks, several studies employed this approach as a feature extractor. Researchers found that the algorithm was quite effective in identifying relevant distinguishing characteristics. Using the SIFT technique, researchers can extract meaningful features from photos, perform a preliminary matching operation, and settle on a suitable mathematical mapping model between two images. The experimental results prove that the algorithm works as intended. Researchers developed a new technique for the categorization of X-ray images of shipping containers, produced in the inspection lines, to further improve the matching accuracy of the described manifest, which lists the claimed substance of the shipping containers, with the exact contents of the container [30]. SIFT feature vectors are used in the proposed method. For the first time, this proposed method considers the most important and conspicuous aspects of feature extraction.

3.6 Strategies for Effective Annotation

When it comes to bone imaging, DL must modify the feature representation capability derived from pre-existing models and data, even if those models and data are not exactly in the same domain or were collected for a different reason. That is because the models and data originate from several programs. This process of integrative learning brings up the possibility of dealing with a variety of different domains, including several different kinds of activities for the very first time.

3.7 Application of Deep Learning to the Detection of Fractures

Accurate identification of fractures may be possible with the help of deep learning, as shown by several research. The authors were interested in whether a deep convolutional neural network trained on data from the general public might be used to automatically identify wrist fractures in plain radiographs (CNN). To compete in the ImageNet Big Visual Recognition Challenge [31], a new version of Inception CNN was developed and trained on non-radiographic images. They retrained the top layer of the inception V3 model to deal with the problem of binary classification using a training data set of roughly 1,389 radiographs that were manually annotated. With a set of roughly 139 radiographs, they were able to get an area under the curve (AUC) of 0.95. This shows that a CNN model trained on general-purpose images may be effectively applied to the plain radiograph fracture detection problem. A sensitivity of 0.88 and a specificity of 0.90 were achieved. The tests have shown a sensitivity and specificity of 75% to 85%, making this technique more accurate than the previously published computer models for automatic fracture diagnosis. This includes techniques like edge recognition, segmentation, and feature extraction. The study provides proof of concept, but it has significant shortcomings. The validation accuracy did not match the training accuracy throughout the training operation. Overfitting is likely to blame for this result. Overfitting may be mitigated using several different approaches. The application of automatic segmentation of the most pertinent feature map is one such strategy. To ensure that only relevant features were used during training, any extra pixels outside of the feature map would be removed. In order to lessen the likelihood of overfitting, sophisticated augmentation methods are proposed by researchers. In addition, [32] suggests using cutting-edge augmentation methods to help reduce overfitting. Furthermore, in machine learning, the size of the population under investigation might act as a barrier to progress. More people in the sample equals a more accurate depiction of the population at large.

Researchers [33] used plain anteroposterior (AP) shoulder radiographs to assess the efficacy of deep learning in the detection and classification of proximal humerus fractures. The results from the deep CNN model were compared to those from humans (general physicians, orthopedic surgeons, and radiologists). Shoulder X-rays from the front and the side were included. Their proximal humerus fracture data were processed via a re-engineered version of the ResNet-152 model. The CNN model performed quite well at differentiating between healthy shoulders and those with fractures. Important results were also seen for classifying fracture types from simple AP (perfect anteroposterior) shoulder radiographs. When compared to general orthopedic surgeons, doctors, and shoulder specialists, the CNN model outperformed all of them. When researchers talk about computer-aided diagnosis, they are referring to the prospect of using plain radiography pictures to identify and categorize musculoskeletal problems like fractures.

In order to determine how well DL works for identifying osteoporotic vertebral fractures (OVFs) from CT scans, researchers [34] carried out a retrospective study and presented an ML-based system, entirely powered by deep neural network architecture, to do so. OVF identification was accomplished through the deployment of a system with two primary components: (1) a feature extraction module based on a convolutional neural network as well as (2) a module based on a recurrent neural network to integrate the collected features and offer the final evaluation. A deep residual model was employed for CT scan analysis and feature extraction (ResNet). There were a total of 1,168 CT scans used in their training set, 135 in their validation set, and 129 in their testing set. Their suggested technique is as accurate and has the same F1 score as those of practicing radiologists when tested on a separate data set. This automated detection technique can reduce the amount of work required by radiologists to manually screen for OVFs, saving both time and effort. Additionally, it helps decrease the number of false-negative diagnoses of vertebral fractures in the pre-symptomatic period.

Cervical spine fractures were identified using CT scan pictures as input. Although CT scans carry more pixel information than X-rays, preprocessing procedures like windowing as well as Hounsfield unit conversion have been utilized to make it simpler to spot anomalies in the intended tissues. If X-ray images are utilized as input for identifying lower and upper limb fractures, the accuracy drops below that observed for cervical spine fractures because of the loss of essential pixel information. When comparing the upper and lower extremities, it is the femur of the upper extremity that has a higher bone density and is therefore better able to support the body's weight.

3.7.1 Upper Limb Fractures

Missing fractures are equally likely to occur in the upper and lower extremities. The missed fracture rates are 1.9% in the shoulder, 6.0% in the elbow, 5.4% in the hand, and 6% in the wrist [35]. The researchers analyzed 1,112 wrist radiographs to train their model and an additional 100 to validate it (containing 50 broken and 50 normal pictures) [36]. They achieved diagnostic performance metrics of 88% selectivity, 90% sensitivity, and AUC of 0.954. One study used 135,409 radiographs to train a CNN-based model to detect wrist fractures. They stated that a 53% reduction in misunderstanding occurred as a result of a rise from 88% to 94% in the doctors' picture reading abilities (both unassisted and with help). Radiographic images of the hand and wrist were used to assess the efficacy of a model established by researchers for distal radius fractures [37]. When compared to the performance of highly skilled orthopedic surgeons, the network was shown to have an excellent sensitivity of 90% and a specificity of 88%. The intricacy of fracture detection and the type of fractures themselves were not defined.

Researchers developed a CNN-based model to detect proximal humerus fractures and classify them according to Neer's classification [33] utilizing data from 1,891 shoulder X-rays. The throughput accuracy of the model was 1, and the mean area under the curve was 1. With a sensitivity of 99% and specificity of 97%, this test is quite reliable. However, the most difficult part is determining how to label broken bones. The predictions were between 65% and 85% accurate. Scientists devised a system using a multiview technique to mimic the radiologists's process of analyzing numerous images of severe pediatric elbow fractures. Twenty-one thousand four hundred fifty-six radiographic examinations, totaling 58,817 radiographic pictures of the elbow, were analyzed by the authors. The model has an accuracy of 88%, a sensitivity of 91%, and a specificity of 84%.

3.7.2 Lower Limb Fractures

Radiographic evidence of osteoporotic fractures occurs in 4–9% of patients having orthopedic surgery, despite 20% of these patients having experienced a hip fracture. Using a CNN-based model, researchers analyzed the ailment of inter-trochanteric hip fractures. A total of 3,346 radiographic pictures of the hip were utilized, including 1,773 photos of fractured hips and 1,573 images of healthy hips. Five orthopedic doctors' opinions were compared to the model's results. Compared to the orthopedic surgeons, the model performed admirably. The claimed results ranged from 96% to 94% accuracy, 97% to 57% specificity, and 94% to 88% sensitivity. Researchers used 25,505 pre-trained images of limb radiography to inform their CNN-based model [38]. This model detects hip fractures with a sensitivity of 98% and a specificity of 91%. The model's 2% false-negative rate makes it a superior screening tool. Researchers developed a model to identify thigh bone breaks with 91% precision and 0.98 AUC [39]. Researchers created a model using convolutional neural networks [40] to identify femoral diaphyseal fractures. To teach the model to distinguish between spiral, transverse, and comminuted femoral diaphyseal fractures, the researchers examined 175 radiographs. In terms of precision, the model's accuracy is 90.7%, while its specificity is 92.3% and its sensitivity is 86.6%.

Fractures of the lower extremities are frequently overlooked, especially in individuals who have suffered trauma. Recent research indicates that radiologists are responsible for 66% of incorrect diagnoses. To this end, researchers are devoting significant time and energy to develop models that can assist radiologists in making more accurate fracture diagnoses. Kitamura *et al.* [41] built a CNN model using only a small sample of ankle X-rays (298 normal and 298 fractured images). The model has been instructed to identify fractures in the proximal forefoot, midfoot, distal tibia, and fibula. The model has 76–81% chance of detecting fractures. Researchers developed two CNN-based algorithms for classifying calcaneal fractures [42] using CT radiography images. The proposed model is a promising tool for the development of future computerized diagnosis, with an accuracy of 0.793%, specificity of 0.729%, and sensitivity of 0.829%. Scholars devised a computer-assisted method for detecting calcaneal fractures in CT scans. They employed the Sanders approach for fracture classification, which used color segmentation to identify and label calcaneus pieces. Overall, the model is accurate 86% of the time.

3.7.3 Vertebral Fractures

According to the findings of several studies, the prevalence of undetected fractures of the spine ranges anywhere from 19.5% to 45%. Lumbar and thoracic CT scans were used to detect, localize, and classify vertebral spine fractures, as well as examine bone density in the lumbar spine, according to the findings of the aforementioned study. Radiology published this study's findings. Compression fractures were diagnosed and localized with a sensitivity of 0.957 and a false-positive rate of 0.29 per patient. The radiographic features of osteoporotic vertebral fractures on CT scans could be extracted with the use of a convolutional neural network model, as described by researchers [43]. With a total of 1,432 CT scans and 10,546 sagittal views used during training, the network was able to reach an accuracy of 89.2%. Researchers [34] created a model to identify vertebrae that are prone to fracture by analyzing 58 CT scans of individuals whose fractures were confirmed to be caused by vertebral insufficiency. The most vulnerable spinal segments were identified using this approach. In total, 120 different factors were considered for the study (60 healthy and 60 unhealthy vertebrae). The accuracy of identifying healthy/unhealthy vertebrae was low though, with an AUC of 0.5.

3.8 Conclusion

It is safe to state that there are numerous techniques for locating and classifying fractures as a result. We can conclude that CNN-based models like InceptionNet and XceptionNet perform well when it comes to identifying fractures. Doctors will be able to recognize and evaluate bone fractures with the use of the SIFT algorithm's data. Expert radiograph analysis and diagnosis is a labor- and time-intensive process that may be automated with the use of fracture detection algorithms. Many of the featured experts concur that the largest challenge to creating a successful classification system is the dearth of labeled training data. There is not yet a standard model that can be applied to the data given.

References

1. Dimililer, K., Neural network implementation for image compression of x-rays. *Electron. World*, 118, 1911, 26–9, 2012 Mar 1.
2. Dimililer, K., Backpropagation neural network implementation for medical image compression. *J. Appl. Math.*, 2013, 1–9, 2013 Dec 1.
3. Gulshan, V., Peng, L., Coram, M., Stumpe, M.C., Wu, D., Narayanaswamy, A., Venugopalan, S., Widner, K., Madams, T., Cuadros, J., Kim, R., Development and validation of a deep learning algorithm for detection of diabetic retinopathy in retinal fundus photographs. *JAMA*, 316, 22, 2402–10, 2016 Dec 13.
4. Roy, S. and Bandyopadhyay, S.K., A new method of brain tissues segmentation from MRI with accuracy estimation. *Proc. Comput. Sci.*, 85, 362–369, 2016 Jan 1.

5. Roy, S., Whitehead, T.D., Li, S., Ademuyiwa, F.O., Wahl, R.L., Dehdashti, F., Shoghi, K.I., Co-clinical FDG-PET radiomic signature in predicting response to neoadjuvant chemotherapy in triple-negative breast cancer. *Eur. J. Nucl. Med. Mol. Imaging*, 49, 1–3, 2022 Jan 1.
6. Sheikh, J.A., Akhtar, S., Parah, S.A., Bhat, G.M., A new method of Haar and Db10 based secured compressed data transmission over GSM voice channel, in: *Intelligent Techniques in Signal Processing for Multimedia Security*, pp. 401–426, 2017.
7. Zhang, J., Chen, G., Jia, Z., An image stitching algorithm based on histogram matching and SIFT algorithm. *Int. J. Pattern Recognit. Artif. Intell.*, 31, 04, 1754006, 2017 Apr 24.
8. Lowe, D.G., Distinctive image features from scale-invariant keypoints. *Int. J. Comput. Vision*, 60, 91–110, 2004 Nov.
9. Meena, T. and Roy, S., Bone fracture detection using deep supervised learning from radiological images: A paradigm shift. *Diagnostics*, 12, 10, 2420, 2022 Oct 7.
10. Krupinski, E.A., Berbaum, K.S., Caldwell, R.T., Schartz, K.M., Kim, J., Long radiology workdays reduce detection and accommodation accuracy. *J. Am. Coll. Radiol.*, 7, 9, 698–704, 2010 Sep 1.
11. Hallas, P. and Ellingsen, T., Errors in fracture diagnoses in the emergency department–characteristics of patients and diurnal variation. *BMC Emerg. Med.*, 6, 1–5, 2006 Dec.
12. Rayan, J.C., Reddy, N., Kan, J.H., Zhang, W., Annapragada, A., Binomial classification of pediatric elbow fractures using a deep learning multiview approach emulating radiologist decision making. *Radiol.: Artif. Intell.*, 1, 1, e180015, 2019 Jan 30.
13. Urakawa, T., Tanaka, Y., Goto, S., Matsuzawa, H., Watanabe, K., Endo, N., Detecting intertrochanteric hip fractures with orthopedist-level accuracy using a deep convolutional neural network. *Skelet. Radiol.*, 48, 239–244, 2019 Feb.
14. Wang, X., Xu, Z., Tong, Y., Xia, L., Jie, B., Ding, P., Bai, H., Zhang, Y., He, Y., Detection and classification of mandibular fracture on CT scan using deep convolutional neural network. *Clin. Oral. Investig.*, 26, 6, 4593–601, 2022 Jun.
15. Krizhevsky, A., Sutskever, I., Hinton, G.E., Imagenet classification with deep convolutional neural networks. *Commun. ACM*, 60, 6, 84–90, 2017 May 24.
16. Zhou, J., Li, Z., Zhi, W., Liang, B., Moses, D., Dawes, L., Using convolutional neural networks and transfer learning for bone age classification, in: *2017 International Conference on Digital Image Computing: Techniques and Applications (DICTA)*, IEEE, pp. 1–6, 2017 Nov 29.
17. Shah, P.M., Ullah, H., Ullah, R., Shah, D., Wang, Y., Islam, S.U., Gani, A., Rodrigues, J.J., DC-GAN-based synthetic X-ray images augmentation for increasing the performance of EfficientNet for COVID-19 detection. *Expert Syst.*, 39, 3, e12823, 2022 Mar.

18. Sanaat, A., Shiri, I., Ferdowsi, S., Arabi, H., Zaidi, H., Robust-deep: A method for increasing brain imaging datasets to improve deep learning models' performance and robustness. *J. Digital Imaging*, 35, 3, 469–481, 2022 Jun.
19. Roy, S., Mitra, A., Roy, S., Setua, S.K., Blood vessel segmentation of retinal image using Clifford matched filter and Clifford convolution. *Multimedia Tools Appl.*, 78, 34839–34865, 2019 Dec.
20. Lin, Q., Li, T., Cao, C., Cao, Y., Man, Z., Wang, H., Deep learning based automated diagnosis of bone metastases with SPECT thoracic bone images. *Sci. Rep.*, 11, 1, 4223, 2021 Feb 19.
21. AlGhaithi, A. and Al Maskari, S., Artificial intelligence application in bone fracture detection. *J. Musculoskelet. Res.*, 5, 4, 2021 Jan 1.
22. Marwa, F., Zahzah, E.H., Bouallegue, K., Machhout, M., Deep learning based neural network application for automatic ultrasonic computed tomographic bone image segmentation. *Multimed. Tools Appl.*, 81, 10, 13537–13562, 2022 Apr.
23. Papandrianos, N., Papageorgiou, E.I., Anagnostis, A., Development of convolutional neural networks to identify bone metastasis for prostate cancer patients in bone scintigraphy. *Ann. Nucl. Med.*, 34, 824–832, 2020 Nov.
24. Rahmaniar, W. and Wang, W.J., Real-time automated segmentation and classification of calcaneal fractures in CT images. *Appl. Sci.*, 9, 15, 3011, 2019 Jul 26.
25. Sarvamangala, D.R. and Kulkarni, R.V., Convolutional neural networks in medical image understanding: A survey. *Evol. Intell.*, 15, 1, 1–22, 2022 Mar.
26. Khashman, A. and Dimililer, K., Image compression using neural networks and Haar wavelet. *WSEAS Trans. Signal Process.*, 4, 5, 330–339, 2008 May 1.
27. Dimililer, K. and Kavalcıoğlu, C., Gaussian noise and Haar wavelet transform image compression on transmission of dermatological images, in: *Advances in Computing and Communications: First International Conference, ACC 2011, Kochi, India, July 22-24, 2011, Proceedings, Part III*, Springer Berlin Heidelberg, 1, pp. 357–364, 2011.
28. Khashman, A., Sekeroglu, B., Dimililer, K., ICIS: A novel coin identification system, in: *Intelligent Computing in Signal Processing and Pattern Recognition: International Conference on Intelligent Computing, ICIC 2006 Kunming*, China, August 16–19, 2006, Springer Berlin Heidelberg, pp. 913–918, 2006.
29. Hua, K.L., Dai, B.R., Srinivasan, K., Hsu, Y.H., Sharma, V., A hybrid NSCT domain image watermarking scheme. *Eurasip J. Image Video Process.*, 2017, 1, 1–7, 2017 Dec.
30. Abdolshah, M., Teimouri, M., Rahmani, R., Classification of X-ray images of shipping containers. *Expert Syst. Appl.*, 77, 57–65, 2017 Jul 1.
31. Russakovsky, O., Deng, J., Su, H., Krause, J., Satheesh, S., Ma, S., Huang, Z., Karpathy, A., Khosla, A., Bernstein, M., Berg, A.C., Imagenet large scale visual recognition challenge. *Int. J. Comput. Vision*, 115, 211–252, 2015 Dec.

32. Lindsey, R., Daluiski, A., Chopra, S., Lachapelle, A., Mozer, M., Sicular, S., Hanel, D., Gardner, M., Gupta, A., Hotchkiss, R., Potter, H., Deep neural network improves fracture detection by clinicians. *Proc. Natl. Acad. Sci. U.S.A.*, 115, 45, 11591–11596, 2018 Nov 6.
33. Chung, S.W., Han, S.S., Lee, J.W., Oh, K.S., Kim, N.R., Yoon, J.P., Kim, J.Y., Moon, S.H., Kwon, J., Lee, H.J., Noh, Y.M., Automated detection and classification of the proximal humerus fracture by using deep learning algorithm. *Acta Orthop.*, 89, 4, 468–473, 2018 Jul 4.
34. Muehlematter, U.J., Mannil, M., Becker, A.S., Vokinger, K.N., Finkenstaedt, T., Osterhoff, G., Fischer, M.A., Guggenberger, R., Vertebral body insufficiency fractures: Detection of vertebrae at risk on standard CT images using texture analysis and machine learning. *Eur. Radiol.*, 29, 2207–2217, 2019 May 1.
35. Tyson, S. and Hatem, S.F., Easily missed fractures of the upper extremity. *Radiol. Clin.*, 53, 4, 717–736, 2015 Jul 1.
36. Kim, D.H. and MacKinnon, T., Artificial intelligence in fracture detection: Transfer learning from deep convolutional neural networks. *Clin. Radiol.*, 73, 5, 439–445, 2018 May 1.
37. Olczak, J., Fahlberg, N., Maki, A., Razavian, A.S., Jilert, A., Stark, A., Sköldenberg, O., Gordon, M., Artificial intelligence for analyzing orthopedic trauma radiographs: Deep learning algorithms—Are they on par with humans for diagnosing fractures? *Acta Orthop.*, 88, 6, 581–586, 2017 Nov 2.
38. Cheng, C.T., Ho, T.Y., Lee, T.Y., Chang, C.C., Chou, C.C., Chen, C.C., Chung, I., Liao, C.H., Application of a deep learning algorithm for detection and visualization of hip fractures on plain pelvic radiographs. *Eur. Radiol.*, 29, 10, 5469–5477, 2019 Oct.
39. Adams, M., Chen, W., Holcdorf, D., McCusker, M.W., Howe, P.D., Gaillard, F., Computer vs human: Deep learning versus perceptual training for the detection of neck of femur fractures. *J. Med. Imaging Radiat. Oncol.*, 63, 1, 27–32, 2019 Feb.
40. Balaji, G.N., Subashini, T.S., Madhavi, P., Bhavani, C.H., Manikandarajan, A., Computer-aided detection and diagnosis of diaphyseal femur fracture, in: *Smart Intelligent Computing and Applications: Proceedings of the Third International Conference on Smart Computing and Informatics*, vol. 1, Springer Singapore, pp. 549–559, 2020.
41. Kitamura, G., Chung, C.Y., Moore, B.E., Ankle fracture detection utilizing a convolutional neural network ensemble implemented with a small sample, de novo training, and multiview incorporation. *J. Digital Imaging*, 32, 672–677, 2019 Aug 15.

42. Pranata, Y.D., Wang, K.C., Wang, J.C., Idram, I., Lai, J.Y., Liu, J.W., Hsieh, I.H., Deep learning and SURF for automated classification and detection of calcaneus fractures in CT images. *Comput. Methods Programs Biomed.*, 171, 27–37, 2019 Apr 1.
43. Tomita, N., Cheung, Y.Y., Hassanpour, S., Deep neural networks for automatic detection of osteoporotic vertebral fractures on CT scans. *Comput. Biol. Med.*, 98, 8–15, 2018 Jul 1.

4

Treatment of Osteoporosis and the Use of Digital Health Intervention

Abstract

Osteoporosis, a disease characterized by decreasing bone mass and microarchitectural deterioration, increases bone fragility and fracture risk. Osteoporotic fractures most commonly occur in the spine, hip, distal forearm, and proximal humerus but can happen elsewhere in the skeleton. Although bone mineral density (BMD) assessed by dual X-ray absorptiometry is the gold standard for the operational diagnosis of osteoporosis, the vast majority of fractures happen at BMD values that are not suggestive of the condition. With the rising prevalence of osteoporosis and fragility fractures, there is an urgent need to improve osteoporosis management throughout healthcare systems. Digital health technologies can be useful in improving the current state of osteoporosis care. Fracture liaison services (FLSs) have been found to considerably improve the quality of life of osteoporosis patients and could benefit from the use of automated solutions. Everything from clinical decision support systems and electronic medical record tools to patient choice aids and patient applications to educational resources and state-of-the-art artificial intelligence (AI) algorithms are all included in the realm of digital health. To pinpoint the most effective areas to work on, this chapter examines AI-based solutions that apply algorithms within health system registries. Using digital health interventions focused on physicians, patients, or healthcare systems may improve the management and prevention of fragility fractures. With the use of digital technology, multidisciplinary teams may be able to provide patients with the best possible care based on the most recent data, and patients may also benefit from these tools for self-management.

Keywords: Osteoporosis, digital health, algorithms, fracture risk, telehealth, mHealth, wearables

4.1 Introduction

Decreased bone mass as well as the microarchitectural degradation of bone tissue characterizes osteoporosis, a systemic skeletal condition. Its effects on

Rishabha Malviya, Shivam Rajput and Makarand Vaidya. Artificial Intelligence for Bone Disorder: Diagnosis and Treatment, (79–104) © 2024 Scrivener Publishing LLC

bone fragility and fracture risk are well documented. Bone mineral density (BMD), determined by dual X-ray absorptiometry (DXA) of the spine, hip, or so-called one-third radius, is used for the operative diagnosis of osteoporosis. The World Health Organization's guidelines [1] are strictly followed. Osteoporosis is diagnosed when a person's BMD falls at least 2.5 standard deviations (or T-score) below the mean normal BMD value of healthy young people. However, because many fractures occur at T-scores of 1.0 to 2.5 (i.e., at osteopenic BMD) or even above 1.0 (i.e., at normal BMD), the sensitivity of this "gold standard" approach and its potential usefulness as a screening tool are compromised [2]. The chance of suffering a second fracture, a lower quality of life, disability, and, apart from distal forearm fracture, an increased risk of death has all been associated with fractures in the spine, shoulder, hip, and wrist [3, 4]. Distal forearm fracture is the only exception to this rule. These kinds of fractures also go by the designation major osteoporotic fractures sometimes. When compared to men, women over the age of 50 have a risk of having a severe osteoporotic fracture that is about half as high over their lifetimes as that of men [5, 6]. Osteoporosis is responsible for around 9 million fractures per year across the world, which equates to one osteoporotic fracture occurring every 3 s.

It is believed that a group of mathematicians, cognitive scientists, and computer scientists at a conference in the middle of the 1950s at Dartmouth College (USA) first used the phrase "artificial intelligence" (AI) in its modern sense. Even though the meeting did not live up to anyone's expectations or expectations in general, it is largely considered the spark that started the subsequent boom in AI research. This growth, on the other hand, was halted at least twice by research slumps, which are also commonly known as "winters of AI research." The first research slump occurred in the middle to late 1970s, and the second research slump occurred in the late 1980s and early 1990s. Both research slumps lasted for several years. In both instances, funding for artificial intelligence-related research programs had already been declining before the arrival of the "winter." After that, thankfully, both research and financing began to pick back up, primarily as a result of the virtually exponential expansion in processing capability. International Business Machine (IBM) Deep Blue® chess computer beat world champion Gary Kasparov in 1997, and IBM's Watson® computer beat the top two humans in Jeopardy! players of all time in 2011 in front of a global audience of millions. Both victories were accomplished by IBM. These and many other important AI accomplishments have, without a shadow of a doubt, paved the way for future AI-based medical research that holds great promise. Throughout the last decade, tremendous progress has been made in a variety of subfields within human medicine [7]. Virtual artificial intelligence, which includes imaging solutions and treatment decision support systems, and physical artificial intelligence, which includes intelligent prosthetics and robot-assisted surgery are the two primary categories of artificial intelligence that are employed in medicine [8]. Virtual AI is currently the most important component of osteoporosis care, with solutions already available (or in development) to aid in the diagnosis, fracture detection, fracture risk assessment, bone quality evaluation, and therapy selection (Figure 4.1) [9].

Digital health interventions aim to link together different treatment facilities to provide the secure and effective electronic interchange of patient records. The following are examples of technology of this type used in the context of bone health:

- Digital health records
- The Role of Clinical Decision Support Systems (CDSSs)
- Patient decision support tools
- The use of e-health technologies to improve doctor–patient dialog
- The use of electronic and mobile applications
- Electronic consultation and triage systems
- Clinicians' access to digitally delivered osteoporosis education
- Patient-oriented resources
- Case-finding strategies that make use of AI

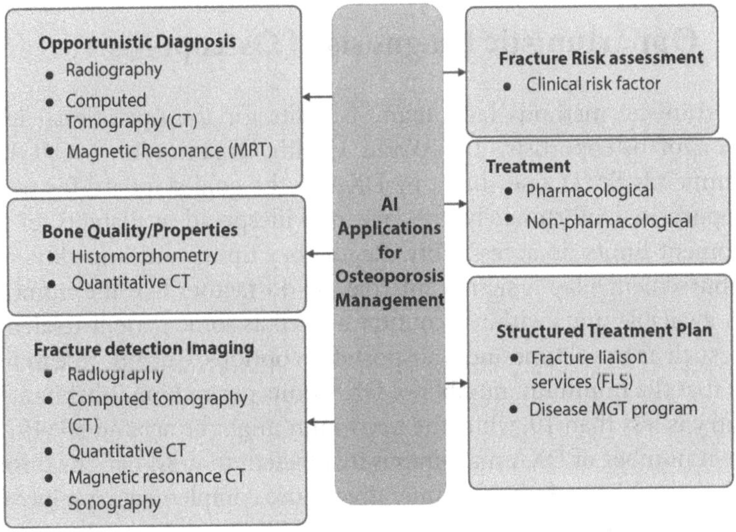

Figure 4.1 Solutions using AI that have been developed and are currently available for the treatment of osteoporosis.

A variety of government policy measures [10] currently support the use of digital technology embedded in healthcare, which is a priority for many nations.

Those with osteoporosis, a disorder marked by decreased bone density, are at a greater risk for suffering from low-impact fractures. There is a strong correlation between fragility fractures and higher mortality and disability rates [11], which poses a significant cost burden on healthcare systems worldwide. One-third of the world's women over the age of 50 and one-fifth of the world's men suffer from fragility fractures.

Meta-analyses [12] show that people with a history of fracture, regardless of the risk because of low BMD or fracture location, have a significantly higher risk of future fracture. The health and economic effect of osteoporosis is on the rise, although this trend may be mitigated by secondary prevention actions done by those who have already experienced a fragility fracture. There is potential for digital health solutions to be quite helpful in this setting. There are many kinds of FLSs, but research shows that even the simplest FLSs help with osteoporosis detection and management, boost long-term treatment adherence, and decrease recurrent fracture rates and hospital expenditures [13–15]. Comprehensive care for the elderly and weak following a hip fracture is just one example of how FLS improves osteoporosis screening and therapy as shown by first-level data like systematic meta-analyses and reviews [16, 17].

4.2 Opportunistic Diagnosis of Osteoporosis

Opportunistic methods have many benefits for the operational identification of osteoporosis. The World Health Organization (WHO) [18] recommends BMD assessment by DXA as the gold standard for treating osteoporosis. Unfortunately, the lack of widespread availability of DXA equipment limits its accessibility. Regulatory limits and impediments to reimbursement play a significant role, as do factors like the number of DXA available units within a country as well as some patient-related barriers, such as travel time and transportation options. Current research suggests that the minimum number of DXA units per million inhabitants in a country is less than 10, while the maximum might be around 50 [19]. The current number of DXA machines is insufficient in most nations throughout the world. Therefore, it is imperative to use complementary approaches that can reach a wider audience, such as traditional radiography.

One area where panoramic radiographs have been employed for a long time to learn about the mandibular bone's quantitative and qualitative qualities is dental medicine, and more specifically dental implantology [20, 21]. Patients who may have osteoporosis based on panoramic radiographs should be referred to medical specialists, it has been suggested. Hence, it is important to develop AI-supported tools to enhance the diagnostic precision of such non-invasive osteoporosis screening procedures. For instance, many distinct CNNs (Convolutional Neural Networks) were used for panoramic radiographs in an unpublished investigation aimed at diagnosing osteoporosis [22]. AUC (area under the curve) values were between 0.98 and 0.99 depending on the CNN employed. Instead of using DXA as the gold-standard reference technology, however, experienced oral and maxillofacial radiologists diagnosed osteoporosis based on identical radiographs. Another study looked at 4 different CNN models and found that their diagnostic performance can be greatly improved through transfer learning and fine-tuning, up to an AUC of 0.86 [23]. The lack of information on the reference technology employed makes the outcomes of this study appear less promising and substantially reduces their therapeutic significance.

There are also artificial intelligence (AI)-based software solutions that may be used with standard hand and wrist radiographs to make an opportunistic diagnosis of osteoporosis. Research using cortical radiogrammetry of the third metacarpal bone shaft as well as cancellous texture analysis of the distal radius, with DXA as the gold standard, resulted in an algorithm that performed well in a test setting [24, 25]. With a demonstrated accuracy of over 89%, the created software may represent a promising candidate for widespread clinical use.

Opportunistic detection of osteoporosis has been proposed utilizing a range of additional diagnostic methods, such as quantitative ultrasonography, computed tomography, and quantitative computed tomography. T-scores are frequently produced as a result of such techniques, and they can be utilized to categorize the bone mineral density as "normal," "osteopenic," or "osteoporotic". T-scores from these other technologies cannot be directly substituted for T-scores produced from DXA [26] because they measure distinct bone characteristics, leading to different gradients of risk. However, it is crucial to keep in mind that opportunistic QCT (quantitative computed tomography) of the spine has been demonstrated to have a greater link with the risk of occurrence of vertebral fractures [27], therefore it is important to remember that T-scores from DXA are the gold standard for evaluating BMD.

Due to these factors, several research projects have introduced AI-supported software tools to boost the sensitivity, specificity, and accuracy of such opportunistic methods. In one study [28], researchers used a completely automated AI method to quantify BMD in the spine using chest CTs (computed tomography) acquired for screening for lung cancer. With an AUC for osteopenia of 0.83 and an AUC for osteoporosis of 0.97, the diagnostic performance was judged to be excellent. Further research revealed that the risk of osteoporosis was reduced by 61% to 80% and the incidence of osteopenia was reduced by 34% to 46% for every 10 HU (Hounsfield unit) increase in CT levels. The researchers found that opportunistic screening for osteopenia and osteoporosis was greatly aided by routine chest CTs combined with AI. Although lumbar vertebrae L1-L4 are used in DXA-based BMD assessment of the spine, the primary focus of chest CT-based BMD measurement is on thoracic vertebrae, limiting the clinical relevance of these findings. One study [29] tried to fix this issue by using a gold-standard method, a DXA of the lumbar spine, to train a CNN model to predict BMD from abdominal CT scans. With an AUC of 0.965 on internal validation data sets and 0.970 on external data sets, the osteoporosis diagnosis accuracy was high. Promising results were also found in an experiment using abdominal/pelvic CT and DXA as the gold standard [30]. An additional attempt was made to create an AI-based method for detecting osteoporosis using abdominal or pelvic CTs [31], however, the results were less clinically relevant because DXA was not used as a reference standard.

A first meta-analysis [32] of imaging-based AI techniques for the opportunistic detection of osteoporosis has been just completed. Seven trials met the inclusion criteria, including nearly 3,000 patients. Overall, the sensitivity was 0.96, as well as the specificity, was 0.95 when using a random effects model. The researchers are spot-on in pointing out the need for caution when interpreting the findings due to the high risk of bias in patient short-listing and the study's substantial heterogeneity. Only three of the seven studies used DXA as the gold standard.

Finally, aberrant bone density has been linked to a high-fat fraction in the bone marrow, as measured by magnetic resonance imaging [33]. But because manual picture segmentation is required, the approach's clinical value is constrained. Data from about 200 healthy volunteers was used to create a fully automated end-to-end radiomics pipeline at Google based on image segmentation with CNN [34]. As contrasted to the gold standard, quantitative computed tomography (QCT) of the lumbar spine, the created bone marrow fat fraction map radiomics showed remarkable accuracy in predicting osteopenia and osteoporosis.

Even though postmenopausal women are disproportionately affected by osteoporosis, the condition is increasingly becoming recognized as a clinical concern in older males. White people have a higher prevalence rate than those of other races [35]. When diagnosing osteoporosis, dual-energy X-ray absorptiometry (DXA) is typically used to estimate BMD in the proximal femur, lumbar spine, and occasionally the forearm. Thereafter, postmenopausal people of the same race and gender are used as a comparison group to evaluate the BMD [36]. The diagnosis is based on how much lower the patient's BMD is compared to a reference group (in terms of standard deviations or the T- score). The WHO classifies individuals as having osteoporosis if their BMD T-score is less than 2.5, as having healthy bone mineral density if it is over 1.0, and as having osteopenia if it is between 1.0 and 2.5. Fragility fractures are more common in those with low bone density [37]. In contrast to the low BMD required for the diagnosis of osteoporosis, the presence of fragility fractures qualifies a patient as having "severe osteoporosis." Half of all women and about 20% of all men will suffer from an osteoporotic fracture at some point in their lives [38].

The BMD assessment is correlated with bone fragility and osteoporosis [39]. However, there are limits to BMD using DXA in terms of modeling due to the use of X-rays, which are a kind of ionizing radiation (although at a very low dosage). Since the DXA test only accounts for the existence of bone and muscle, fat will always confound the results. As a 2D projection method, it also has limitations concerning bone form, size, and microstructure [40]. As a result, many people have not gotten the care they needed from doctors. According to population-based studies, osteopenia is present in most women who suffer from fragility fractures [41]. According to the National Osteoporosis Risk Assessment (NORA), 82% of osteoporotic fractures occurred in women who did not match the diagnostic parameters for osteoporosis according to DXA [42]. This study was conducted in the United States and included slightly under 150,000 postmenopausal women.

4.3 Predictive Models

Fragility fracture risk is influenced not only by BMD but also by age, a family medical history of hip fractures, a past of fragility fractures, as well as taking corticosteroids [43]. Several factors are considered by the widely used fracture risk assessment tool (FRAX) [44], including age, body mass index, sex, height, rheumatoid arthritis, previous fracture, use of glucocorticoids, parental fracture history, alcohol consumption, secondary osteoporosis, and smoking. The credibility of the 10-year fracture probability it generates has been questioned. Concerns have been raised about the model's assumptions (for instance, in FRAX most factors are input dichotomously, like smoking, regardless of their intensity) and its potential use as a tool to support pharmaceutical therapy for increasing BMD. It has been suggested [45] that other simpler models may be more effective.

Scrutinizing models is a breeze. All models are erroneous, but some are useful, to quote the great statistician George Box [46]. Recently, with the use of AI approaches, many models have been constructed to quantify the probability of fragility fracture, with the eventual goal of delivering more accurate projections. Linear and nonlinear combinations of all input risk variables, including those of linear and Poisson regression, are inadequate in comparison to the predictive power of these models. AI technologies can learn from data, which means they might potentially catch underlying trends and patterns that were previously hard to understand.

4.3.1 Machine Learning and Deep Learning

The AI toolkit is extensive, and it is still expanding. A more thorough and good description may be discovered in the introductory chapters of well-known textbooks [47], which the investigator will refer to briefly here as the investigator provides a high-level review of the models and approaches. Algorithms are often grouped into two broad categories: supervised and unsupervised. Supervised models are the most common type of model, and they work by transforming input data into a measurable value. During training, the prediction distance from the result might rise or decrease, allowing for a corresponding adjustment in the weights assigned to these input variables. Without these metrics, unsupervised models attempt to describe the many classes of inputs. Semisupervised algorithms are the ones that occasionally exhibit the characteristics of both categories. Classification refers to the process of dividing a population into two groups—those with and without osteoporosis—based on the model's predictions of the presence or absence of the disease. When the model is asked to forecast each subject's BMD in the osteoporosis dataset, for example, the job is referred to as regression if the result is quantitative. The third approach involves making predictions based on ordered categorical variables of outcome, such as the proportion of people with normal, osteopenia, and osteoporosis T-scores.

4.3.2 The AI Algorithms

Traditional methods of modeling and predicting continue to make use of linear and logistic regression. However, in recent decades, there has been an explosion in the number of models from which to choose. These days, deciding on a machine learning algorithm depends on factors like the job at hand, the quality of the data, and the amount of time you must run the algorithm. Although naive Bayes is one of the easiest classifiers to implement, it often displays strong bias and low variance, making it a good fit only for very small datasets. A classifier of association, k-nearest neighbor (kNN) is a straightforward technique for determining which entities are most like another set of entities based on their distances. In order to categorize information into two categories, the support vector machine (SVM) employs hyperplanes, which are n-inside-n geometric subspaces. SVMs are quite good at dealing with nonlinear and complex circumstances and seldom overfit. Predictions in classification and regression trees are more efficient than kNN at avoiding extraneous features, but they are also more susceptible to overfitting, which may be alleviated via ensemble learning. Ensemble learning takes the best features of multiple simpler base models and combines them into a single model by using techniques like boosting (in which the learners evolve to produce a weighted result) and bootstrap aggregation (that considers several decision trees and averages their predictions).

"Deep learning" refers to a set of methods that are based on the use of neural networks to facilitate the learning process [48, 49]. The term "(artificial) neural network" (or "NN") refers to a group of nonlinear statistical algorithms inspired by the way neurons in the human brain process data. The model's characteristics are the strengths and directions of the links between the network's nodes. The output is presented as a nonlinear combination of input parameters called "derived parameters," which are linear combinations of those inputs. They are computationally demanding despite their ability to efficiently process many inputs.

The convolutional neural net (CNN) is a well-known deep learning technique because it allows for the sharing or convolving of some of the weights.

4.3.3 Treatment Decision Support

Several people have argued over the past 30 years about the ideal timing to begin therapy and the most effective osteoporosis medication for reducing fracture risk. Treatment with osteoporosis drugs that have been proven to minimize the probability of future fractures [50] is recommended by most scientific groups concerned with osteoporosis for individuals who have had a low-trauma fracture. The rationale behind this method is that, in the first 12 to 24 months following a fracture, the risk of a second fracture is highest. The term "sentinel fracture" is often used to describe this idea. People who have experienced an osteoporotic fracture within the past year to 2 years are therefore at an extremely high risk [51]. Current guidelines recommend bone anabolic medications such as teriparatide or romosozumab as first-line therapy in these patients because of their earlier and more obvious anti-fracture effectiveness compared to antiresorptive therapies [52]. Treatment for osteoporosis is currently accepted for anyone whose fracture prediction is at least the same as a patient of the same age and sex [53]. This is because if a patient with a prevalent fracture is mandated to receive treatment for osteoporosis, then everyone is mandated to receive treatment. However, there is less consensus about how soon a patient with no obvious fracture should start treatment. Moreover, different risk classifications (such as high and extremely high) may be assigned to patients based on different standards and/or guidelines [54], and different calculators are available to help physicians evaluate their patients' fracture risks. However, even after receiving "sufficient" therapy with established anti-fracture effectiveness, a sizeable percentage of individuals with osteoporosis do not react [55, 56].

The proliferation of electronic medical records across healthcare systems and providers has resulted in a wealth of big data that has prompted an uptick in efforts by software developers to make use of this information. One recent AI system created to predict treatment-related BMD response included data from over 15,000 individuals with osteoporosis who were tracked for a decade [57]. Total alkaline phosphatase was the sole meaningful laboratory marker concerning bone turnover, but the algorithm took into account over 3,500 medicines and 5,200 ICD codes. Bone resorption and bone formation indicators like vitamin D were left out. The top-performing ML model for estimating treatment response as measured by BMD growth attained a receiver operating characteristic of 0.70 and an accuracy of 0.69 out of a possible 1.00. As an illustration, this AI-powered application may generate a report detailing probable qualifying prescriptions, which of these drugs is most likely associated with the biggest BMD rise, and any relevant clinical information.

In conclusion, several artificial intelligence algorithms have been designed in recent years to aid with osteoporosis therapy. Diagnosis, evaluation of bone quality, risk assessment, detection of fractures, and treatment selection are all part of this process. When compared to human medical professionals, such solutions have similar outcomes and, in some cases, even perform better than the AI system. Evidence suggests that combining clinical data with radiomics, which comprises AI-supported opportunistic techniques for BMD testing, can effectively identify individuals at a high risk of fracture. Even though the results of a newly developed AI algorithm appear good at first glance, it is crucial to always study the technique behind the results and critically evaluate them. Two major problems with AI development research are the selection of irrelevant or unimportant characteristics (i.e., variables) and the use of poor reference standards. Furthermore, there is no assurance that the AI algorithm selected or developed will produce results that are superior to those obtained by using traditional statistical methods. This makes the need for rigorous clinical studies of AI as a therapy for osteoporosis abundantly evident. To this end, it would be helpful to produce universally applicable recommendations for best practices that can be used by everyone from healthcare regulators and those in charge of approval processes to AI researchers, osteoporosis experts, and the scientific organizations that represent them all. Once these criteria are met, AI may be able to alter osteoporosis therapy, and its benefits to doctors, patients, and the healthcare system are likely to become more apparent and applicable in the years to come.

4.3.4 AI and Machine Learning in EHRs to Predict Falls and Fractures

It is possible to evaluate the likelihood of a fracture by employing several data sources and several computer-based methodologies or prediction algorithms. A patient's 5- or 10-year risk of fracture can be determined with their use by doctors. The highest levels of discrimination were seen with the combination of QFracture and BMD, the FRAX and BMD, and Garvan and BMD [58]. Much information on the general population's health is already collected by the administrative healthcare system, making it an ideal resource for assessing fracture risk. Risk assessment could be provided at the site of treatment by automating data entry and putting it into electronic health records (EHRs), thereby guiding physician management. The best solution is to have this in a centralized location where it can be utilized as a screening tool for numerous individuals. Data collected during normal healthcare for a community is drawing a lot of interest to improve fracture risk estimations. Large datasets and AI with machine learning make it necessary to detect patients at a high risk of fracture using routinely collected data. This research details the creation and testing of a predictive model "FREX" for spotting those who are likely to suffer from osteoporotic fractures or hip fractures. In this study, only administrative ICD-10 data from public health registries for people aged 45 and over were employed [59]. For this reason, FREX is well suited to automation; no data entry is needed at the point of service because it only uses routinely collected administrative data. According to FREX, age is the most important risk factor for osteoporotic fractures, followed by a history of multiple previous osteoporotic fractures and fragility or a high risk of falls. In order to determine whether the FREX tool and others like it can be seamlessly incorporated into EHRs and national patient information registries, experiments are now being conducted. Fewer workers are needed to perform the task when integration is used to automate it [60].

4.4 Assessment of Fracture Risk and Osteoporosis Diagnosis by Digital Health

Tools to measure fracture risk, such as the free online FRAX calculator, are the most visible example of digital health's use for osteoporosis. The primary goal of calculating a patient's 10-year risk of fractures is to locate those who might gain from osteoporosis treatment. Human limitations, such as clinicians' propensity to routinely enter clinical data manually and turn results into clinical practice, limit FRAX's applicability, adoption, and, by extension, effectiveness in identifying osteoporosis cases. The FRAX digital health approach [16] has been improved thanks to the work of the National Osteoporosis Guidelines Group (NOGG) in electronically incorporating 10-year fracture risk data to accepted treatment criteria. This provides physicians with a clearer picture of whether to propose therapy or merely comfort patients. QFracture is a web-based substitute for FRAX that detects fracture risk automatically and with no user input [61]. It is a part of the larger digital health system used for primary care. There is no connection to national guidelines, and bone density information is not accepted. Nonetheless, it does try to help patients visualize their risk by using "smiley" face grids of 100 that are simple to interpret, with colored "unhappy" faces showing unfavorable outcomes.

4.4.1 Advances in FLS Models and Digital Health

Since the original demonstration of the clinical efficacy of this paradigm in 1999 [62], at least 225 FLSs have been constituted in over 35 countries (statistics from the International Osteoporosis Foundation). A selected person or people, generally clinical nurse specialists, manage such programs [63]. These individuals conduct case findings, follow defined protocols with some form of support, and refer patients to specialized physicians. Reminders, risk assessments, and education provided by digital health technologies have been proven to increase BMD screening rates and drug initiation times for osteoporosis patients, thereby decreasing the occurrence of secondary fractures [64]. Tools with numerous components (such as reminders and education) that are designed to reach both physicians and patients are more likely to enhance the results [65, 66]. Few evaluative randomized controlled trials (RCTs) [67] describe using acceptable procedures of randomization and concealing, blinding, and following up on study participants.

The Fracture Liaison Service Database (FLS-DB) is a national patient-level audit that exemplifies the promise of digital health to enhance care following a fracture and reduce risk. FLS-DB will begin with a hip fracture database to assess the scope and quality of secondary fracture prevention services in England and Wales (which correlated financial incentives with better hip fracture care). Audits of both facilities and individual patients help determine where there may be room for improvement in the quality of treatment provided. Recently, the Hospital Quality Improvement Partnership (HQIP) commissioned the Royal College of Physicians (RCP) to conduct a new nationwide audit dubbed the Fragility Fracture Audit Programme (FFFAP) [68, 69]. From all around England and Wales, 69 different FLSs were represented in the annual database report from the 2020 RCP. The findings of this analysis can be used by local commissioners and FLSs to enhance post-fracture care provision by service enhancement and/ or increased commissioning, hence reducing the frequency of unnecessary fragility fractures [70]. Users of FLS DB will find it inconvenient to enter patient-level data manually due to the large number of variables already captured in individual hospitals' electronic medical records (EMRs). The value of EMRs would increase dramatically if they were linked to FLS-DB.

4.5 Clinical Decision Support Tools, Reminders, and Prompts for Spotting Osteoporosis in Digital Health Settings

A clinical decision support system (CDSS) is a useful resource for medical professionals. Online apps, EHRs, and computerized physician order entry (CPOE) are frequently used at the point of care because they allow doctors to combine their knowledge with data from other sources. It is common practice to use a variety of devices, including a computer, tablet, smartphone, and others, to gain entry to a CDSS [71]. Digital health is a new technology that helps in the treatment process (Figure 4.2). The Icelandic Osteoporosis Advisor (OPAD) is a wonderful example of a CDSS; it uses in-depth recommendations and risk variables to assist in identifying those who have a high probability of breaking a bone. The physician is prompted

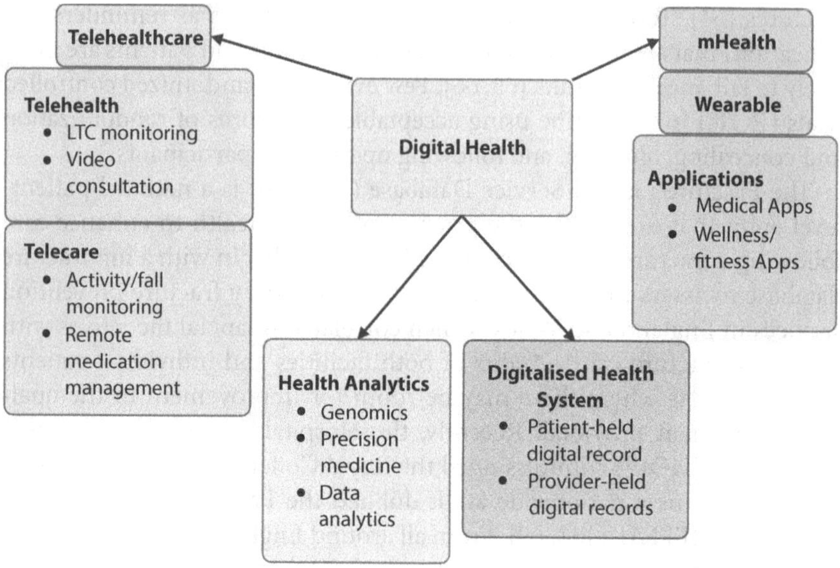

Figure 4.2 Sub-categories of digital health.

by OPAD to provide primary preventive guidance, evidence-based treatment suggestions, and follow-up advice [72]. Through the usage of EHR, prompts or alerts have become standard procedures in primary care. A CDSS has built-in prompts for when you need to do anything. Using them has been shown to improve follow-through on guidelines. Logic-based AI techniques might work well with CDSSs as well. The high cost and complexity of integrating CDSS with legacy and existing EHRs are two obstacles to its widespread adoption [73].

To better execute guidelines, notifications are effective in a meta-analysis of five separate randomized controlled studies [74]. The positive impact of alerts, reminders, and prompts on practitioner practice and patient outcomes can be maximized, but there is a lack of data to guide their selection and deployment [75]. However, there are cases when computerized system warnings significantly improved osteoporosis management [76]. The electronic health record (EHR) evaluation method used in primary care incorporates Canadian osteoporosis recommendations to enhance the screening and management of patients at the time of service. Better management of fragility fractures supported by proactive therapy and continuous monitoring following Canadian best practices standards [77] are made possible through the early identification and alerting of doctors to individuals at risk of developing osteoporosis.

4.6 The Role of Digital Health in Facilitating Patient Education, Decision, and Conversation

4.6.1 Decision Tools for Patients and Shared Decision Making

The need for shared decision-making in the management of osteoporosis has never been higher. Rather than relying solely on the "wild west" of clinical and quasi-clinical information available online, patients, family members, or carers are increasingly consulting with one or more healthcare experts before making decisions about a patient's care [78]. Although patients are always provided with informational pamphlets about their medications, such as those published by the Royal Osteoporosis Society, they are increasingly likely to "conduct their research online," particularly regarding the rare and very rare adverse effects of osteoporosis medicines. As a result, decision aids, which are based on evidence, can assist in bringing about collaborative decision-making [79]. In the context of osteoporosis treatment, these instruments have been found to increase patients' realism of their own risk. How someone perceives their risk of suffering a painful occurrence that is in part attributable to chance is crucial in determining whether they will seek out and adhere to a therapy designed to prevent osteoporosis (fragility fracture). Tools that exist on the web may be easily spread and updated. Suitable use of such tools has been shown to increase patient–clinician rapport, which, in turn, leads to the creation of a more appropriate and transparent treatment plan, most frequently concerning the initiation of pharmacological therapy. In 2008, a choice aid called "The Osteoporosis Choice Decision Aid" was created. With its help, patients and doctors may make educated decisions together. A patient's anticipated 10-year fracture risk utilizing the FRAX online calculator and the contributing factors are provided. Utilizing the FRAX fracture risk assessment tool led to less disagreement over care decisions, earlier treatment initiation, and greater patient understanding and participation, according to a randomized controlled trial [80].

Not all decision support tools are created equal; some have been found to have little effect on the number of healthcare professionals who adhere to guidelines [81], while others fall short of even the most basic quality requirements. Patients are not always keen on decision aids; some continue to put their faith in their doctors or specialists to do all the heavy lifting when it comes to making important healthcare decisions. Such aids must utilize the finest information available and/or have represented it well if they are to enhance osteoporosis therapy, but basic problems with current patient decision aids have been recognized [82].

4.6.2 Patient Interaction Enabled by Digital Health

Patients having osteoporosis seek education regarding their disease, fracture risk, treatment options, and the value of BMD testing so that they may take charge of their care [51]. A role for interactive voice response (IVR) systems and other kinds of multimedia technology in inspiring and educating patients is possible. Interventions in digital health can range from the rudimentary, like a phone call, to the complex, such as the use of many media types. According to a new analysis, elderly patients with fragility fractures can benefit from a patient-centered, integrated model of treatment that is supported by digital health technology solutions. Integration of pain management, exercise, nutritional, slumber–hygiene, and psychological health-enhancing resources is possible. Providing health information without instruction is not enough. Constant progress reporting and evaluation are essential. Behavioral modification strategies and motivational interviewing should be standard practice.

Poorer post-fracture outcomes are a direct result of patients being left to navigate the healthcare system on their own once they are discharged. Studies in digital health should target individuals with a wider range of conditions, including those that need a more individualized and coordinated treatment [83]. In the United States, a 4- to 5-min-long script was used in an IVR system to evaluate postmenopausal women who are at an increased risk for osteoporosis. The results of a RCT comparing patients who received educational packets in the mail in addition to their regular therapy showed no significant improvement [84]. Due to the wide variety of options, it might be tough to zero down on the best method.

4.6.3 Expert Clinical Instruction Aided by Digital Health Technologies

Project Extension for Community Healthcare Outcomes (ECHO) is a US proposal for a technology-enabled, collaborative learning program for medical practitioners to employ in the treatment of bone illnesses. The purpose of the weekly video conferences conducted by Bone Health TeleECHO is to enable a discourse between healthcare professionals with various degrees of experience and knowledge regarding osteoporosis [85]. Consistent users of Bone Health TeleECHO demonstrated statistically significant increases in self-efficacy across 20 categories of osteoporosis management. Video conferencing facilitates the exchange of information and expert opinion, allowing for the exploration of individualized treatment options that may fall outside of institutional norms or individual preferences [86].

4.6.4 Digital Health-Supported Patient Education

The Activating Patients at Risk for Osteoporosis (APROPOS) research created and tested a patient-centered, personalized, video-based behavioral intervention to increase the detection and treatment of osteoporosis. Intervention materials, including personalized movies, were delivered by DVD and emailed to a custom webpage. Telephone follow-up and automated voice reminders were also incorporated into the intervention to ensure that the films were seen. Similar percentages of self-reported treatment initiation and follow-up were found at 6 and 18 months [87]. Multimedia, in the form of a series of dramatized video segments, can be just as effective as a printed pamphlet in educating patients about osteoporosis and its risk factors, prevention, and management [88].

4.6.5 Smart, Portable Applications for Smartphones

Mobile health (mHealth) is a fast-growing industry that shows promise as an adjunct to standard medical procedures. More than a hundred thousand apps have been developed for mobile devices, and a large percentage of them are related to healthcare. There is some evidence to show that mHealth applications can help people with chronic conditions better manage their symptoms and have a positive impact on their health outcomes [89]. However, there is a dearth of apps that are designed to treat osteoporosis, and there is no oversight or regulation of app creators. The benefit of mHealth applications for osteoporosis is underappreciated, despite their growing popularity [90]. Apps tend to be well liked by their users, and there is some proof that those 65 and over are open to trying them out.

4.7 Conclusion

The development and implementation of digital technologies have accelerated dramatically. To improve patient care, healthcare administrations are looking to collaborate with the academic community, private sector, and other industries. Evidence shows that digital technologies can aid interdisciplinary teams in providing patients with the best possible care based on the best available evidence and can also aid patients in self-management.

First, the methodological quality of several of the studies evaluating these technologies has been low; second, the majority of the investigations have been conducted in a diverse set of worldwide locations. Thus, especially in mHealth, we still need robust randomized controlled studies to assess the efficacy and cost-effectiveness of these technologies. Finally, the successful adoption and integration of these technologies into practice depends on having a workforce that is digitally literate and able to make good use of them.

References

1. Dimai, H.P., Use of dual-energy X-ray absorptiometry (DXA) for diagnosis and fracture risk assessment; WHO-criteria, T- and Z-score, and reference databases. *Bone*, 104, 39–43, 2017 Nov 1.
2. Dyer, O., Covid-19: Many poor countries will see almost no vaccine next year, aid groups warn. *BMJ: Brit. Med. J. (Online)*, 371, 2020 Dec 11.
3. Öz, O.K., Zerwekh, J.E., Fisher, C., Graves, K., Nanu, L., Millsaps, R., Simpson, E.R., Bone has a sexually dimorphic response to aromatase deficiency. *J. Bone Miner. Res.*, 15, 3, 507–514, 2000 Mar.
4. Johansson, H., Siggeirsdóttir, K., Harvey, N.C., Odén, A., Gudnason, V., McCloskey, E., Sigurdsson, G., Kanis, J.A., Imminent risk of fracture after fracture. *Osteoporosis Int.*, 28, 775–780, 2017 Mar.
5. Johnell, O. and Kanis, J., Epidemiology of osteoporotic fractures. *Osteoporosis Int.*, 16, S3–7, 2005 Mar.
6. Johnell, O. and Kanis, J.A., An estimate of the worldwide prevalence and disability associated with osteoporotic fractures. *Osteoporosis Int.*, 17, 1726–1733, 2006 Dec.
7. Topol, E.J., High-performance medicine: The convergence of human and artificial intelligence. *Nat. Med.*, 25, 1, 44–56, 2019 Jan.
8. Hamet, P. and Tremblay, J., Artificial intelligence in medicine. *Metabolism*, 69, S36–S40, 2017.
9. Smets, J., Shevroja, E., Hügle, T., Leslie, W.D., Hans, D., Machine learning solutions for osteoporosis—A review. *J. Bone Miner. Res.*, 36, 5, 833–851, 2021 May.
10. Mathews, S.C., McShea, M.J., Hanley, C.L., Ravitz, A., Labrique, A.B., Cohen, A.B., Digital health: A path to validation. *NPJ Digital Med.*, 2, 1, 38, 2019 May 13.
11. Svedbom, A., Hernlund, E., Ivergård, M., Compston, J., Cooper, C., Stenmark, J., McCloskey, E.V., Jönsson, B., Kanis, J.A., EU review panel of the IOF. Osteoporosis in the European Union: A compendium of country-specific reports. *Arch. Osteoporos.*, 8, 1–218, 2013 Dec.
12. Kanis, J.A., Johnell, O., De Laet, C.E., Johansson, H., Odén, A., Delmas, P., Eisman, J., Fujiwara, S., Garnero, P., Kroger, H., McCloskey, E.V., A

meta-analysis of previous fracture and subsequent fracture risk. *Bone*, 35, 2, 375–382, 2004 Aug 1.

13. Mitchell, P.J., Best practices in secondary fracture prevention: Fracture liaison services. *Curr. Osteoporos. Rep.*, 11, 1, 52–60, 2013 Mar.
14. Åkesson, K., Marsh, D., Mitchell, P.J., McLellan, A.R., Stenmark, J., Pierroz, D.D., Kyer, C., Cooper, C., Fracture Working Group, I.O.F., Capture the fracture: A best practice framework and global campaign to break the fragility fracture cycle. *Osteoporos. Int.*, 24, 2135–2152, 2013 Aug.
15. Nakayama, A., Major, G., Holliday, E., Attia, J., Bogduk, N., Evidence of effectiveness of a fracture liaison service to reduce the re-fracture rate. *Osteoporos. Int.*, 27, 873–879, 2016 Mar.
16. Geusens, P., Bours, S.P., Wyers, C.E., van den Bergh, J.P., Fracture liaison programs. *Best Pract. Res. Clin. Rheumatol.*, 33, 2, 278–289, 2019 Apr 1.
17. Wu, C.H., Tu, S.T., Chang, Y.F., Chan, D.C., Chien, J.T., Lin, C.H., Singh, S., Dasari, M., Chen, J.F., Tsai, K.S., Fracture liaison services improve outcomes of patients with osteoporosis-related fractures: A systematic literature review and meta-analysis. *Bone*, 111, 92–100, 2018 Jun 1.
18. Shuhart, C.R., Yeap, S.S., Anderson, P.A., Jankowski, L.G., Lewiecki, E.M., Morse, L.R., Rosen, H.N., Weber, D.R., Zemel, B.S., Shepherd, J.A., Executive summary of the 2019 ISCD position development conference on monitoring treatment, DXA cross-calibration and least significant change, spinal cord injury, peri-prosthetic and orthopedic bone health, transgender medicine, and pediatrics. *J. Clin. Densitom.*, 22, 4, 453–471, 2019 Oct 1.
19. Wen, J., Thibeau-Sutre, E., Diaz-Melo, M., Samper-Gonzalez, J., Routier, A., Bottani, S., Dormont, D., Durrleman, S., Burgos, N., Colliot, O., Alzheimer's Disease Neuroimaging I, Australian Imaging B, and Lifestyle flagship study of a 2020, Convolutional neural networks for classification of Alzheimer's disease: Overview and reproducible evaluation. *Med. Image Anal.*, 63, 101694, 2020.
20. Yasar, F. and Akgunlu, F., The differences in panoramic mandibular indices and fractal dimension between patients with and without spinal osteoporosis. *Dentomaxillofac. Radiol.*, 35, 1, 1–9, 2006 Jan.
21. White, S.C., Taguchi, A., Kao, D., Wu, S., Service, S.K., Yoon, D., Suei, Y., Nakamoto, T., Tanimoto, K., Clinical and panoramic predictors of femur bone mineral density. *Osteoporos. Int.*, 16, 339–346, 2005 Mar.
22. Lee, J.S., Adhikari, S., Liu, L., Jeong, H.G., Kim, H., Yoon, S.J., Osteoporosis detection in panoramic radiographs using a deep convolutional neural network-based computer-assisted diagnosis system: A preliminary study. *Dentomaxillofac. Radiol.*, 48, 1, 20170344, 2019 Jan.
23. Lee, K.S., Jung, S.K., Ryu, J.J., Shin, S.W., Choi, J., Evaluation of transfer learning with deep convolutional neural networks for screening osteoporosis in dental panoramic radiographs. *J. Clin. Med.*, 9, 2, 392, 2020 Feb 1.
24. Areeckal, A.S., Kamath, J., Zawadynski, S., Kocher, M., Combined radiogrammetry and texture analysis for early diagnosis of osteoporosis using

Indian and Swiss data. *Comput. Med. Imaging Graphics*, 68, 25–39, 2018 Sep 1.

25. Areeckal, A.S., Jayasheelan, N., Kamath, J., Zawadynski, S., Kocher, M., David, S.S., Early diagnosis of osteoporosis using radiogrammetry and texture analysis from hand and wrist radiographs in Indian population. *Osteoporos. Int.*, 29, 665–673, 2018 Mar.
26. Rosen, H.N., Vokes, T.J., Malabanan, A.O., Deal, C.L., Alele, J.D., Olenginski, T.P., Schousboe, J.T., The official positions of the international society for clinical densitometry: Vertebral fracture assessment. *J. Clin. Densitom.*, 16, 4, 482–488, 2013 Oct 1.
27. Löffler, M.T., Jacob, A., Valentinitsch, A., Rienmüller, A., Zimmer, C., Ryang, Y.M., Baum, T., Kirschke, J.S., Improved prediction of incident vertebral fractures using opportunistic QCT compared to DXA. *Eur. Radiol.*, 29, 4980–4989, 2019 Sep 1.
28. Yang, S., Yin, B., Cao, W., Feng, C., Fan, G., He, S., Diagnostic accuracy of deep learning in orthopaedic fractures: A systematic review and meta-analysis. *Clin. Radiol.*, 75, 9, 713–e17, 2020 Sep 1.
29. Yasaka, K., Akai, H., Kunimatsu, A., Kiryu, S., Abe, O., Prediction of bone mineral density from computed tomography: Application of deep learning with a convolutional neural network. *Eur. Radiol.*, 30, 3549–3557, 2020 Jun.
30. Krishnaraj, A., Barrett, S., Bregman-Amitai, O., Cohen-Sfady, M., Bar, A., Chettrit, D., Orlovsky, M., Elnekave, E., Simulating dual-energy X-ray absorptiometry in CT using deep-learning segmentation cascade. *J. Am. Coll. Radiol.*, 16, 10, 1473–1479, 2019 Oct 1.
31. Fang, Y., Li, W., Chen, X., Chen, K., Kang, H., Yu, P., Zhang, R., Liao, J., Hong, G., Li, S., Opportunistic osteoporosis screening in multi-detector CT images using deep convolutional neural networks. *Eur. Radiol.*, 31, 1831–1842, 2021 Apr.
32. Gao, L., Jiao, T., Feng, Q., Wang, W., Application of artificial intelligence in diagnosis of osteoporosis using medical images: A systematic review and meta-analysis. *Osteoporos. Int.*, 32, 1279–1286, 2021 Jul.
33. Zhao, Y., Huang, M., Ding, J., Zhang, X., Spuhler, K., Hu, S., Li, M., Fan, W., Chen, L., Zhang, X., Li, S., Prediction of abnormal bone density and osteoporosis from lumbar spine MR using modified dixon quant in 257 subjects with quantitative computed tomography as reference. *J. Magn. Reson. Imaging*, 49, 2, 390–399, 2019 Feb.
34. Zhao, Y., Zhao, T., Chen, S., Zhang, X., Sosa, M.S., Liu, J., Mo, X., Chen, X., Huang, M., Li, S., Zhang, X., Fully automated radiomic screening pipeline for osteoporosis and abnormal bone density with a deep learning-based segmentation using a short lumbar mDixon sequence. *Quant. Imaging Med. Surg.*, 12, 2, 1198, 2022 Feb.
35. US Preventive Services Task Force*, Screening for osteoporosis: US preventive services task force recommendation statement. *Ann. Intern. Med.*, 154, 5, 356–364, 2011 Mar 1.

36. Kanis, J.A. and Kanis, J.A., Assessment of fracture risk and its application to screening for postmenopausal osteoporosis: Synopsis of a WHO report. *Osteoporos. Int.*, 4, 368–381, 1994 Nov.
37. Peck, W.A., Consensus development conference: Diagnosis, prophylaxis, and treatment of osteoporosis. *Am. J. Med.*, 94, 6, 646–650, 1993.
38. US D. Bone health and osteoporosis: A report of the Surgeon General, 2004, http://www. surgeongeneral. gov/library/bonehealth/content. html.
39. Marshall, D., Johnell, O., Wedel, H., Meta-analysis of how well measures of bone mineral density predict occurrence of osteoporotic fractures. *BMJ*, 312, 1254–1259, May. 1996.
40. Chang, G., Honig, S., Brown, R., Deniz, C.M., Egol, K.A., Babb, J.S., Regatte, R.R., Rajapakse, C.S., Finite element analysis applied to 3-T MR imaging of proximal femur microarchitecture: Lower bone strength in patients with fragility fractures compared with control subjects. *Radiology*, 272, 2, 464–474, 2014 Aug.
41. Wainwright, S.A., Marshall, L.M., Ensrud, K.E., Cauley, J.A., Black, D.M., Hillier, T.A., Hochberg, M.C., Vogt, M.T., Orwoll, E.S., Study of Osteoporotic Fractures Research Group. Hip fracture in women without osteoporosis. *J. Clin. Endocrinol. Metab.*, 90, 5, 2787–2793, 2005 May 1.
42. Siris, E.S., Chen, Y.T., Abbott, T.A., Barrett-Connor, E., Miller, P.D., Wehren, L.E., Berger, M.L., Bone mineral density thresholds for pharmacological intervention to prevent fractures. *Arch. Intern. Med.*, 164, 10, 1108–1112, 2004 May 24.
43. Kanis, J.A., Diagnosis of osteoporosis and assessment of fracture risk. *Lancet*, 359, 9321, 1929–1936, 2002 Jun 1.
44. Kanis, J.A., Johnell, O., Odén, A., Johansson, H., McCloskey, E.F., FRAX™ and the assessment of fracture probability in men and women from the UK. *Osteoporos. Int.*, 19, 385–397, 2008 Apr.
45. Rubin, K.H., Friis-Holmberg, T., Hermann, A.P., Abrahamsen, B., Brixen, K., Risk assessment tools to identify women with increased risk of osteoporotic fracture: Complexity or simplicity? A systematic review. *J. Bone Miner. Res.*, 28, 8, 1701–1717, 2013 Aug.
46. Box, G.E., Science and statistics. *J. Am. Stat. Assoc.*, 71, 356, 791–799, 1976 Dec 1.
47. Hastie, T., Tibshirani, R., Friedman, J., *The elements of statistical learning*, Springer Series in Statistics, New York, NY, USA, 2001.
48. Le, Q.V., A tutorial on deep learning part 2: Autoencoders, convolutional neural networks and recurrent neural networks. *Google Brain*, 20, 1–20, 2015 Oct 20.
49. 摇LeCun, Y., Bengio, Y., Hinton, G., Deep learning. *Nature*, 521, 7553, 436–444, 2015.
50. Camacho, P.M., Petak, S.M., Binkley, N., Diab, D.L., Eldeiry, L.S., Farooki, A., Harris, S.T., Hurley, D.L., Kelly, J., Lewiecki, E.M., Pessah-Pollack, R., American Association of Clinical Endocrinologists/American College of Endocrinology

clinical practice guidelines for the diagnosis and treatment of postmenopausal osteoporosis—2020 update. *Endocr. Pract.*, 26, 1–46, 2020 May 1.

51. Kanis, J.A., Harvey, N.C., McCloskey, E., Bruyère, O., Veronese, N., Lorentzon, M., Cooper, C., Rizzoli, R., Adib, G., Al-Daghri, N., Campusano, C., Algorithm for the management of patients at low, high and very high risk of osteoporotic fractures. *Osteoporos. Int.*, 31, 1–2, 2020 Jan.
52. Kanis, J.A., Johansson, H., Harvey, N.C., Gudnason, V., Sigurdsson, G., Siggeirsdottir, K., Lorentzon, M., Liu, E., Vandenput, L., McCloskey, E.V., Adjusting conventional FRAX estimates of fracture probability according to the recency of sentinel fractures. *Osteoporos. Int.*, 31, 1817–1828, 2020 Oct.
53. Kanis, J.A., McCloskey, E.V., Johansson, H., Cooper, C., Rizzoli, R., Reginster, J.Y., Scientific Advisory Board of the European Society for Clinical and Economic Aspects of Osteoporosis and Osteoarthritis (ESCEO) and the Committee of Scientific Advisors of the International Osteoporosis Foundation (IOF), European guidance for the diagnosis and management of osteoporosis in postmenopausal women. *Osteoporos. Int.*, 24, 1, 23–57, 2013 Jan.
54. Shoback, D., Rosen, C.J., Black, D.M., Cheung, A.M., Murad, M.H., Eastell, R., Pharmacological management of osteoporosis in postmenopausal women: An endocrine society guideline update. *J. Clin. Endocrinol. Metab.*, 105, 3, 587–594, 2020 Mar.
55. Díez-Pérez, A., Adachi, J.D., Adami, S., Anderson Jr., F.A., Boonen, S., Chapurlat, R., Compston, J.E., Cooper, C., Gehlbach, S.H., Greenspan, S.L., Hooven, F.H., Risk factors for treatment failure with antiosteoporosis medication: The global longitudinal study of osteoporosis in women (GLOW). *J. Bone Miner. Res.*, 29, 1, 260–267, 2014 Jan.
56. Francis, R.M., Non-response to osteoporosis treatment. *Br. Menopause Soc. J.*, 10, 2, 76–80, 2004 Jun 1.
57. Lundberg, S.M. and Lee, S.I., A unified approach to interpreting model predictions. *Advances in neural information processing systems*, p. 30, 2017.
58. Beaudoin, C., Moore, L., Gagné, M., Bessette, L., Ste-Marie, L.G., Brown, J.P., Jean, S., Performance of predictive tools to identify individuals at risk of non-traumatic fracture: A systematic review, meta-analysis, and meta-regression. *Osteoporos. Int.*, 30, 721–40, 2019 Apr 1.
59. Rubin, K.H., Möller, S., Holmberg, T., Bliddal, M., Søndergaard, J., Abrahamsen, B., A new fracture risk assessment tool (FREM) based on public health registries. *J. Bone Miner. Res.*, 33, 11, 1967–1979, 2018 Nov.
60. Yang, S., Leslie, W.D., Morin, S.N., Lix, L.M., Administrative healthcare data applied to fracture risk assessment. *Osteoporos. Int.*, 30, 565–71, 2019 Mar 5.
61. Kanis, J.A., Harvey, N.C., Johansson, H., Odén, A., McCloskey, E.V., Leslie, W.D., Overview of fracture prediction tools. *J. Clin. Densitom.*, 20, 3, 444–450, 2017 Jul 1.
62. McLellan, A.R., Gallacher, S.J., Fraser, M., McQuillian, C., The fracture liaison service: Success of a program for the evaluation and management of patients with osteoporotic fracture. *Osteoporos. Int.*, 14, 1028–1034, 2003 Dec.

63. Ganda, K., Puech, M., Chen, J.S., Speerin, R., Bleasel, J., Center, J.R., Eisman, J.A., March, L., Seibel, M.J., Models of care for the secondary prevention of osteoporotic fractures: A systematic review and meta-analysis. *Osteoporos. Int.*, 24, 393–406, 2013 Feb.
64. Halldorsson, B.V., Bjornsson, A.H., Gudmundsson, H.T., Birgisson, E.O., Ludviksson, B.R., Gudbjornsson, B., A clinical decision support system for the diagnosis, fracture risks and treatment of osteoporosis. *Comput. Math. Methods Med.*, 2015, 1–8, 2015 Mar 1.
65. Britnell, M., Bakalar, R., Shehata, A., Digital health: Heaven or hell, KPMG International, 2016.
66. Stacey, D., Légaré, F., Lewis, K., Barry, M.J., Bennett, C.L., Eden, K.B., Holmes-Rovner, M., Llewellyn-Thomas, H., Lyddiatt, A., Thomson, R., Trevena, L., Decision aids for people facing health treatment or screening decisions. *Cochrane Database Syst. Rev.*, 4, 1–287, 2017.
67. Gadkari, A.S. and McHorney, C.A., Medication nonfulfillment rates and reasons: Narrative systematic review. *Curr. Med. Res. Opin.*, 26, 3, 683–705, 2010 Mar 1.
68. Mitchell, P.J., Cooper, C., Fujita, M., Halbout, P., Åkesson, K., Costa, M., Dreinhöfer, K.E., Marsh, D.R., Lee, J.K., Chan, D.C., Javaid, M.K., Quality improvement initiatives in fragility fracture care and prevention. *Curr. Osteoporos. Rep.*, 17, 510–520, 2019 Dec.
69. Gallagher, C., Vasilakis, N., Javaid, K., Fracture Liaison Services in England and Wales, inequity of access and quality of care after a fragility fracture. *Clin. Med.*, 19, Suppl 2, 77, 2019 Mar.
70. Boulton, C., Gallagher, C., Rai, S., Tsang, C., Vasilakis, N., Javaid, M.K., Royal College of Physicians. Fracture Liaison Service Database (FLS-DB) clinical audit, *FLS forward: Identifying high-quality care in the NHS for secondary fracture prevention*, Programme FaFFA (Ed.), pp. 1–70, Royal Collge of Physicians, London, 2017.
71. Dias, D. and Paulo Silva Cunha, J., Wearable health devices—Vital sign monitoring, systems and technologies. *Sensors*, 18, 8, 2414, 2018 Jul 25.
72. Gudmundsson, H.T., Hansen, K.E., Halldorsson, B.V., Ludviksson, B.R., Gudbjornsson, B., Clinical decision support system for the management of osteoporosis compared to NOGG guidelines and an osteology specialist: A validation pilot study. *BMC Med. Inf. Decis. Making*, 19, 1, 1–8, 2019 Dec.
73. Sutton, R.T., Pincock, D., Baumgart, D.C., Sadowski, D.C., Fedorak, R.N., Kroeker, K.I., An overview of clinical decision support systems: Benefits, risks, and strategies for success. *NPJ Digital Med.*, 3, 1, 17, 2020 Feb 6.
74. Brown, V.T., Underwood, M., Mohamed, N., Westwood, O., Morrissey, D., Professional interventions for general practitioners on the management of musculoskeletal conditions. *Cochrane Database Syst. Rev.*, 5, 1–147, 2016.
75. Backman, R., Bayliss, S., Moore, D., Litchfield, I., Clinical reminder alert fatigue in healthcare: A systematic literature review protocol using qualitative evidence. *Syst. Rev.*, 6, 1, 1–6, 2017 Dec.

76. Goldshtein, I., Shamai-Lubovitz, O., Guindy, M., Shalev, V., Chodick, G., Lerner, U., Rouach, V., Development and efficacy of a computerized decision support system for osteoporosis management in the community. *Arch. Osteoporos.*, 15, 1–7, 2020 Dec.
77. Hawarden, A., Bullock, L., Chew-Graham, C.A., Herron, D., Hider, S., Jinks, C., De Silva, R.E., Machin, A., Paskins, Z., Incorporating FRAX® into a nurse-delivered integrated care review: A multi-method qualitative study. *BJGP Open*, 7, 1–10, 2023 Feb 3.
78. Légaré, F., Adekpedjou, R., Stacey, D., Turcotte, S., Kryworuchko, J., Graham, I.D., Lyddiatt, A., Politi, M.C., Thomson, R., Elwyn, G., Donner-Banzhoff, N., Interventions for increasing the use of shared decision making by health-care professionals. *Cochrane Database Syst. Rev.*, 7, 1–385, 2018.
79. Paskins, Z., Torres Roldan, V.D., Hawarden, A.W., Bullock, L., Meritxell Urtecho, S., Torres, G.F., Morera, L., Espinoza Suarez, N.R., Worrall, A., Blackburn, S., Chapman, S., Quality and effectiveness of osteoporosis treatment decision aids: A systematic review and environmental scan. *Osteoporos. Int.*, 31, 10, 1837–1851, 2020 Oct.
80. LeBlanc, A., Wang, A.T., Wyatt, K., Branda, M.E., Shah, N.D., Van Houten, H., Pencille, L., Wermers, R., Montori, V.M., Encounter decision aid vs. clinical decision support or usual care to support patient-centered treatment decisions in osteoporosis: The osteoporosis choice randomized trial II. *PLoS One*, 10, 5, e0128063, 2015 May 26.
81. Fønhus, M.S., Dalsbø, T.K., Johansen, M., Fretheim, A., Skirbekk, H., Flottorp, S.A., Patient-mediated interventions to improve professional practice. *Cochrane Database Syst. Rev.*, 9, 2018.
82. Paskins, Z., Worrall, A., Chapman, S., Patient and public views of bisphosphonate decision aids: Not fit for purpose, in: *Osteoporosis International*, vol. 29, pp. S374–S374, Springer London Ltd, Springer Nature Switzerland AG., 2018 Apr 1.
83. Yadav, L., Haldar, A., Jasper, U., Taylor, A., Visvanathan, R., Chehade, M., Gill, T., Utilising digital health technology to support patient-healthcare provider communication in fragility fracture recovery: Systematic review and meta-analysis. *Int. J. Environ. Res. Public Health*, 16, 20, 4047, 2019 Oct.
84. Heyworth, L., Kleinman, K., Oddleifson, S., Bernstein, L., Frampton, J., Lehrer, M., Salvato, K., Weiss, T.W., Simon, S.R., Connelly, M., Comparison of interactive voice response, patient mailing, and mailed registry to encourage screening for osteoporosis: A randomized controlled trial. *Osteoporos. Int.*, 25, 1519–1526, 2014 May.
85. Lewiecki, E.M., Jackson, A., Lake, A.F., Carey, J.J., Belaya, Z., Melnichenko, G.A., Rochelle, R., Bone Health TeleECHO: A force multiplier to improve the care of skeletal diseases in underserved communities. *Curr. Osteoporos. Rep.*, 17, 474–482, 2019 Dec.

86. Lewiecki, E.M., Rochelle, R., Bouchonville, M.F., Chafey, D.H., Olenginski, T.P., Arora, S., Leveraging scarce resources with bone health TeleECHO to improve the care of osteoporosis. *J. Endocr. Soc.*, 1, 12, 1428–1434, 2017 Dec 1.
87. Danila, M.I., Outman, R.C., Rahn, E.J., Mudano, A.S., Thomas, T.F., Redden, D.T., Allison, J.J., Anderson, F.A., Anderson, J.P., Cram, P.M., Curtis, J.R., A multi-modal intervention for Activating Patients at Risk for Osteoporosis (APROPOS): Rationale, design, and uptake of online study intervention material. *Contemp. Clin. Trials Commun.*, 4, 14–24, 2016 Dec 15.
88. Danila, M.I., Outman, R.C., Rahn, E.J., Mudano, A.S., Redden, D.T., Li, P., Allison, J.J., Anderson, F.A., Wyman, A., Greenspan, S.L., LaCroix, A.Z., Evaluation of a multimodal, direct-to-patient educational intervention targeting barriers to osteoporosis care: A randomized clinical trial. *J. Bone Miner. Res.*, 33, 5, 763–772, 2018 May.
89. Whitehead, L. and Seaton, P., The effectiveness of self-management mobile phone and tablet apps in long-term condition management: A systematic review. *J. Med. Internet Res.*, 18, 5, e97, 2016 May 16.
90. Slomian, J., Appelboom, G., Ethgen, O., Reginster, J.Y., Bruyère, O., Can new information and communication technologies help in the management of osteoporosis? *Women's Health*, 10, 3, 229–232, 2014 May.

5

Utilizing AI to Improve Orthopedic Care

Abstract

Over the past few years, artificial intelligence has had an impact on society. A subject called machine learning (ML), which defines a computer's capacity to recognize patterns in data without being explicitly programmed to do so, is fostering innovation across a wide range of disciplines. Throughout the past 10 years, scientists have worked to advance orthopedics to support surgeons and medical professionals in their work. With the use of algorithms controlled by pattern recognition and self-correction on vast amounts of data to restrict possibilities and lower the risk of making mistakes, artificial intelligence (AI) enables machines to do tasks. AI has already had an impact on orthopedic surgery in several areas, including image identification, risk prediction, patient-specific payment models, and clinical decision-making. Its application is only anticipated to increase. This chapter seeks to serve as a reference, offering the most recent research and achievements in orthopedics connected to these new technologies, outlining the key concepts of various applications, and addressing the most important problems the technology is currently confronting.

Keywords: Artificial intelligence, orthopedic, algorithm, machine learning, deep learning, natural language processing, Internet of Things, surgery prediction

5.1 Introduction

John McCarthy first used the term "artificial intelligence" (AI) to describe his notion that machines may be taught to execute human activities by automatically recognizing patterns with minimal involvement from input [1]. Due to the exponential growth of extraordinarily big datasets ("big data") and the falling cost of computing power, artificial intelligence has gonc from a theoretical concept to practical use on a massive scale [2]. Several aspects of modern life rely on AI because of its ability to analyze vast amounts of data quickly and accurately. This includes everything from self-driving cars as well as Netflix suggestions to product recommendations on Amazon and Facebook ads and even fraud detection.

Rishabha Malviya, Shivam Rajput and Makarand Vaidya. Artificial Intelligence for Bone Disorder: Diagnosis and Treatment, (105–132) © 2024 Scrivener Publishing LLC

Machine learning (ML) is a subfield of AI [3, 4]. The goal of AI is to give computers capabilities that were formerly thought to be unachievable for a machine. Modern developments in data storage, computer power, and the availability of large amounts of data have all contributed to the introduction of AI into the medical field. AI-based techniques are beginning to address several challenges unique to orthopedics, including image identification, clinical decision-making, preoperative risk assessment, and the processing of huge datasets.

While orthopedic surgeons have always taken great satisfaction in the quality of their clinical work, they can no longer afford to resist the inexorable advance of technology. Opportunities for the implementation of computer-assisted and AI applications into everyday practices are becoming increasingly apparent as clinicians try to further improve the quality and results of the services [5]. A growing amount of information is being gathered before, during, and then after surgical procedures [6, 7], making this a task well suited for automation. Although patient-generated health data (PGHD) is on the rise [8], the sheer volume of data collected from a single patient [9] provides more information than any human brain can interpret. Wearables, even those that are "off-the-shelf" [10], can record millions of data points [11], making them perfect for long-term studies of small cohorts or even single patients. "Big data" means the massive amounts of information that can be stored digitally [12]. Computers (and computer software) are ideally equipped for the task of categorizing, receiving, and objectively evaluating such massive amounts of patient- and care-related documents. Before orthopedic surgeons can confidently hand off data management to computers and overcome the inherent biases against such a technique, they need to have at least a foundational understanding of the potentially useful function of computers in life, healthcare, and surgery. Included in this knowledge should be the evolution of these technologies, the range of tasks they can reasonably be expected to complete, and the means by which their future contributions can be assured of their quality.

5.2 What is AI?

Artificial intelligence (AI) has been seen as a metaphor for a mental state called "cognitive emptying". This is a state in which humans can delegate tasks to a computer that require them to examine enormous amounts of data in time frames that are incomprehensible to the conscious human mind. Algorithms (sets of computational instructions) are used as guides by these computers as they carry out very specialized tasks. Some elements may be given weight in the decision-making analysis [13] by "categorizing," "identifying," or "connecting" them. The ability to quickly sort through massive amounts of data is the practical advantage of such job delegation [14, 15]. One or more computers, depending on the tasks they have been assigned, may find patterns or trends in the collected data that can be used to prove the existence of an attribute connection. To summarize, the computer is given a dataset that is designated as "training" [16, 17] (usually just a small portion of the whole body of knowledge that exists). Ordinarily, training datasets in clinical orthopedics will include information on thousands of patients [18]. The computer "learns" [19] to recognize traits with the use of detailed code (instructions). Many people then compare the computer's results with the established "gold standard" to assess its reliability (historically a human-defined standard). AI systems can be fed large amounts of data to "pattern recognition" at high speeds and with high repeatability, typically to predict some predetermined consequence or set of occurrences. Adjustments to the algorithm allow for a steadily more precise evaluation of the dataset, hence improving the system's accuracy. An established gold standard is used once more to evaluate the new result's accuracy, and metrics for reducing errors are fed back into the index calculation. Essentially, this process "teaches" the AI system to become more accurate and exact. This has been compared to the way humans learn, where knowledge is built up over time by repeated exposure to the material.

When the AI training cycle has reached the desired degree of accuracy, it can be repeated multiple times with minor adjustments to the underlying algorithms. The discriminating AI algorithm can be fine-tuned with each whole learning cycle (or "epoch"), resulting in an ever-more-precise system. Many traditional AI systems will iterate for 10–1,000 epochs [20], with the exact number based on the complexity and size of the training dataset and the intended final system "accuracy" criterion. Machine learning refers to the process of "teaching" a computer to perform a task with varying degrees of automation [21, 22]. It is possible to get a very precise and repeatable result for some jobs, but setting up such a system takes a lot of time and effort. Predictive modeling based on a complex multivariate analysis allows the AI system to be used autonomously on future (unseen) information, allowing for the identification of a projected outcome. After a "final algorithm" is decided upon, this will be achievable (to a suitable degree of accuracy for the purpose at hand).

Artificial intelligence methods have been used in arthroplasty component identification from plain radiographs [23]. The system is fed data on distinguishing imaging features between implant types and brands that a "human" interpretation may utilize. Size/length, proximal body-to-stem segment ratio, deformations, neck-shaft angle, collar status, etc., could all fall under this category. The system is shown a training set of images (implant radiography in which the manufacturer and the kind of implant are specified). The AI then analyzes the photos by comparing the radial features to the parameters of the implant. Image assessment [24] is then performed to determine how well the system performs in comparison with the actual answers. In cases when the system has been off, the training epoch can be restarted with the addition of new information (i.e., data entered by hand). This loop can be continued, with new data being added to the algorithm one by one until an "acceptable" level of precision is reached. After that, the AI system can be used in the "real world."

As computational power and the ability to refine algorithms continue to advance, AI systems may eventually be "trained" to assess their performance and refine their own sets of algorithmic codes. With more data in the training set, the index AI algorithm gets smarter, increasing accuracy with each iteration and boosting predicting ability to its highest level. This new technique, despite its apparent similarities to the ML processes that have been detailed in the past, requires a fundamentally different iterative programming basis. As a major step towards true "automation" [25], this framework requires the program to have the ability and autonomy to "self-write" its own coding instruction. When this is done, the amount of time needed to design a functional system may frequently be cut down by a significant amount, and the demand for human input can be removed from the process of improving the algorithm. This sort of artificial intelligence is referred to as "deep learning" (DL) [26] (note: DL is an abbreviation for "deep learning"). The system is based on a set of fixed outcomes and a set of connected, associative variables that are already known at the outset. Its potential for cluster association is progressively re-refined with the passing of each epoch, resulting in an increased level of accuracy. Because of the algorithmic functionality of modern DL neural networks, it is now possible to build artificial multilayered "evolutionary plexuses" that are conceptually identical to human neurons [27]. Most DL systems are supported by artificial neural networks (ANNs) [28], which are comprised of a series of layers between an initial "input" layer (which is where the data to be processed are inputted) and a final "output" layer. Input variables and data points can be connected to several evaluation criteria in subsequent layers. Next, each piece of discrete information in the second layer can be connected to a specific evaluation procedure in the third layer and so on. When there are more levels of brain processing between the input and output stages, it may conclude that there are "hidden layers" involved (the higher the demand will be placed upon the capacity of the computer's processor). Because of the way data points buried inside particular layers can be impacted in a selectively disproportionate manner by nearby data points, deep convolutional neural networks (CNNs) are complicated systems that are usually referred to as CNNs [29–31] (The effect of these points can, in a sense, be weighted more strongly in the sense that they can influence the final product.).

5.3 Introduction to Machine Learning: Algorithms and Applications

XGBoost (Extreme Gradient Boosting), CNNs, DCNNs, and EfficientNet, all of which use supervised learning [32] to hone a model with a large amount of data, are compared in this study.

Supervised machine learning primarily focuses on classification and regression. It is the goal of a classification problem to identify which of several possible categories the input best fits into [33]. Such a model could be used, for example, to spot bone fractures in X-rays (binary classification). As a result, the output is erratic and has a low dynamic range. On the other hand, regression is employed to predict a constant quantity [34]—for instance, one could develop a model to predict a patient's post-operative recovery period provided their age, height, and weight.

Once the problem is defined, training must then aim to minimize a loss function. The loss function estimates how close the model's result is to the target output by using the error as input. To minimize the error and loss function, the learning process makes changes to the gain values ("weights") on nodes [35] across layers. Hyper-parameters are crucial to education and growth [36]. A model's loss function [37] or the number of feature mappings in a convolution layer might be related to the network's topology and regularization. Pursuing the best possible performance, as measured by several different metrics, requires playing around with the values of many different controls. CNNs rely heavily on convolution [38] as a key operational step. For the sake of pattern recognition, CNNs use convolutional filters to extract relevant image features [39]. It is common practice to perform a series of computations on an input image, which is represented as a matrix (table) of values with different values stored for each pixel (cell), by first layering a set of filters, also matrices but with predetermined cell values, over the top of the input image. You can use the numbers you just crunched to do things like sharpen or blur an image or pull out specific characteristics from a video (Human eyes, for instance, are made up of more basic geometric shapes like circles, ellipses, and edges).

The following is a typical operation of this neural network: The data is collected in the first layer, then processed in the second, and finally presented in the third. CNNs consist of convolutional, pooling, and fully connected layers. The convolution of matrices ("convolutional filters") is carried out on the picture near the input by the convolutional layers. A convolutional operator is performed among the elements of the matrix representing the region and the value of the convolution filter whenever these filters are moved across the image and assigned to new regions. As it learns, the approach adjusts the convolution matrix's parameters. A "feature map" [40] is the output of a convolutional procedure. To perform calculations quickly, pooling layers will down-sample the input along its spatial dimensions. The mappings of the features become a single-column vector after passing through the pooling and convolution layers (in the flattened layer). Classes are determined by CNN's interconnected layers.

As the complexity of the studied pattern or study goal increases, so does the size of the training dataset necessary for CNN models. This massive sum is required to prevent overfit problems: Overfitting happens when a model is too dependent on a small subset of training datasets, making it incapable of uncovering underlying patterns in the data. Overfitting is more common in complicated models, which contain many parameters when trained on small datasets [41]. On the other hand, simpler models have lesser parameters and are unable to discern artificial patterns and correlations. Data augmentation approaches adjust the qualities of images (such as saturation, contrast, brightness, or geometric elements like scale or orientation) to make "altered" duplicates of the same image to increase the total number of training instances. As CNNs work with rectangular parts of the picture that have set dimensions, they are not great at compensating for rotation and scaling.

CNN performance may be evaluated using test sets or internal validation. However, this information must be consistent with the data used to train and build the model (i.e., it must come from the same hospital and time frame). Most algorithms fail when assessed in the real world; hence, internal validation is usually done first (i.e., with datasets from various universities [42]). If different hospitals use a different labeling system for their radiographs, a different radiation dosage, or different machines or if the same hospital changes these characteristics over time, an internally validated ML model (trained on a certain type of data) in the orthopedic sector may not be suitable for generalization. The XGBoost method [43] uses decision trees that boost gradients. The purpose of boosting techniques is to combine numerous mediocre learners (models) into a formidable one. Specifically, these inept students use decision trees, which are defined as "a supervised machine learning technique utilized for predictive modeling of a dependent variable (objective) on the input of a big number of independent variables." Their topiary shape originates at the base [44].

5.3.1 Machine Learning Performance Indexes

One class is typically designated as "positive" and the other as "negative" when tackling a basic two-class categorization issue. The positive class is typically the focus of research, even though this has little bearing on the advantages or values of the topic at hand. The training samples used to train the model are the first step in this differentiation. A fractured bone, for diagnostic purposes, would be a positive sample, while a healthy bone could be a negative sample. After the model has been trained with both positive as well as negative examples, its predictions can be put into four groups: true positives (TP), which are estimations of a positive result for a positive sample; true negatives (TN), which are estimations of a positive result for a negative sample; false positives (FP), which are projections of a positive and negative result; and false negatives (FN), which are projections of a positive and negative result.

The concepts form the basis for the calculations used to calculate key performance indicators. Because, likely, a single index is not enough to show how well a model works, it is important to talk about key performance measures right away so that readers can get a good idea of how well the models that will be talked about later work. Despite the fact that the formulas presented here are tailored towards a binary classifier, the principles at play there can just as easily be applied to problems with more than two categories [45].

Accuracy: Because, likely, a single index will not be sufficient to reflect the effectiveness of a model, it is essential to propose key performance measures right off the bat (Equation 5.1). This will allow readers to get a solid understanding of the effectiveness of the models that will be discussed in the following sections.

$$Accuracy = \frac{TP+TN}{TP+FP+FN+TN} \tag{5.1}$$

Sensitivity: As a measure of the model's accuracy in making predictions about positive samples, sensitivity quantifies the proportion of correct classifications made (Equation 5.2). As a metric of the model's success in making accurate predictions, it goes by the name "true positive rate" (all of the sick people who were labeled as sick by the model).

$$Sensitivity = \frac{TP}{TP + FN} \tag{5.2}$$

Specificity: The degree to which a model can correctly identify negative results concerning the total number of projections made for truly negative results is measured by a parameter known as "specificity." It is also referred to as the true negative rate since it demonstrates the number of patients for whom the model properly predicted that they did not have a particular condition (Equation 5.3).

$$Specificity = \frac{TN}{TN + FP} \tag{5.3}$$

Precision: When attempting to reduce the number of false positives, one may employ a metric called "precision," which calculates what percentage of positive predictions turned out to be correct (Equation 5.4).

$$Precision = \frac{TP}{TP + FP} \tag{5.4}$$

F1 Score: The F1 score is the average of how accurate and responsive the system is (Equation 5.5).

$$F1\ Score = 2 \times \frac{Precision \times Sensitivity}{Precision + Sensitivity} \tag{5.5}$$

ROC: ROC curve, which stands for receiver operator characteristic curve: Figure 5.1 depicts this curve, which can be derived by plotting the "true positive rate" (also known as "sensitivity") along the y-axis while simultaneously plotting the "false positive rate" (also known as "specificity") along the x-axis. These are tested at a variety of thresholds so that it can be determined how the differences in the two rates would impact the effectiveness of the model. The compromise between detection ability and target identification is depicted by this curve as well.

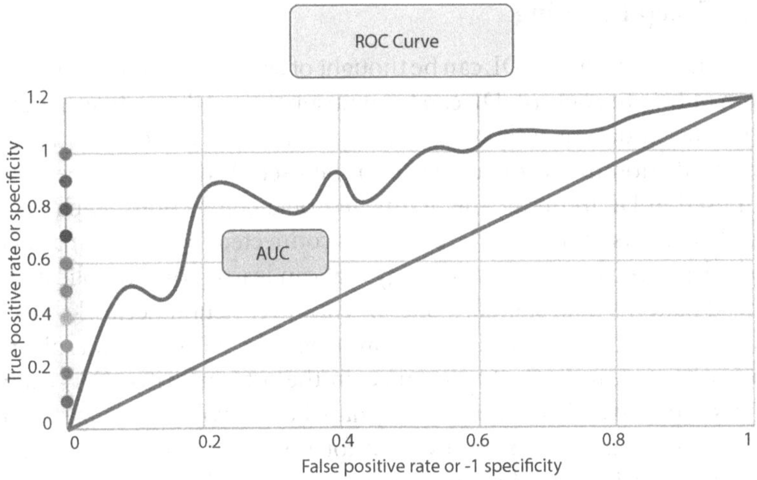

Figure 5.1 The ROC curve is in red, and AUC is the area between red and green.

AUC: The term "area under the curve" refers to the region that can be found among the ROC curve as well as the bisector (AUC). The area under the receiver operating characteristic curve is a useful tool for quickly assessing the ability of a classifier to differentiate between several different classes (ROC). The value of the area under the curve, also known as AUC, can be anything between 0 and 1, with 0 indicating that all the inputs were misclassified (all positives were interpreted as negatives and *vice versa*) and 1 indicating that all the inputs were correctly identified. Classifiers that have a curve that is closer to the top left corner perform better than those that have a curve that is closer to the 45° diagonal. This is because this strategy generates great sensitivity while maintaining a low false positive rate.

In the case of an unbalanced dataset, accuracy may be the first reported performance indicator; nevertheless, it should not be the sole statistic relied upon (which is often the case in the orthopedic field). When there are significantly more instances of one category than the other, it means that the dataset is imbalanced. The ability to appropriately categorize one of the two classes is where sensitivity and specificity come into play. When the goal is to maximize the fraction of correctly categorized positive instances, sensitivity is more essential, while when the goal is to reduce the fraction of wrongly identified negative examples, specificity is more critical. Remember that there is typically an inverse relationship between sensitivity and specificity, so if you try to improve one, you will end up hurting the other.

5.3.2 Deep Learning

To put it more succinctly, DL can be thought of as an improved and expanded version of ML. In contrast, DL can train unsupervised through unstructured and unlabeled data as well as discard inputs that are not highly important to the prediction that is of relevance to the user. ANNs are a type of algorithm used in DL to mimic the brain's neuronal connections. Each node in an ANN consists of multiple layers and is connected to others *via* a specific set of rules. Deep learning is a strategy that can learn more complicated and nuanced patterns than standard one- or two-layer neural networks [46, 47]. This is due to the approach's intricate layering, which is why it was given the moniker "deep learning"—for instance, in the osteoarthritis (OA) example that was supplied earlier, one node may have been involved for edge contrast, another node may have been involved for pixilation density, a third node may have been involved for breadth, and so on [48]. The only nodes that will serve to establish the radiographic diagnosis of osteoarthritis are those that are clinically connected to subchondral sclerosis, cysts, joint space constriction, or other as-yet-unknown characteristics of OA. Clinically, ML OA algorithms may be most beneficial as a screening, teaching, or referral tool for general care physicians, PAs, internists, and radiologists who do not concentrate on orthopedics. This is because these types of medical professionals do not have extensive training in orthopedics. DL has been successfully used for a variety of difficult problems, including handwriting recognition, facial identification, and autonomous driving vision systems.

5.4 Natural Language Processing

Natural language processing (NLP) seeks to generate structured data from unstructured free text; hence, NLP experts explore how computers interpret human language. Because of the potential therapeutic value it possesses, the ability to create order out of the huge amounts of patient data that are preserved in the written language of emails, electronic medical records (EMR), and the spoken word is currently the subject of research. Clinic schedulers might use this information, for instance, to aid in triage and practitioner assignment or to determine whether non-operative therapy has failed. This may be the case with the rise of digital scribes that may interface with an electronic medical record (EMR) and take notes in the office in real time, with the potential to aid in pre- and post-operative patient education, and in other similar scenarios. Connecting the exponentially growing body of medical knowledge and individual health data in real time during every patient visit is both a formidable challenge and an enormous potential [49].

Let us take the previous knee OA example one step further and apply it to a real-world scenario: a first-time patient visit. Preoperative planning and medical optimization for a total knee arthroplasty can be delivered instantaneously by auto-populating a note from past referrals to use as a template for the clinical visit, as will be described in more detail below. To get started, the plan requires access to the patient's EMR so that any imaging associated with radiographic knee OA can be analyzed. In addition, any primary care notes that reflect pain, functional deterioration, or previous attempts at non-operative therapy must also be reviewed. To understand what "NSAIDs" are and account for small typographical errors, many natural language processing algorithms possess direct access to medical dictionaries and related acronyms. The medical records of a patient who has been treated with nonsteroidal anti-inflammatory medications (NSAIDs) and physical therapy (PT) for radiographic OA symptoms would benefit from indicating this as "treatment," with the understanding that PT and rehab are similar words. Without a doubt, the doctor will record their findings from the history and exam, but the NLP might "suggest" sentences that conform to coding requirements. To simplify or elaborate on a statement, the machine may employ many algorithms.

Although the EMR example is extremely simplified, it is not impossible. Most importantly, it shows promise in easing the burden of paperwork on orthopedic surgeons and freeing up valuable clinical time. Imagine a future where doctors can walk into a room and start a conversation with a patient while using a NLP-assisted EMR that is organized and responsive to tasks and instructions like "bring up all CT images on person's shoulder," "graph the structure of all CRPs (C-reactive proteins) since explant of infected TKA (total knee arthroplasty)," and "book for left carpal tunnel release." This type of environment would be ideal. These types of virtual assistants are now being researched [50, 51] and developed at institutions like Vanderbilt and Rochester. With the aid of NLP, it could be possible to generate a clinic note and treatment result prediction that considers the whole biopsychosocial profile of the patient as well as the information in the medical record. This will help researchers make significant strides towards the ultimate objective of precision medicine.

5.5 The Internet of Things

The Internet of Things (IoT) is, in a nutshell, a system of "smart" devices that can collect and send data to connect people, places, and ecosystems [52].

Computing gadgets, intraoperative tools, mobile phones, clothing, sleeves, and braces are all examples of orthopedic-related equipment [53]. Mobile health, or mHealth for short [54], is the application of such cutting-edge technology in the medical field. Artificial intelligence and mobile health are creating exciting new opportunities in orthopedics. McClelland draws parallels between the human brain and the Internet of Things [55]. In the same way that the brain uses information from the body's peripheral organs to make sense of a broad range of sensory inputs [56], the Internet of Things collects data that is sent to an artificial intelligence system to make sense of clinical situations. Wearable sensors that connect to a smartphone and send data to a remote patient monitoring platform after a total knee replacement are examples of AI in the IoT that has already been tested [57]. Data collection and analysis can be done on a wide range of outcomes, including but not restricted to opioid use, range of motion, compliance with home exercises, and the Visual Analogue Score for Pain. The validity of using a smart orthotic for remote monitoring of the shoulder range of motion has also been established by the same authors [58]. This opens a whole new world of possibilities for pre- and post-operative patient involvement in orthopedic research and treatment. This technology has also made it possible to collect a huge amount (about 18,000 data points per person) of real-time information about rehabilitation starting on day 0 and going on for 12 weeks after TKA [59]. Having access to this information could help determine which patients, based on either internal or external circumstances, are most likely to experience difficulties during their recovery. It can also be used to gauge whether a patient has reached his or her full rehabilitative capacity and can stop engaging in physical therapy.

5.6 Prospective AI Advantages in Orthopedics

There may be many advantages to incorporating AI into standard orthopedic practice. Diagnosis, technique selection and use, and managerial logistics are all potential contributors. Artificial intelligence technologies have already been used to enhance the precision of or shorten the duration of crucial diagnostic processes before surgery. This may involve diagnosing and categorizing pathology, or it may need to identify the appropriate implant type or model for use in each situation. Such applications are well suited to the digital image-based AI systems' outstanding discriminative capacity [60]. In the case of revision surgery, when the patient's existing implant must be identified (frequently reflecting versions no longer in regular use) to arrange salvage alternatives and get essential equipment, this has apparent and immediate implications. AI systems have been demonstrated to accurately recognize *in situ* hip and knee replacement structures in preoperative imaging in several high-quality studies. These studies claimed near-perfect accuracy in identifying a small set of implant types, with some reports claiming an accuracy of 99.6% or higher. Every single clinical application of automatic implant recognition that I could find also mentioned significant time savings. Patient anteroposterior (AP) pelvic radiographs were taken, and the researchers observed an average implant identification time of just 0.96 s using a commercially available but antiquated iPhone 6. Clinicians' time is a major cost driver; thus, any reduction in that time spent on similar "manual identification" chores is being heralded as a huge potential cost saver [61]. In the following section, the authors will examine numerous additional "real-world" therapeutic applications of AI technologies.

Artificial intelligence applications can be used to supplement or take over routine decision-making tasks. Evidence-based risk mitigation can be achieved prospectively, thanks to the ability to connect and assess a wide range of important patient parameters within the context of a robust and trained AI system [62]. Artificial intelligence can be trained to analyze or incorporate data from postoperative patient-described outcome measures in order to pattern-recognize significant elements (singly or multifactorially) that attribute to optimum clinician- and/or patient-reported outcome measurements (PROM). This data, if used properly, can provide objective feedback on the quality of care provided, and it can also be fed back into the patient screening and decision-making processes to help with preoperative expectation management [63]. There is evidence that suggests both can improve treatment outcomes [64]. The capacity to segment patients depending on their perceived risk profile is intrinsically linked to the ability to estimate risk in advance which is essential for estimating the overall cost of a treatment session. In the case of total knee arthroplasty (TKA), such analyses have already been used in cohorts with close to 150,000 patients [65].

Artificial intelligence algorithms have already proven to be quite useful in the field of information management. At the heart of this matter are two interrelated ideas: enhanced data management accuracy and time savings (mostly by reducing the requirement for human time commitment). Both have the potential to significantly reduce healthcare expenditures [14]. Developed health systems are struggling under the weight of nearly oppressive data collection volumes caused by the widespread adoption of electronic medical records (EMRs) for patient care. How can a single physician make sense of the vast amounts of volumetric data and extract the information they need to make timely, informed decisions at the point of care? Initial endeavors into synthesizing and extracting EMR data have shown promising results in the literature [18]. During quite short training cycles, such applications have been shown to deliver quicker and more precise key information recovery than "manual" record searches. In a non-academic healthcare setting, researchers used AI to extract EMR data from a cohort of roughly 550 patients with excellent accuracy of over 95% [25].

5.7 Diagnostic Application of AI

Throughout the past decade, those interested in artificial intelligence's application to orthopedics have concentrated on diagnostics and, more specifically, image analysis [66]. Conventional neural network apparatuses (CNNs) are frequently used for computer vision, which is a significant function application in such an activity.

5.7.1 The Diagnosis of Hip-Related Conditions

In order to identify hip fractures in anterior pelvic X-rays, scientists trained a diffusion convolution neural network (DCNN). The initialization of the model involved 25,505 limb radiographs. This process is carried out so that the final model's recognition capacity can be improved upon, as training on the required task will now begin with weights that have already been calibrated to perform a similar task rather than with randomly selected weights. After training on 2,804 frontal pelvic radiographs, the model achieved 91% accuracy, 98% sensitivity, 84% specificity, and an F1 score of 0.916 when testing its ability to identify hip fractures. Although the model was taught to distinguish between healthy bones and fractures in the background of the skeletal architecture on radiographs, it may not be able to identify other abnormalities relevant to routine diagnostics [35]. The model's sole responsibility was to affirm the presence or absence of a fracture on the X-ray without adding any other context. Given the gender, age, and injury severity rating discrepancies between those with fractures and those without [8], bias is to be expected. Although the results fell just short of those achieved by radiologists and orthopedic surgeons, they were nonetheless encouraging.

Alternatively, a researcher-trained CNN fared better than the experts in the field. The neural network Park and his colleagues created can identify proximal femur bone cancers. The radiographs had all text removed and were split vertically down the middle. After inverting the right side of each image, the researchers had 538 femoral images that were all facing the same direction (the left), giving the computer a more stable foundation upon which to perform its analysis. From among the various trained models, investigators settled on three distinct iterations of the Efficient Net model (EfficientNet-b1, EfficientNet-b2, and EfficientNet-b3). Both general orthopedic surgeons and musculoskeletal tumor specialists, whose diagnostic accuracy was compared with that of the EfficientNet-b2 model, found that the latter was more accurate [45]. The model's sensitivity, accuracy, and F1 scores were superior when compared to those of both rival models and human doctors. Because of the standardized hip radiographs, image pre-processing was necessary, yet the leading model outperformed the others because of its lower number of weights, which is helpful when operating with sparse data because it reduces the model's capacity to infer irrelevant patterns and associations.

5.7.2 The Diagnosis of Knee-Related Conditions

In this study, researchers compared the accuracy and speed with which a convolutional neural network (CNN) was trained to detect tibial plateau fracture (TPF) in X-ray images to that of orthopedic specialists. A total of 916 JPEG images were used to teach the algorithm, while 84 images were used to verify its performance. The test required the program to identify possible fracture zones and label them with rectangles. Although the machine took 16 times longer on average per sample than human radiologists, there was no statistically significant difference in accuracy (0.91 vs. 0.92 0.03), which is encouraging (8.44 s. vs. 3.26 s.). The doctors were evaluated in a low-pressure setting, which is not typical of a real-world ER. That is why the researchers behind that study speculated that their AI system might thrive in a healthcare facility [67]. While the trained system achieved remarkable results overall, it was unable to correctly label the fracture line. The researchers have promised that the algorithm will be updated to include this functionality. The lack of normal knee radiographs in the dataset was another flaw in this study, as it prevented the calculation of sensitivity and specificity. Furthermore, it is possible that anteroposterior films alone are not sufficient for making a definitive diagnosis of a TPF.

Meniscal tears, which are a common consequence of TPF because of the menisci's location and role in the knee, have also become commonplace. There is bone and soft tissue involved, making it more difficult to diagnose. While magnetic resonance imaging (MRI) is a helpful diagnostic technique due to its high resolution for soft tissues and absence of patient pain, the final image can occasionally appear fuzzy due to micro-movements of the limbs generated by the patient, breathing, and/or heartbeat. In order to improve MRI scans, the researchers considered employing a machine learning strategy. Specifically, they applied a CNN-based algorithm to the scan reconstruction phase to eliminate "shadowy" regions and blurriness in the under-sampled images, leading to fully sampled, cleaner scans. These photos were used to make diagnoses, which were then verified during surgery. Although the study found encouraging outcomes (95.3% accuracy and 96.9% sensitivity), the sample size employed must be considered because the dataset is not large enough to reinforce the conclusions of the investigation. Tibial plateau fracture with meniscus injury may benefit from this CNN-based MRI optimizing approach [68].

Researchers have trained a convolutional neural network to distinguish between different types of total knee implants; this knowledge can be used to better prepare for partial knee replacement surgery and is thus another example of AI (in which only one or two parts of the implant needs to be changed). Although humans with sufficient experience can generalize quite well the characteristics of objects, situations, and conditions from across domains of knowledge and identify them with a high degree of accuracy, they are unable to process large amounts of data like machines can, making this a task well suited to artificial intelligence. The manufacturer, model, and factory defaults for the implant can all be found here. Surgeons generally send a radiograph of the individual to a medical representative at the implant manufacturer through email if they are unsure of the manufacturer and model of the implant. An 878-image dataset spanning six models and five manufacturers was utilized to train and verify a CNN for this challenge. The sample size was increased through data augmentation, and a contrast was performed [69]. To improve the photos' contrast, the researchers employed limited adaptive histogram equalization. Despite there being a small sample size of radiographs for each implant type, the model was able to complete the assignment with a success rate of 96.66%. In addition, no genuine external validation was undertaken because of the challenges in getting external clinical data, with samples from the data available coming from only two distinct institutions as well as from different textbooks.

5.7.3 Other Orthopedic-Related Diagnosis

Distal radial fracture (DRF) was studied, and a deep learning method was designed to detect DRF in AP and lateral radiographs. Image analysis software (ViDi Suite 2.0) was utilized for model construction. Two models (designated M1 and M2 from here on) were chosen after determining to have the highest AUC values after being subjected to extensive testing with a wide range of hyper-parameter combinations. Each resulting model was required to provide a value between -1 and 1, where 0 indicated no anomalous features were present in the image and 1 indicated the presence of a flaw. In addition to the score, a heatmap of the ROI (area of interest) was superimposed on the image to show where the computer thought the fracture was most likely to be located; this red zone was the subject of the highest score. The final region was compared to the ROI determined by two expert radiologists using two test datasets, one consisting of radiographs from the institution and the other from outside sources, as is customary practice. M1's DRF fracture diagnostic performance was nearly human, with an AUC of 93% when trained on anteroposterior perspectives, 94% when taught on lateral views, and 95% when training on a composite version of both views [70]. M2 achieved similar results, with AUCs of 95%, 94%, and 96% when training on anteroposterior, lateral, and combined views. When tested on radiographs from many institutions, the model's AUC, sensitivity as well as specificity for detecting DRF were marginally reduced. The possible explanation for the marginal improvement in radiologists' performance on the external dataset is that higher-quality images were more likely to be included in the external dataset.

Researchers created another model for determining the severity of distal radial fractures. The distal radiuses in anteroposterior wrist radiographs were initially chosen as the area of interest (ROI) for training a region-based CNN by a team of two professional radiologists. Thereafter, the enhanced and cropped images were sent to an Inception-V4 model for analysis. This model was trained on 2,040 images and then put through its paces on 300 images, split evenly between radiographs with and without DRFs. The AUC was 0.96, the accuracy was 93%, and the sensitivity was 90%; these numbers are on par with those obtained by the tested orthopedists and represent an improvement over the performance of the tested radiologists. Many of the misdiagnoses occurred because of a lack of apparent fracture traits on the corresponding anteroposterior radiographs, traits that were instead readily apparent on the lateral radiographs [71]. This is why the authors argue that providing the model with both types of radiographs will improve its sensitivity.

5.8 Prediction Application With AI

Prediction capabilities are another crucial component of AI and one of the most typical uses for an ML model—for example, in orthopedics, ML approaches have been used to predict hospitalization charges, discharge disposition, and length of stay [72]. Effectively addressing these concerns may lead to enhanced patient care, decreased physician burnout, and better budget management [73]. This method is especially useful for musculoskeletal surgeries, including the selection of appropriate patients for knee arthroplasty and the subsequent referral to the most qualified orthopedic surgeon.

5.8.1 Prediction Related to Surgery

In a study, an EfficientNet-b4 was utilized to identify candidates for TKA as well as medial unicompartmental knee arthroplasty (MUKA).

Before any data enhancement was done, radiographs of the anteroposterior, weight-bearing lateral, and patellar views were taken on each of the 2,767 patients. With only these three images, which are typically required by primary care physicians, the system was able to complete the task with an accuracy of 87.8%. Given that anterior–medial osteoarthritis is the most common cause of unicompartmental knee arthroplasty (UKA) [74], the fact that this result was reached without first determining whether the patient had this disease is even more impressive (So, without having to use a valgus stress perspective, that would have needed a staff that knew what they were doing.). It should be noted that the follow-up information of the people who were used to fill the training set showed that they had very few problems after surgery. Because of this, the decisions made were thought to be good enough to represent t. The study had this flaw because the information used to train the model heavily relied on the decisions made by the surgeons who did the surgeries in the training set, and their choices were then treated as the "perfect choice."

Because of financial incentives, knee surgeons who treat patients who could benefit from TKA "cherry pick" the healthier patients and "lemon drop" the ones with more difficult cases and other medical needs. This leaves a gap for those who need TKA but cannot get it. Researchers made an artificial neural network and used it to look at 15 key patient characteristics to predict the length of stay, costs, and how the patient would be treated. The mortality risk for all patients refined (APR), the severity of the illness, the number of other chronic conditions as well as diagnoses, whether the patient was admitted on the weekend or during the week, the type of hospital, the patient's income quartile, and whether they were transferred were among the 15 factors that were looked at. In its place, each type only had two outputs. To make the model more generalizable, it needed to know if the predicted value for the patient's length of stay, charges, and expenses was above or below the 50th percentile and if the patient would have been cared for at home after surgery. Investigators further used a patient-specific risk-based payment model to assess the potential for financial over-cost linked with APR risk of death. The All Patient Refined-Diagnosis Linked Group (APR-DLG) method [75] created by 3M contains the APR score, which simplifies the process to look at outcomes for a specific diagnosis across large cohorts.

The testing data came from the Orthopedic Minimal Dataset Episode of Care (OME), which had information from 11 hospitals, and the training data came from the National Inpatient Sample database, which has information from a wide range of hospitals. The second database did not include any inpatient charges, so only the first two results might be independently verified. The model improved from an accuracy of 75.3% and an AUC of 74.8% for estimating the length of stay after training to an accuracy of 80% and an AUC of 83.2% after being exposed to external validation. The results were the same for inpatient discharges but the lowest for discharge disposition, highlighting the need to incorporate additional patient-level data. The model's dependability, generalizability, and responsiveness all fell below 90% after being applied to the external OME dataset, even though accuracy and AUC improved. According to the risk-based patient-specific payment model, the cost of surgery is expected to increase by over 83% for patients with extremely high APR death risk and by roughly 22% for persons with moderate APR mortality risk. When all parties involved in a knee replacement procedure have a common knowledge of these considerations, it is much easier to get everyone on the same page before surgery [26]. The authors suggested a wide variety of additional research that could help the model produce more precise time and cost estimates [76].

5.8.2 Prediction Related to Post-Operative Complications

The increased complexity, higher costs, and poorer success rates of a later-revision TKA have a significant financial impact on the patient if issues arise after the initial TKA (as they do after many other types of arthroplasties). Therefore, the ability to predict which patients may need a revision is becoming increasingly important. Researchers explored the issue of anticipating post-operative problems and unpredictable lengths of the surgery. The dataset used to train the XGBoost algorithm included 864 patients, 54 of whom experienced problems and 99 of whom experienced unexpectedly long or short surgical times. To compensate for the disparity in sample sizes between the two classes, a loss weighting was implemented. To solve it, researchers turned it into a binary classification problem in which the investigator sought to determine whether a certain patient had any complications at all. Projections of complications had a sensitivity of 34.8 and a specificity of 95.8%, whereas predictions of irregular operation time had a sensitivity of 74.1% and a specificity of 96.3%. In contrast to the first problem, where only 6.3% of the cases were correctly classified, in the second problem, 11.5% of the instances were classified correctly. Also, a "feature significance" was determined by ranking the major features utilized by the model to categorize the inputs according to how well they predicted a target, providing some insight into the relative relevance of each input variable in the ML model. However, this does not imply any objective or causal connections [36].

Dislocation of the prosthetic hip joint after total hip arthroplasty (THA) is the most common immediate complication and a major reason for a subsequent surgical intervention. After a THA, complications like the one described are very possible. A CNN was developed and tested on a dataset of 97,934 anteroposterior pelvic radiographs obtained at least 1 day after surgery and at least 1 day before the potential dislocation to predict the risk of hip dislocation. For this evaluation, the researcher used a 10-fold cross-validation technique, in which the dataset was divided into 10 equal portions and used, in turn, as a test dataset and a training dataset at each stage of the process. Model efficacy was measured using sum totals. By utilizing YOLO-V3 (You Only Live Once) (a CNN), the model was able to achieve a mean average precision of 99.2% between the right and left pelvis, indicating that it successfully detected the presence of dislocation in nearly 99% of all instances. One possible explanation for the discrepancy in performance between the sexes is that the model used a different set of imaging features for male and female patients. This, in addition to the differing number of dislocations in the dataset, could explain the results. A saliency map was used as the basis for making decisions, and it was suggested that additional context and X-ray angles be used in the future [37].

5.9 Conclusion

Readers should have a better knowledge of AI and the possible advantages it might have for the area of orthopedics after reading this brief introduction to the subject. This chapter analyzed many studies on the application of AI in orthopedics, stressing the distinctive elements, benefits, and drawbacks of each study and, more broadly, the technology. The potential applications of this powerful technology are nearly endless, ranging from helping physicians to anticipating surgical results. As a result, to avoid unfavorable outcomes, future applications of AI in orthopedics must be carefully considered without losing sight of their downsides.

References

1. Liu, P., Chen, Y., Zhang, J., Fang, Y., Xue, M., Wang, H., Hu, J., Sun, B., Jiao, R., Yang, J., Huo, T., Artificial intelligence as the clinical assistant for detection of femoral neck fracture: Intelligent medicine brings the bright future.
2. Topol, E., *Deep medicine: How artificial intelligence can make healthcare human again*, Hachette UK, New York City, 2019 Mar 12.
3. Scarlat, A., Machine learning primer for clinicians.
4. Chollet, F., *Deep learning with Python*, First, Manning Publications Co, Shelter Island in New York, 2018.
5. Bini, S.A., Artificial intelligence, machine learning, deep learning, and cognitive computing: What do these terms mean and how will they impact health care? *J. Arthroplasty*, 33, 8, 2358–2361, 2018 Aug 1.
6. Cao, Z., Yang, W., Yang, M., Kong, X., Wang, Y., Guo, R., Chen, J., Chai, W., Application of preoperative digital-template planning in total hip arthroplasty via direct anterior approach. *Zhongguo Xiu Fu Chong Jian Wai Ke Za Zhi= Zhongguo Xiufu Chongjian Waike Zazhi= Chin. J. Reparative Reconstr. Surg.*, 33, 11, 1374–1378, 2019 Nov 1.
7. Karnuta, J.M., Churchill, J.L., Haeberle, H.S., Nwachukwu, B.U., Taylor, S.A., Ricchetti, E.T., Ramkumar, P.N., The value of artificial neural networks for predicting length of stay, discharge disposition, and inpatient costs after anatomic and reverse shoulder arthroplasty. *J. Shoulder Elbow Surg.*, 29, 11, 2385–2394, 2020 Nov 1.
8. Borjali, A., Chen, A.F., Muratoglu, O.K., Morid, M.A., Varadarajan, K.M., Detecting total hip replacement prosthesis design on plain radiographs using deep convolutional neural network. *J. Orthop. Res.*, 38, 7, 1465–1471, 2020 Jul.
9. Harris, A.H., Kuo, A.C., Weng, Y., Trickey, A.W., Bowe, T., Giori, N.J., Can machine learning methods produce accurate and easy-to-use prediction models of 30-day complications and mortality after knee or hip arthroplasty? *Clin. Orthop. Relat. Res.*, 477, 2, 452, 2019 Feb.
10. Van de Meulebroucke, C., Beckers, J., Corten, K., What can we expect following anterior total hip arthroplasty on a regular operating table? A validation study of an artificial intelligence algorithm to monitor adverse events in a high-volume, nonacademic setting. *J. Arthroplasty*, 34, 10, 2260–2266, 2019 Oct 1.
11. Fu, S., Wyles, C.C., Osmon, D.R., Carvour, M.L., Sagheb, E., Ramazanian, T., Kremers, W.K., Lewallen, D.G., Berry, D.J., Sohn, S., Kremers, H.M., Automated detection of periprosthetic joint infections and data elements using natural language processing. *J. Arthroplasty*, 36, 2, 688–692, 2021 Feb 1.
12. Leopold, S.S., Editor's Spotlight/Take 5: Can machine learning algorithms predict which patients will achieve minimally clinically important differences

from total joint arthroplasty? *Clin. Orthop. Relat. Res.*, 477, 6, 1262–1266, 2019 Jun 1.

13. Ramkumar, P.N., Karnuta, J.M., Navarro, S.M., Haeberle, H.S., Scuderi, G.R., Mont, M.A., Krebs, V.E., Patterson, B.M., Deep learning preoperatively predicts value metrics for primary total knee arthroplasty: Development and validation of an artificial neural network model. *J. Arthroplasty*, 34, 10, 2220–2227, 2019 Oct 1.
14. Ampadi Ramachandran, R., Chi, S.W., Srinivasa Pai, P., Foucher, K., Ozevin, D., Mathew, M.T., Artificial intelligence and machine learning as a viable solution for hip implant failure diagnosis—Review of literature and *in vitro* case study. *Med. Biol. Eng. Comput.*, 26, 1–7, 2023 Jan.
15. Lu, Y., Khazi, Z.M., Agarwalla, A., Forsythe, B., Taunton, M.J., Development of a machine learning algorithm to predict nonroutine discharge following unicompartmental knee arthroplasty. *J. Arthroplasty*, 36, 5, 1568–1576, 2021 May 1.
16. Helm, J.M., Swiergosz, A.M., Haeberle, H.S., Karnuta, J.M., Schaffer, J.L., Krebs, V.E., Spitzer, A.I., Ramkumar, P.N., Machine learning and artificial intelligence: Definitions, applications, and future directions. *Curr. Rev. Musculoskelet. Med.*, 13, 69–76, 2020 Feb.
17. Shah, R.F., Bini, S.A., Martinez, A.M., Pedoia, V., Vail, T.P., Incremental inputs improve the automated detection of implant loosening using machine-learning algorithms. *Bone Joint J.*, 102, 6 Supple A, 101–106, 2020 Jun.
18. Kunze, K.N., Polce, E.M., Sadauskas, A.J., Levine, B.R., Development of machine learning algorithms to predict patient dissatisfaction after primary total knee arthroplasty. *J. Arthroplasty*, 35, 11, 3117–3122, 2020 Nov 1.
19. Pua, Y.H., Kang, H., Thumboo, J., Clark, R.A., Chew, E.S., Poon, C.L., Chong, H.C., Yeo, S.J., Machine learning methods are comparable to logistic regression techniques in predicting severe walking limitation following total knee arthroplasty. *Knee Surg. Sports Traumatol. Arthrosc.*, 28, 3207–3216, 2020 Oct.
20. Schwartz, A.J., Clarke, H.D., Spangehl, M.J., Bingham, J.S., Etzioni, D.A., Neville, M.R., Can a convolutional neural network classify knee osteoarthritis on plain radiographs as accurately as fellowship-trained knee arthroplasty surgeons? *J. Arthroplasty*, 35, 9, 2423–2428, 2020 Sep 1.
21. Bloomfield, R.A., Williams, H.A., Broberg, J.S., Lanting, B.A., McIsaac, K.A., Teeter, M.G., Machine learning groups patients by early functional improvement likelihood based on wearable sensor instrumented preoperative timed-up-and-go tests. *J. Arthroplasty*, 34, 10, 2267–2271, 2019 Oct 1.
22. Shah, A.A., Devana, S.K., Lee, C., Kianian, R., van der Schaar, M., SooHoo, N.F., Development of a novel, potentially universal machine learning algorithm for prediction of complications after total hip arthroplasty. *J. Arthroplasty*, 36, 5, 1655–1662, 2021 May 1.
23. El-Galaly, A., Grazal, C., Kappel, A., Nielsen, P.T., Jensen, S.L., Forsberg, J.A., Can machine-learning algorithms predict early revision TKA in the Danish knee arthroplasty registry? *Clin. Orthop. Relat. Res.*, 478, 9, 2088, 2020 Sep.

24. Navarro, S.M., Wang, E.Y., Haeberle, H.S., Mont, M.A., Krebs, V.E., Patterson, B.M., Ramkumar, P.N., Machine learning and primary total knee arthroplasty: Patient forecasting for a patient-specific payment model. *J. Arthroplasty*, 33, 12, 3617–3623, 2018 Dec 1.
25. Murphy, M., Killen, C., Burnham, R., Sarvari, F., Wu, K., Brown, N., Artificial intelligence accurately identifies total hip arthroplasty implants: A tool for revision surgery. *HIP Int.*, 32, 6, 766–770, 2022 Nov.
26. Karhade, A.V., Thio, Q.C., Ogink, P.T., Shah, A.A., Bono, C.M., Oh, K.S., Saylor, P.J., Schoenfeld, A.J., Shin, J.H., Harris, M.B., Schwab, J.H., Development of machine learning algorithms for prediction of 30-day mortality after surgery for spinal metastasis. *Neurosurgery*, 85, 1, E83–91, 2019 Jul 1.
27. Karnuta, J.M., Haeberle, H.S., Luu, B.C., Roth, A.L., Molloy, R.M., Nystrom, L.M., Piuzzi, N.S., Schaffer, J.L., Chen, A.F., Iorio, R., Krebs, V.E., Artificial intelligence to identify arthroplasty implants from radiographs of the hip. *J. Arthroplasty*, 36, 7, S290–4, 2021 Jul 1.
28. Ramachandran, R.A., Chi, S.W., Pai, P.S., Foucher, K., Ozevin, D., Mathew, M.T., Artificial intelligence and machine learning as a viable solution for hip implant failure diagnosis-review of literature and *in vitro* case study. *Med. Biol. Eng. Comput.*, 61, 1239–1255, 2023.
29. Jayakumar, P., Moore, M.G., Furlough, K.A., Uhler, L.M., Andrawis, J.P., Koenig, K.M., Aksan, N., Rathouz, P.J., Bozic, K.J., Comparison of an artificial intelligence–enabled patient decision aid vs educational material on decision quality, shared decision-making, patient experience, and functional outcomes in adults with knee osteoarthritis: A randomized clinical trial. *JAMA Netw. Open*, 4, 2, e2037107–, 2021 Feb 1.
30. Jacofsky, D.J. and Allen, M., Robotics in arthroplasty: A comprehensive review. *J. Arthroplasty*, 31, 10, 2353–2363, 2016 Oct 1.
31. Zhao, J.X., Su, X.Y., Zhao, Z., Xiao, R.X., Zhang, L.C., Tang, P.F., Radiographic assessment of the cup orientation after total hip arthroplasty: A literature review. *Ann. Transl. Med.*, 8, 4, 1–20, 2020 Feb.
32. Marotta, N., De Sire, A., Marinaro, C., Moggio, L., Inzitari, M.T., Russo, I., Tasselli, A., Paolucci, T., Valentino, P., Ammendolia, A., Efficacy of Transcranial Direct Current Stimulation (tDCS) on balance and gait in multiple sclerosis patients: A machine learning approach. *J. Clin. Med.*, 11, 12, 3505, 2022 Jun 17.
33. Hallinan, J.T., Zhu, L., Yang, K., Makmur, A., Algazwi, D.A., Thian, Y.L., Lau, S., Choo, Y.S., Eide, S.E., Yap, Q.V., Chan, Y.H., Deep learning model for automated detection and classification of central canal, lateral recess, and neural foraminal stenosis at lumbar spine MRI. *Radiology*, 300, 1, 130–138, 2021 Jul.
34. Pinto, M., Marotta, N., Caracò, C., Simeone, E., Ammendolia, A., de Sire, A., Quality of life predictors in patients with melanoma: A machine learning approach. *Front. Oncol.*, 12, 843611, 2022 Mar 25.

35. Cheng, C.T., Ho, T.Y., Lee, T.Y., Chang, C.C., Chou, C.C., Chen, C.C., Chung, I., Liao, C.H., Application of a deep learning algorithm for detection and visualization of hip fractures on plain pelvic radiographs. *Eur. Radiol.*, 29, 10, 5469–5477, 2019 Oct.
36. Hinterwimmer, F., Lazic, I., Langer, S., Suren, C., Charitou, F., Hirschmann, M.T., Matziolis, G., Seidl, F., Pohlig, F., Rueckert, D., Burgkart, R., Prediction of complications and surgery duration in primary TKA with high accuracy using machine learning with arthroplasty-specific data. *Knee Surg. Sports Traumatol. Arthrosc.*, 8, 1, 2022 Apr.
37. Rouzrokh, P., Ramazanian, T., Wyles, C.C., Philbrick, K.A., Cai, J.C., Taunton, M.J., Kremers, H.M., Lewallen, D.G., Erickson, B.J., Deep learning artificial intelligence model for assessment of hip dislocation risk following primary total hip arthroplasty from postoperative radiographs. *J. Arthroplasty*, 36, 6, 2197–2203, 2021 Jun 1.
38. Bezdan, T. and Džakula, N.B., Convolutional neural network layers and architectures, in: *Data Science and Digital Broadcasting Systems, International Scientific Conference on Information Technology and Data Related Research*, vol. 10, 2019 Jan.
39. O'Shea, K. and Nash, R., An introduction to convolutional neural networks. *Neural and Evolutionary Computing, arXiv preprint arXiv:1511.08458*, 2, 1–11, 2015 Nov 26.
40. LeCun, Y. and Bengio, Y., Convolutional networks for images, speech, and time series, in: *The Handbook of Brain Theory and Neural Networks*, vol. 3361(10), 1995 Apr.
41. Müller, A.C. and Guido, S., *Introduction to machine learning with Python: A guide for data scientists*, O'Reilly Media, Inc., Mumbai, India, 2016 Sep 26.
42. Carmo, L.O.E., van den Merkhof, A., Olczak, J., Gordon, M., Jutte, P.C., Jaarsma, R.L., IJpma, F.F., Doornberg, J.N., Prijs, J., Machine Learning Consortium, An increasing number of convolutional neural networks for fracture recognition and classification in orthopaedics: Are these externally validated and ready for clinical application? *Bone Jt. Open*, 2, 10, 879, 2021 Nov.
43. Bentéjac, C., Csörgő, A., Martínez-Muñoz, G., A comparative analysis of gradient boosting algorithms. *Artif. Intell. Rev.*, 54, 1937–1967, 2021 Mar.
44. Jain, I., Malik, S., Agrawal, S., Automatic railway barrier system, railway tracking and collision avoidance using IOT. *Int. J. Comput. Appl.*, 975, 8887, 2017 Oct.
45. Park, C.W., Oh, S.J., Kim, K.S., Jang, M.C., Kim, I.S., Lee, Y.K., Chung, M.J., Cho, B.H., Seo, S.W., Artificial intelligence-based classification of bone tumors in the proximal femur on plain radiographs: System development and validation. *PLoS One*, 17, 2, e0264140, 2022 Feb 24.
46. Hashimoto, D.A., Rosman, G., Rus, D., Meireles, O.R., Artificial intelligence in surgery: Promises and perils. *Ann. Surg.*, 268, 1, 70–76, 2018 Jul 1.

47. Shi, L., Wang, X.C., Wang, Y.S., Artificial neural network models for predicting 1-year mortality in elderly patients with intertrochanteric fractures in China. *Braz. J. Med. Biol. Res.*, 46, 993–999, 2013 Nov 18.
48. LeCun, Y., Bengio, Y., Hinton, G., Deep learning. *Nature*, 521, 7553, 436–444, 2015.
49. Kohane, I.S., Ten things we have to do to achieve precision medicine. *Science.*, 349, 6243, 37–8, 2015.
50. Myers, T.G., Ramkumar, P.N., Ricciardi, B.F., Urish, K.L., Kipper, J., Ketonis, C., Artificial intelligence and orthopaedics: An introduction for clinicians. *J. Bone Joint Surg. Am. Vol.*, 102, 9, 830, 2020 May 5.
51. Qi, Y., Vrooman, J.C., Almansa, J., Ots, P., Brouwer, S., Reijneveld, S.A., A capital-based approach to better understand health inequalities: Theoretical and empirical explorations. *SSM-Popul. Health*, 21, 101309, 2023 Mar 1.
52. Morgan, J., A simple explanation of'the Internet of Things'. Retrieved November. 2015, 20, 2014 May 13, https://www.forbes.com/sites/jacobmorgan/2014/05/13/simple-explanation-internet-things-that-anyone-can-understand/?sh=75958b361d09" and not published in any journal. Accessed date, March 2023.
53. Ramkumar, P.N., Haeberle, H.S., Navarro, S.M., Sultan, A.A., Mont, M.A., Ricchetti, E.T., Schickendantz, M.S., Iannotti, J.P., Mobile technology and telemedicine for shoulder range of motion: Validation of a motion-based machine-learning software development kit. *J. Shoulder Elbow Surg.*, 27, 7, 1198–1204, 2018 Jul 1.
54. Ramkumar, P.N., Muschler, G.F., Spindler, K.P., Harris, J.D., McCulloch, P.C., Mont, M.A., Open mHealth architecture: A primer for tomorrow's orthopedic surgeon and introduction to its use in lower extremity arthroplasty. *J. Arthroplasty*, 32, 4, 1058–1062, 2017.
55. McClelland, C., The difference between artificial intelligence, machine learning, and deep learning, Medium.
56. Ravì, D., Wong, C., Deligianni, F., Berthelot, M., Andreu-Perez, J., Lo, B., Yang, G.Z., Deep learning for health informatics. *IEEE J. Biomed. Health Inf.*, 21, 1, 4–21, 2016 Dec 29.
57. Ramkumar, P.N., Haeberle, H.S., Ramanathan, D., Cantrell, W.A., Navarro, S.M., Mont, M.A., Bloomfield, M., Patterson, B.M., Remote patient monitoring using mobile health for total knee arthroplasty: Validation of a wearable and machine learning–based surveillance platform. *J. Arthroplasty*, 34, 10, 2253–2259, 2019 Oct 1.
58. Sabetian, P.W., Ouyang, V.W., Fox, J.D., Jimenez, A.E., Ankem, H.K., Saks, B.R., Maldonado, D.R., Lall, A.C., Domb, B.G., Telemedicine: An effective tool for patient–physician communication. *Orthopedics*, 1, 1–6, 2023 Jan.
59. Ramkumar, P.N., Haeberle, H.S., Bloomfield, M.R., Schaffer, J.L., Kamath, A.F., Patterson, B.M., Krebs, V.E., Artificial intelligence and arthroplasty at a single institution: Real-world applications of machine learning to big

data, value-based care, mobile health, and remote patient monitoring. *J. Arthroplasty*, 34, 10, 2204–2209, 2019 Oct 1.
60. Karnuta, J.M., Luu, B.C., Roth, A.L., Haeberle, H.S., Chen, A.F., Iorio, R., Schaffer, J.L., Mont, M.A., Patterson, B.M., Krebs, V.E., Ramkumar, P.N., Artificial intelligence to identify arthroplasty implants from radiographs of the knee. *J. Arthroplasty*, 36, 3, 935–940, 2021 Mar 1.
61. Chen, T.L., Buddhiraju, A., Seo, H.H., Subih, M.A., Tuchinda, P., Kwon, Y.M., Internal and external validation of the generalizability of machine learning algorithms in predicting non-home discharge disposition following primary total knee joint arthroplasty. *J. Arthroplasty*, 2023 Feb 9.
62. Magan, A.A., Kayani, B., Chang, J.S., Roussot, M., Moriarty, P., Haddad, F.S., Artificial intelligence and surgical innovation: Lower limb arthroplasty. *Br. J. Hosp. Med.*, 81, 10, 1–7, 2020 Oct 2.
63. Kunze, K.N., Jang, S.J., Li, T., Mayman, D.A., Vigdorchik, J.M., Jerabek, S.A., Fragomen, A.T., Sculco, P.K., Radiographic findings involved in knee osteoarthritis progression are associated with pain symptom frequency and baseline disease severity: A population-level analysis using deep learning. *Knee Surg. Sports Traumatol. Arthrosc.*, 31, 2, 586–595, 2023 Feb.
64. Tibbo, M.E., Wyles, C.C., Fu, S., Sohn, S., Lewallen, D.G., Berry, D.J., Kremers, H.M., Use of natural language processing tools to identify and classify periprosthetic femur fractures. *J. Arthroplasty*, 34, 10, 2216–9, 2019 Oct 1.
65. Farooq, H., Deckard, E.R., Ziemba-Davis, M., Madsen, A., Meneghini, R.M., Predictors of patient satisfaction following primary total knee arthroplasty: Results from a traditional statistical model and a machine learning algorithm. *J. Arthroplasty*, 35, 11, 3123–3130, 2020 Nov 1.
66. Corban, J., Lorange, J.P., Laverdiere, C., Khoury, J., Rachevsky, G., Burman, M., Martineau, P.A., Artificial intelligence in the management of anterior cruciate ligament injuries. *Orthop. J. Sports Med.*, 9, 7, 23259671211014206, 2021 Jul 2.
67. Liu, P.R., Zhang, J.Y., Xue, M.D., Duan, Y.Y., Hu, J.L., Liu, S.X., Xie, Y., Wang, H.L., Wang, J.W., Huo, T.T., Ye, Z.W., Artificial intelligence to diagnose tibial plateau fractures: An intelligent assistant for orthopedic physicians. *Curr. Med. Sci.*, 41, 6, 1158–1164, 2021 Dec.
68. Xie, X., Li, Z., Bai, L., Zhou, R., Li, C., Jiang, X., Zuo, J., Qi, Y., Deep learning-based MRI in diagnosis of fracture of tibial plateau combined with meniscus injury. *Sci. Program.*, 2021, 1–8, 2021 Dec 20.
69. Ghose, S., Datta, S., Batta, V., Malathy, C., Gayathri, M., Artificial intelligence based identification of total knee arthroplasty implants, in: *2020 3rd International Conference on Intelligent Sustainable Systems (ICISS)*, IEEE, pp. 302–307, 2020 Dec 3.
70. Blüthgen, C., Becker, A.S., de Martini, I.V., Meier, A., Martini, K., Frauenfelder, T., Detection and localization of distal radius fractures: Deep learning system versus radiologists. *Eur. J. Radiol.*, 126, 108925, 2020 May 1.

71. Gan, K., Xu, D., Lin, Y., Shen, Y., Zhang, T., Hu, K., Zhou, K., Bi, M., Pan, L., Wu, W., Liu, Y., Artificial intelligence detection of distal radius fractures: A comparison between the convolutional neural network and professional assessments. *Acta Orthop.*, 90, 4, 394–400, 2019 Jul 4.
72. Lee, L.S., Chan, P.K., Wen, C., Fung, W.C., Cheung, A., Chan, V.W., Cheung, M.H., Fu, H., Yan, C.H., Chiu, K.Y., Artificial intelligence in diagnosis of knee osteoarthritis and prediction of arthroplasty outcomes: A review. *Arthroplasty*, 4, 1, 16, 2022 Mar 5.
73. Li, W., Xu, S.M., Zhang, D.B., Bi, H.Y., Gu, G.S., Research advances in the application of AI for preoperative measurements in total knee arthroplasty. *Life*, 13, 2, 451, 2023 Feb.
74. Houserman, D.J., Berend, K.R., Lombardi Jr., A.V., Fischetti, C.E., Duhaime, E.P., Jain, A., Crawford, D.A., The viability of an artificial intelligence/machine learning prediction model to determine candidates for knee arthroplasty. *J. Arthroplasty*, 2022 Apr 8.
75. Baram, D., Daroowalla, F., Garcia, R., Zhang, G., Chen, J.J., Healy, E., Riaz, S.A., Richman, P., Use of the All Patient Refined-Diagnosis Related Group (APR-DRG) risk of mortality score as a severity adjustor in the medical ICU. Clinical medicine. *Circ. Respir. Pulm. Med.*, 2, CCRPM–S544, 2008 Jan.
76. Neubauer, M., Moser, L., Neugebauer, J., Raudner, M., Wondrasch, B., Führer, M., Emprechtinger, R., Dammerer, D., Ljuhar, R., Salzlechner, C., Nehrer, S., Artificial-intelligence-aided radiographic diagnostic of knee osteoarthritis leads to a higher association of clinical findings with diagnostic ratings. *J. Clin. Med.*, 12, 3, 744, 2023 Jan 17.

6
Significance of Artificial Intelligence in Spinal Disorder Treatment

Abstract
Artificial intelligence (AI) and machine learning (ML) techniques are revolutionizing many fields of industry and science, including computer vision, natural language processing, autonomous driving, and speech recognition. In many fields where automation is already having a major impact, the availability of automated solutions has the potential to increase the accuracy and reliability with which crucial operations are completed. In the first part of this chapter, readers get a high-level summary of the numerous methods that are currently in development, with an emphasis on those that are used in spine research. Examples of AI and ML applications to spine-related issues include localizing vertebrae and discs in radiological images, computer-aided diagnosis, image segmentation, prediction of clinical outcomes as well as complications, decision support systems, biomechanics, content-based image retrieval, and motion analysis.

Keywords: Spinal disorder, artificial neural networks, deep learning, outcome prediction, segmentation, biomechanics

6.1 Introduction

The last 10 years have seen a rapid rise in the popularity of machine learning and artificial intelligence. Millions of smartphones have virtual assistants that can understand natural language and carry out basic activities such as accessing a calendar, navigating a home automation system, or making an online purchase. Self-driving vehicles can recognize their surroundings using a combination of computer vision and other sensors and then use automated control systems to make judgments and drive themselves.

Machine learning (ML) is sometimes used interchangeably with "artificial intelligence" (AI), although ML is essentially merely a subsection of AI that examines ways to allow a machine to "learn" or improve its performance in specific tasks depending on its exposure to similar examples

Rishabha Malviya, Shivam Rajput and Makarand Vaidya. Artificial Intelligence for Bone Disorder: Diagnosis and Treatment, (133–168) © 2024 Scrivener Publishing LLC

or data [1, 2]. ML may be the most potential AI discipline for medical research, notwithstanding the significant contributions of abstract thinking, heuristics, and evolutionary algorithms to the advancement of science and technology (Figure 6.1).

Machine learning is data-driven. Applications like picture categorization, which employ input data to construct an output depending on a portion of the inputs, are ideal use cases for ML. Research into image processing has been given a major boost by ML. Because of technological progress, a deep neural network won the ImageNet Large Scale Visual Recognition Competition [3] for the first time in 2015. A computer may now be able to outperform humans in tasks such as picture labeling, object detection (including face recognition and detection), and landmark localization. Experts in the field of radiology concur that ML is a game-changing innovation that has the potential to revolutionize the way imaging data is analyzed and applied in diagnostic and therapeutic processes [4]. Although ML and AI are having an increasing impact in fields such as movement analysis and mechanical characterization of tissues, their influence on other fields of basic medical research has been more muted. Figure 6.2 depicts various sub-fields of AI.

As evidenced by a growing body of literature, AI and ML are increasingly being applied to the study of spine problems, most frequently not only in radiological imaging but also in other domains such as treatment

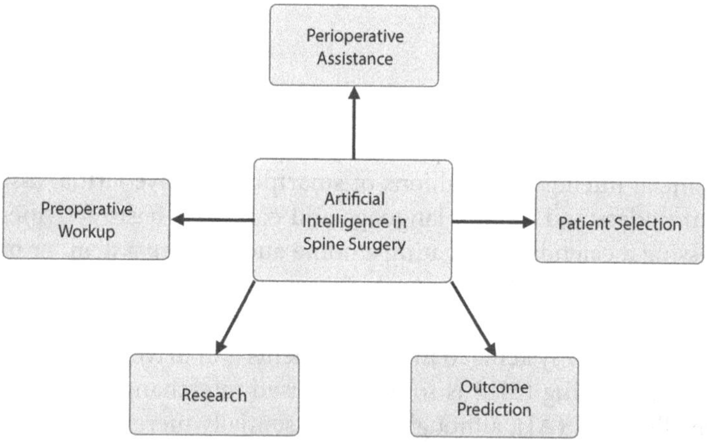

Figure 6.1 AI will cause a shift in the spine care industry by enhancing the standard of treatment and decreasing wait times for patients. AI helps in this regard by improving (1) preoperative patient workup, patient selection, and result prediction; (2) the quality and reproducibility of spine research; (3) perioperative surgical support and data tracking optimization; and (4) intraoperative surgical performance.

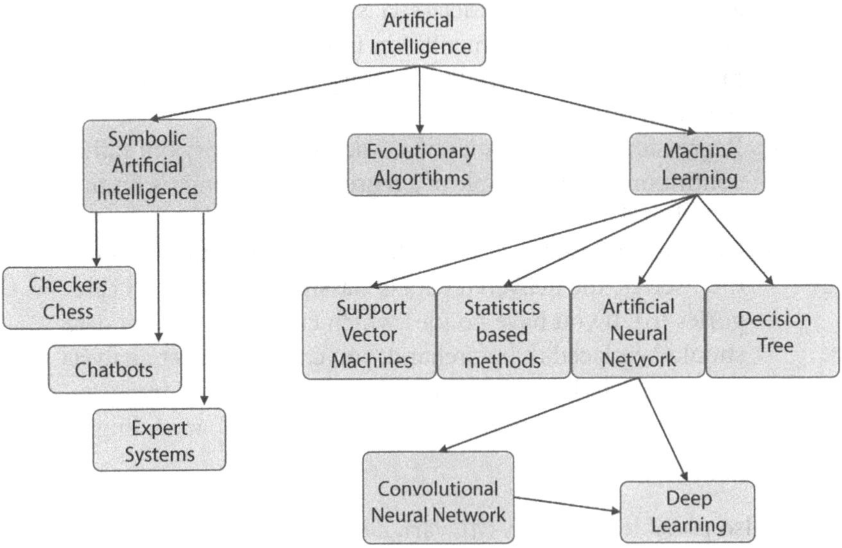

Figure 6.2 The major subfields of AI, like machine learning techniques, and how they are influencing spinal research.

success prediction. Intervertebral disc degradation on magnetic resonance imaging (MRI) scans may now be reliably graded using machine learning techniques. More benefits are anticipated as a result of technological progress.

6.2 Machine Learning

Arthur Samuel first used the term "machine learning" (ML) in 1959 to refer to the research into providing computers with the capability to learn without being explicitly programmed [14].

To forecast the value of the intended output given the input, ML relies on the automatic acquisition of features by either the model developer or the model itself. Some of ML's many applications include the following:

- Classification: The input is categorized into two or more groups. Histopathological image-based automated cancer diagnosis uses binary classification to determine if an image has pathological traits like texture and color. Assigning an MRI scan category between 1 (healthy disc) and 5 (severe disc degeneration) using the Pfirrmann grading system automatically is a multiclass classification task [5]. In the context of images, segmentation is a subset of classification problems that involves the labeling of pixels according to region or anatomical structure.

- Regression: The outcomes of a task are not binary but rather continuous. One example of a regression challenge is finding a landmark on a radiograph.
- Clustering: Based on the attributes learned from the inputs themselves, the delivered data is classified into distinct categories [6]. If you have no idea which categories a set of data should be placed in beforehand, you can use cluster analysis to organize it. Patients with osteoporotic vertebral fractures, for instance, have been clustered into groups according to their pain levels [7].

It is also possible to classify ML variants according to the kinds of work they are expected to do as follows:

- Supervised learning: When a computer is given a series of inputs for which the expected outcome (ground truth) is known, the computer can acquire the ability to forecast the output. In supervised learning, the objective is often to minimize a loss function that quantifies how far off the machine's predictions are from the actual data. These days, this kind of schooling is the norm in the healthcare industry. Estimating a function that maps an input (such as an image or set of patients' clinical data) to an output value is the foundation of supervised learning [8]. To clarify, the input and the expected output are both part of the training data. After the mapping function has been established, it can be used with unanticipated inputs to determine their corresponding outputs. The algorithm ought to be capable to adapt or give accurate results when displayed with inputs that are comparable to but different from those used during training if the training data is sufficiently extensive and the appropriate learning technique is employed. Underfitting depicts the opposite issue, where the learning model is too simplistic to capture the features of the input data while overfitting characterizes the outcomes that perfectly approximate the input data but are unable to offer trustworthy predictions in a few cases [9].

- Unsupervised learning: The machine is taught by being fed data for which it has no context. Extracting new information from existing data is the goal of this type of learning assignment, which is accomplished by spotting patterns and characteristics in the inputs. An example of unsupervised learning is cluster analysis.
- Reinforcement learning: In this scenario, ground truth data is not provided before the activity begins; feedback regarding the accuracy of the performance is instead provided after the activity has been completed and might be seen as either a reward or a punishment. The most common applications of reinforcement learning are in dynamic or interactive settings, such as video games. The field of clinical decision-making is another that is seeing rapid growth. Using models of reinforcement learning can considerably improve the understanding of how organisms of all kinds (including humans) learn the basic patterns of behavior necessary to complete tasks and make sense of occurrences.

There must be large datasets provided both for training the algorithm as well as verifying its accuracy before ML can be properly applied.

6.3 Methods Derived From Statistics

Simple functions that map inputs like numbers or vectors of values to outputs can be created with linear regression. Linear regression can be used to analyze any dataset where the variables are discrete numbers (a.k.a. features). Features are what set one dataset apart from another. Simple and human-readable information, such as a patient's sex and age, can be retrieved from images using specific algorithms like scale-invariant feature transform (SIFT) [10] and oriented FAST and rotated BRIEF (ORB) [11] or texture and form analyses. Even without any feature extraction, a radiograph can be viewed as an array of integer values, where each member represents the color value of a single pixel (gray level). Because of this, linear regression may be performed with ease, even when dealing with complex and large inputs.

The least squares method fits the linear regression function, making it the learning algorithm. By comparing the predicted value to the actual value, linear regression attempts to reduce the mean squared error (MSE) of the prediction or input. In ML literature, the L2 loss of MSE is more prevalent than the L1 loss of mean absolute error (MAE), which may be better for regression problems. Linear regression underfits due to its simplicity and inability to capture nonlinear behavior, making it unsuitable for difficult ML regression applications.

Logistic regression is linear regression for classification issues. The logistic sigmoid function, a nonlinear curve, is used to fit one or more continuous integers to a binary output (0 or 1). If the output probability is higher than 0.5, the anticipated value is 1; else, it is 0. Logistic regression can also predict multiclass outcomes. Logistic regression loss functions like cross-entropy are better than MSE. Most ML classification problems outperform logistic regression, like linear regression.

The Bayes classifier [12] is another statistical inference approach used in ML that is founded on Bayes' theorem of conditional probability. The naive Bayes classifier, which assumes feature independence, is simple to develop, can be trained quickly even on massive training datasets, and may be beneficial in settings where this assumption is plausible. Vertebral fracture classification and computer-assisted diagnosis are two applications of Bayes classifiers found in spine research [13].

6.3.1 Support Vector Machines

A classification issue can be viewed as the task of finding a partition of a multidimensional space in such a way that the training data points are separated into their appropriate classes, where each training data input is assumed to be a multidimensional vector. To split the points effectively and optimally into their respective classes, a support vector machine (SVM) constructs the hyperplane (or hyperplanes) to partition the space [14] (Figure 6.3).

Multiclass linear classification problems, such as image segmentation, can be accomplished with ease using support vector machines. SVMs have been around since at least 1963 [15], yet they are nevertheless commonly employed today and may even outperform the most cutting-edge algorithms in some cases, especially if the dataset available for training is limited. Disc degeneration grading [16] and the identification of scoliosis curve types [17] are only two examples of the many ways SVMs have been used in the study of the spine. The SVM can be used for unsupervised learning and nonlinear classification/regression issues (e.g., for clustering).

6.3.2 Classification and Regression Decision Trees

Since Arthur Samuel's original checker systems, artificial intelligence has frequently made use of tree-like structures. The first applications of the

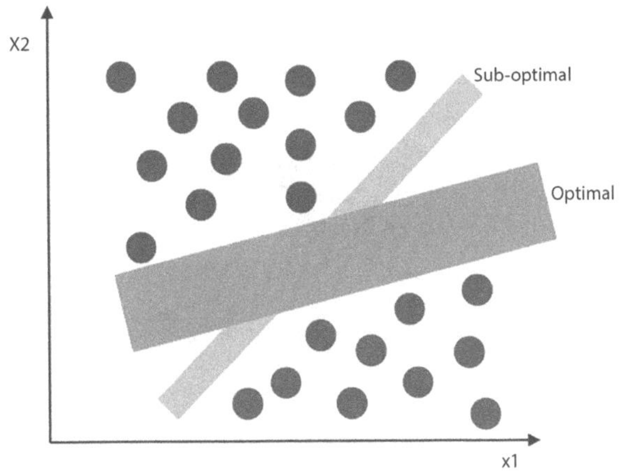

Figure 6.3 A simplified support vector machine (SVM) for binary classification, depicted in a schematic form. In a nutshell, the SVM constructs the green optimal hyperplane that most effectively divides the two groups. An alternative hyperplane (illustrated in orange) is also presented, which appropriately divides the groups but does so with a narrower gap. The SVM performs its operations in the feature space ("×1" and "×2" in the diagram).

decision tree in the fields of classification and regression date back to the 1950s [18]. In addition to their widespread use in today's healthcare system, decision trees are finding increasing applications in fields like economics as well as the military.

Classification and regression decision trees (CARTs) in machine learning connect feature values to potential outcomes using a predetermined set of constraints, thus realizing either a classification or regression job [19]. As the tree grows with each condition, the terminal nodes on the branches reflect the decision's conclusions, making CARTs more approachable to humans than other ML methods. For very big datasets, which are required for CART training, specialized approaches [20] are frequently not computationally costly. Pruning, which limits the size of the tree, and random forests [21], which use several decision trees based on random subsets of the data to generate an average forecast, are two methods that can be used to combat CART's proneness to overfit. To learn more about the spine, both CARTs and random forests have been implemented in various forms. Decision trees, a type of clinical decision support system, have been employed in the preoperative assessment of individuals with adult spinal deformity [22] and the therapy of low back pain [23]. Further uses include prognosticating proximal junctional failure [24] and gauging the primary fixation strength of pedicle screws [25] (Figure 6.4).

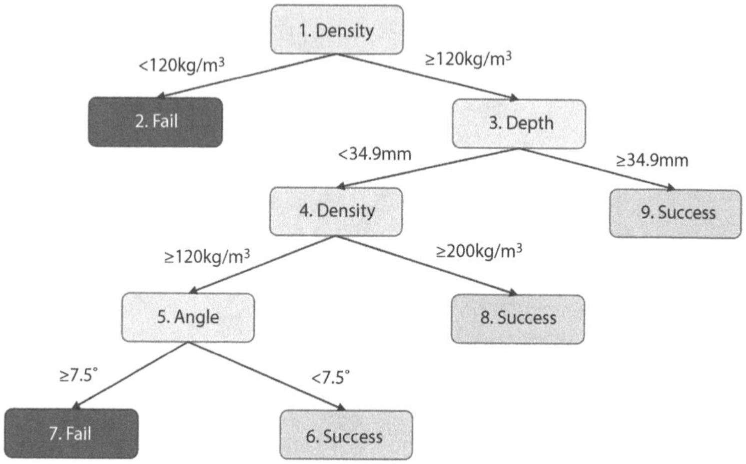

Figure 6.4 A decision tree that has been trained to predict the likelihood of a pedicle screw failing is shown as an example [25].

6.3.3 Artificial Neural Networks

Nonlinear problems in the field of medicine have seen the widespread application of artificial neural network (ANN) models, which are mathematical representations of the human nervous system [26]. A form of machine learning, artificial neural networks can efficiently learn the relationships between input and output variables.

Prediction and classification tasks typically utilize neural networks due to their superior pattern recognition capabilities [27]. There are already well-documented accounts of the development and theory behind ANNs. Researchers have also previously reported the benefits and drawbacks of ANN [28]. A decision support tool with several medical applications, ANN offers cost-effective strategies for managing time and resources [29]. There have been remarkable advancements in the evaluation of spinal illnesses in recent years, thanks in a large part to the use of artificial intelligence and related algorithms. Moreover, ANNs are applied in biomechanical assessments of spinal disorders, clinical diagnoses, and prognoses [30]. Few clinical applications of ANN have been made in the field of spine medicine. In light of current developments in spinal illness management and the critical role of decision, the purpose of this article is to provide an overview of the ANN-aided decision support system for the diagnosis, prognosis, and outcome prediction of spinal disorders.

ANNS have been evaluated and developed as predictive models for common adverse events following spinal anesthesia as well as the diagnosis of low back pain [31], the automatic estimation (and identification of risk factors) of complications following posterior lumbar spine fusion surgical operation [32], and other fields. Several clinical outcomes [33] following spine surgery are amenable to prediction using ANNs, including the return to work, physical disability, readmission rates, risk of complications, discharge, mobility capacity, and disposition. In addition, it is used to automatically quantify muscle fat infiltration after whiplash injury [34], to evaluate clinically relevant improvement in leg pain, back pain, and functional disability following lumbar disc herniation (LDH) surgery [35], and to develop prediction models for postoperative complications following anterior cervical discectomy as well as fusion [36]. ANNs have also been shown to accurately predict survival, hospital discharge, and hospital readmission rates after spinal metastasis surgery [37], rehabilitation discharge, as well as unexpected readmission rates in patients undergoing spinal fusion [38], and prolonged opioid prescription following surgery for LDH [39]. Finally, artificial neural networks have been used to predict four types of major problems, including cardiac issues, venous thromboembolism, wound complications, and mortality in individuals undergoing spine fusion, with better results than the routinely used clinical rating methods [40].

6.3.4 CNN or ConvNets

One of the most widespread uses of ANNs is in image processing and other forms of computer vision. Observations of the visual cortex in cats and monkeys have informed the architecture of convolutional neural networks (CNNs or ConvNets) [41]. Hubel and Wiesel saw in the 1960s that certain regions of the visual cortex are activated and subsequently extracted features and information from only very tiny portions of the visual field. There are specific networks of neurons in the brain that are tuned in to specific features, such as edge orientation. By integrating the data from these different sets of neurons and making use of prior knowledge about their organization, researchers can build an accurate mental image.

CNNs are designed to look like neurons [42]. A convolutional layer is a prime part of a CNN, and it works by multiplying the values of the input layer's elements by the weights of a tiny filter (usually $3 \times 3 \times 3$ or $5 \times 5 \times 3$) as it slides over the input image. This produces a number for each conceivable point in the image. The "activation map" is the cumulative result. A large number of filters utilized in a convolutional layer causes the resulting matrix to be three-dimensional, with each layer being an activation map. Dense (completely connected) layers are the standard non-convolutional layers used in ANNs to generate an output and hence execute a classification or a regression operation; pooling layers [43] down sample the input and help in decreasing the risk of overfitting. To prevent overfitting, CNNs will sometimes use dropout layers, which involve the intentional removal of a certain percentage of virtual neurons. This encourages the network to learn alternative paths to the same output. The goal of training the convolutional layer, like that of ordinary ANNs, is to find the optimal values for the filter weights by optimization methods [44].

6.3.5 Deep Learning

Deep learning uses many layers of processing units to understand different levels of abstraction. Multilayer ANNs, often known as deep neural networks, are commonly used in deep learning. Convolutional neural networks (CNNs) and similar multi-layered ANNs were invented in the 1970s, but they were never extensively adopted due to the high processing power needed for training and the lack of effective learning methods. LeNet-1, developed by a researcher and his team in 1989, is a backpropagation-trainable network consisting of two convolutional layers and two pooling layers. LeNet-5 and other recent developments demonstrated that increasing the network's layer count has the potential to significantly improve prediction accuracy [45]. Because of these early efforts and improvements in computing power, deep learning has emerged as the cutting edge of machine learning—for instance, deep recurrent neural networks are used in speech recognition and natural language processing [46], while deep Boltzmann machines are used to make recommendations for media on the web.

The accuracy of picture recognition is rising, thanks to the use of deep architectures. With its five convolutional layers and three dense layers, AlexNet (a convolutional neural network that is eight layers deep) [47] proved to be the most successful deep CNN in 2012 research, showing that this type of network holds the most promise for further advancements in computer vision, yet there are notable designs from much later eras out there as well. The VGG architecture [48] developed by the Visual Geometry Group (VGG) at Oxford is a huge network with 138 million trainable parameters, 13 convolutional layers, and two dense layers. GoogLeNet, developed by Google in 2014, is a 22-layer neural network architecture (including nine inception layers, a unique design) with 11 million parameters that significantly lessens the computer resources required for training [49]. There are 152 unconnected layers in Microsoft's ResNet (residual neural network) 2015. When it comes to image categorization, ResNet was the first network to achieve human-level accuracy. Some state-of-the-art designs make advantage of residual learning, which bypasses layers to make the deep network easier to train.

Due to the widespread availability of powerful graphics processing units (GPUs) and cloud computing platforms delivering AI goods and services, cutting-edge deep learning software is now being used in many academic domains. Although deep learning is still in its infancy, it has the potential to disrupt long-standing businesses like spine imaging.

6.4 Applications of Machine Learning in Spine Surgery

6.4.1 Degenerative Disease

A prevalent form of degenerative back pain, lumbar degeneration, may benefit from computer-aided MRI interpretation. Degenerative intervertebral discs in spinal MRI T2-weighted images were segmented and categorized using a method developed in 2009. Based on a modest, consistent dataset, this method was validated using 10 traditional imaging processing approaches. Researchers [50] used probabilistic computer vision to classify lumbar discs as deteriorated or normal. Further work used ML approaches instead of probabilistic computer vision. A support vector machine was employed to automatically extract intensity, shape, and texture information from disc images by the research group [51]. In consideration of these results, a classifier was developed [52] to place lumbar discs into one of five Pfirrman categories [53]. This data was then passed to a proprietary classifier that employed a more conventional image processing technique based on the disc's intensity, shape, and texture as extracted by a segmentation algorithm. Researchers in research [54] were the first to use an ANN to extract disc characteristics from a midsagittal T2-weighted picture using automatic segmentation training. Due to their use of an artificial segmentation approach and a limited number of training images, previous investigations had questionable internal validity. When using a CNN, the segmentation step before classification is unnecessary. It was novel that so many MRIs were employed by researchers [55]. Convolutional neural networks were used to analyze 12,018 discs from 2009 patients to automatically extract features without segmentation. Researchers in this study employed a grading method very similar to how humans would grade the severity of disc narrowing, lumbar disc degeneration, upper/lower endplate abnormalities, upper/lower marrow alterations, spondylolisthesis, and central canal stenosis. Based on these observations, the DeepSPINE framework trained a CNN to differentiate between the central canal and foraminal stenosis [56] by analyzing 22,796 lumbar disc levels from 4,075 people. These investigators had a higher rate of accuracy than previously reported studies in grading lumbar spinal and foraminal stenosis at 84.5% and 89.0%, respectively. As with human beings, DeepSPINE was able to detect and rate the severity of lumbar spinal as well as foraminal stenosis.

Although some research has looked at cervical degeneration in the spine, lumbar disease has been the primary focus of automated evaluation of degenerative spinal imaging. Degenerative cervical myelopathy patients who undergo surgery were studied [57] using diffusion tensor imaging (DTI) measures. Predicting surgical success using these DTI metrics using ML algorithms was difficult due to a small patient sample. Fatty infiltration in the paraspinal musculature was measured using a convolutional neural network [58], and the researchers found clinical relevance. It was proposed by these authors that their metric be used to assess people with degenerative cervical myelopathy. Age-related increases in spinal degenerative disease have been documented [59, 60]. The results of these studies demonstrate that ML technology may automate the analysis of MRI scans, hence relieving the workloads of radiologists. Furthermore, the results of these trials demonstrate that ML models can produce quantitative parameters from imaging data far more quickly than radiologists can. To aid in decision-making, future ML models may incorporate quantitative imaging metrics with demographic and neurologic examination data. The use of an ML-powered decision-making tool could improve pre-operative planning and help surgeons identify the patients most likely to benefit from their surgery.

6.4.2 Spinal Deformity

Automated spinal deformity image analysis uses ML algorithms. Initially, ML techniques were employed to categorize scoliotic curves using non-invasive surface topography scans. Researchers [61] classified scoliotic individuals into mild, moderate, and severe curves using surface topography data. Using radiology-interpreted radiographs as a gold standard, an SVM predicted scoliotic curve severity with 85% accuracy. Researchers [62] predicted the Lenke class in 97 scoliosis patients using trunk surface topography data. Their researchers outperformed radiograph-based radiologist classifications by 72.7%. Automatic extraction of spinal features from scoliosis radiographs has been attempted recently. Researchers [63] predicted Cobb angles using coronal radiographs and an SVM. This classifier outperformed human-derived metrics with 92.76% accuracy. The model suited the training data well with a 21.6% root mean squared error. Researchers [64] trained a coronal radiograph-based ANN to estimate Cobb angles. They were 3° off from human-derived measures.

Researchers created an automated idiopathic scoliosis assessment framework [65]. Model View Controller network (MVC-Net) employs anteroposterior and lateral radiographs to determine vertebral levels and calculate the Cobb angle between them. When compared with radiologists' hand-annotated radiographs, the mean absolute error of this system was 4. Using two-plane radiographs, researchers [66] developed an automated method for estimating spinal parameters. Markers such as hip joint centers, endplate centers, and the S1 end plate angle were easily located by their CNN trained on 493 patients. This caused kyphosis from T4 to T12, lordosis from L1 to L5, a scoliotic Cobb angle, a scoliotic pelvic incidence, a scoliotic sacral slope, and a scoliotic pelvic tilt. The model's produced parameters were generally consistent with radiologist readings, with standard errors ranging from 2.7 for pelvic tilt to 11.5 for L1-5 lordosis.

Quantitative spine metrics including pelvic incidence, T4–T12 kyphosis, and pelvic tilt have been the subject of research into automatically extracting these measurements from radiographs. It takes a lot of time and leads to inconsistencies when spinal parameters are annotated by hand. The foregoing findings suggest that ML learning models could speed up and improve spinal radiograph interpretation. A larger dataset might be used to compare the spinal parameters generated by an ML model to those labeled by human raters. In the future, it may be possible to automatically categorize adult spinal deformity using the Scoliosis Research Society (SRS)–Schwab criteria, which are accurate. It is possible that, in the future, a patient's responses to surgery and the best way to approach the procedure could be predicted using a model of spinal traits that was generated autonomously.

6.4.3 Spine Trauma

Spine trauma patients require prompt and accurate volumetric MRI interpretation. Hence, computerized image analysis can improve spine trauma care.

Thoracolumbar injuries have been the primary focus of most ML-based spine trauma imaging analyses [67]. Scientists have developed a system that can detect thoracolumbar fractures automatically. The method used here effectively flattened the three-dimensional spinal column into one. These scientists educated a panel of SVMs to identify fracture patterns in 2D images. This investigation employed a sophisticated method with inadequate data for training. The same research methods were used on 104 patients by this team [68]. In this dataset, they were just 0.81% sensitive and 2.7% false positive. This group of scientists devised a mechanism for classifying thoracolumbar fractures caused by osteoporosis using the Genant system [69]. The researchers recruited 75 thoracolumbar fracture patients and 75 matched CT scan-negative individuals. They detected patient-level compression fractures with 98.7% sensitivity and 77.3% specificity. Their approach also classified each fracture in their imaging data into one of the four Genant classes. The Genant categorization accuracy was 68%.

Researchers [70] employed 90 CT scans tagged by two raters to train a CNN to detect thoracolumbar osteoporotic fractures. This group used a 3D CNN to match earlier reports. Researchers [71] used 2D CNNs to automatically detect osteoporotic fractures in thoracolumbar imaging. The largest dataset was used by [72] researchers; it included 1,432 CT scans, 713 of which showed osteoporotic compression fractures and 719 did not. These experts educated a CNN on images taken in the middle of the sagittal plane, which is not always indicative of any specific spot. This model obtained an F1 score of 90% and an accuracy of 89.2% on the holdout dataset.

Osteoporotic compression fractures have been studied in smaller datasets. This research is new, and no studies have reached human-level performance. Emergency CT scans are collected in enormous numbers, which could be used in future research. This project aims to create a machine learning model that can diagnose any spinal fracture better than humans. If developed, this methodology could minimize radiologists' efforts and boost sensitivity to minor discoveries.

6.4.4 Spine Oncology

Although machine learning methods have been studied extensively for their application in other areas of spine surgery, this field of study has yet to catch on in spinal oncology. Using CT scan data from 114 patients, a support vector machine system was trained to identify spinal metastases [73]. Both the current study and a previous one by researchers [74] were constrained by the modest size of the available imaging data. One recent study used a novel method: a segmentation algorithm to separate images into sections with comparable signal characteristics [75]. The segmented sections were then classified using a support vector machine to find potentially cancerous spots. The training sample size of 49 patients was, again, too small, and the algorithm exhibited a high percentage of false positives. To identify metastatic lesions, researchers [76] utilized a convolutional neural network (CNN) educated on MRI data from 26 patients. In this instance, the performance of the model could not be evaluated by using a different set of test photos.

As a possible future avenue for spinal oncology research beyond tumor diagnosis, the automatic generation of clinically relevant characteristics from MRI scans is discussed. Among these features are an evaluation of spinal instability and a Bilsky grade. The parameters obtained by ML models can help clinicians choose individuals who might benefit from surgery when used in conjunction with other clinical information such as degree of impairment, patient demographics, and oncologic information.

6.5 Application of AI and ML in Spine Research

6.5.1 Spinal Structure Localization and Labeling

Planar radiographs, CT scans, and MRI data have all been mined with ML techniques to extract vertebrae, discs, and spinal form. The process of identifying anatomical structures in an image database is often the first step in creating an automated system for identifying and classifying abnormalities or predicting the results of a treatment.

The use of ML-based localization methods, such as thresholding and heuristic search, is not new [77]. When Schmidt used a classification tree to construct a probability map of each intervertebral disc centroid in MRI scans, he was able to feed that map into a probabilistic graphical model and reduce the average localization error to 6.2 mm [78]. Researchers used a support vector machine trained using the pyramidal histogram of directed gradients to locate discs [79], with average localization errors between 2.6 and 3.6 mm. A rectangular section called a "sliding window" was employed in this method to traverse a multiscaled replica of the source image. Each candidate window position is given a feature descriptor and transmitted to the SVM, which then decides whether the window in question includes an intervertebral disc. Once the most likely locations for each disc have been determined, a graphical model is utilized to infer their actual locations. Similar authors also implemented vertebral localization, which resulted in a decrease in average errors to 4 mm. When attempting to localize vertebrae in computed tomography (CT) datasets of diseased spines with sagittal deformity, severe scoliosis, and fixation devices, the average localization error was between 6 and 8.5 mm [80]. Classification random forests were trained using a variety of methods for generating training data and suppressing false positive predictions to locate the vertebral centroid.

Current research has used ANNs as well as deep learning to pinpoint spinal structures. To power a deep convolutional neural network, researchers used a random forest classifier for an initial coarse localization [81]. The approach they developed improved upon the prior state of the art by increasing the intervertebral disc's center point by 1.6–2 mm [82]. Researchers used both 3D and 2D convolutional neural networks [83]. As part of a regression challenge, the researchers used a six-layer neural network to vote on the vector connecting each voxel to the centroid. Voting provided a statistically reliable method for determining the most likely location of the vertebral centroid [84]. Regression heatmaps of landmark sites were created using 2D and 3D CNNs [85], but spinal images were excluded. Some articles in [86] employed graphical models to mark vertebral or disc centroids after locating them. Without resorting to coarse localization or sliding window methods, complex models that use the complete 3D dataset to pinpoint landmarks and vertebral centroids have shown promising results. Researchers employed a wide range of fields of view and image resolution [87] to detect the vertebral centroid among 6.9 and 9 mm in CT scans of individuals with varied diseases and surgical equipment.

Modern techniques for identifying and labeling the spinal column are on par with those of trained human observers. Although commercial picture archiving and communication system (PACS) and clinical imaging software offer identification and labeling features, their underlying technical implementations are kept secret.

6.5.2 Segmentation

Image analysis has a significant challenge in determining what each pixel in a picture represents. This is known as pixel-level segmentation. Semantic segmentation, which can be performed by hand or by machine, has generated a large body of research because of its centrality to fields as diverse as computer vision and autonomous driving [88]. Typically, a segmentation algorithm in medical imaging should do more than just detect whether a given pixel is part of a disc (e.g., either L1–L2 or L2–L3). Hence, researchers identify instance segmentation as the best method for researching the spine [89].

Defining quantitative criteria to assess a segmentation algorithm's quality may be difficult, in contrast to the localization error used in localization jobs. The Dice similarity coefficient (DSC), which quantifies the degree of spatial overlap between the segmented image and the ground truth, as well as the mean surface distance (MSD), which characterizes the average distance among each voxel of the segmented surface and its nearest voxel of the ground truth, are two of the most widely used metrics introduced in the prior research.

Some research articles [90, 91] and researchers [92] proposed approaches for spine segmentation that did not involve ML techniques, and some of them even required human interaction. Other approaches used optimization techniques to adapt deformable anatomical models to the pictures [93, 94]. Several methods have been published; among them, those based on graphs and normalized cuts, as well as their derivatives [95], proved to be the most effective [96–98]. As an example, the DSC values obtained by researchers were 0.88 and the MSD was 2.7 mm due to the standardization of the incisions [99]. To segment an object, marginal space learning takes for granted that its pose and shape can be quantized in a small set of parameters [100]. Then, many hypotheses are generated to describe the parameter space or all the possible configurations of the item, and a classifier is used to choose the most promising one.

The use of convolutional neural networks tailored to instance segmentation tasks has become commonplace in recent years. To calculate the likelihood that a voxel belongs to a certain location, researchers [101] used a deep convolutional neural network with 3D convolutional layers. The segmentation was fine-tuned using post-processing methods like thresholding and smoothing. Researchers [102] built a 3D convolutional neural network with a memory component to maintain track of the tagged vertebrae. The technique uses a 3D sliding windows strategy to deal with large datasets; first, the position inside the window containing a whole vertebra is identified; next, pixel-level segmentation is conducted using a deep classifier. When looking for the next set of vertebrae, if a segment from an earlier set is recognized, the memory is adjusted so that it is ignored. Researchers obtained impressive precisions with this method, having a mean DSC of 0.94 and a mean standard deviation of 0.2 mm.

6.5.3 Diagnostic Imaging and Computer-Aided Diagnostics

The first ML tests were developed in the 1980s. As early as 1988, a multilayer perceptron was successfully trained to outperform human doctors in the diagnosis of low back pain and sciatica. Based on common medical data and symptoms, the ANN separated cases of back pain into four categories: basic radicular pain, spinal pathology (tumor, infection, inflammation), back pain, and back pain with severe psychological overlay. Automatic imaging-based diagnosis of spinal illness has recently been reported in the literature. Diagnoses of spinal anomalies, degenerative diseases, and cancer are all made with ML.

Early studies of medical imaging-based computer-aided diagnosis used non-ML techniques based on classical image processing [103] or primitive ML approaches like Bayesian classifiers [104]. In the new millennium, perceptrons were used for osteophyte detection [105]. In 2009, researchers published two binary classification methods for identifying degenerative intervertebral discs within T2-weighted MRI scans. Two studies were conducted, one using a Bayesian binary classifier trained on a dataset of 34 MRI scans from patients and the other using a simple statistical model built on a dataset of 30 MRI scans from the same patients [106]. Signal strength and disc texture were considered in both analyses. Several classifiers, including a support vector machine, were applied to 35 MRI stacks in 2011 and achieved accuracies between 80% and 94% [107]. There was a clear victor, and that victor was the SVM. To classify damaged discs with 91.6% accuracy, researchers [108] proposed an SVM-based approach that incorporated texture, intensity, and disc shape. T1-weighted MRI data was added by researchers [109] to improve this method. The researcher's categorization system [110, 111] is widely used in clinical practice and was developed by Ruiz and Castro. This system classifies disc degeneration into five distinct stages, each corresponding to a different degree of degeneration. The intensity and form characterizing features were retrieved in both investigations and fed into a classifier; however, in one case, a customized solution was used, while in the other a simple ANN was employed. The discs were automatically partitioned before feature extraction in both works. Using a convolutional neural network as a classifier, the researchers [112] collected 12,018 disc images from 2,009 patients for training and testing, while most previous work relied on fewer than 100 MRI datasets. Thus, pre-classification segmentation was unnecessary. Like the inter-rater agreement of 70% found between professional radiologists, the approach achieved 70% agreement with human observations. This technique was also successful in detecting lesions on the endplates and alterations in the bone marrow. Using a deep convolutional neural network and a larger training set, researchers have increased the accuracy of automatic degeneration grading using the Pfirrmann classification strategy to 97% [113].

ML has been used to analyze spinal abnormalities and deteriorating spines. ML has had the greatest influence on noninvasive adolescent idiopathic scoliosis severity assessment using surface topography. As such techniques do not directly visualize the spine, inference algorithms that can leverage minor patterns in the data that may not be evident to humans can help extract therapeutically useful results. Researchers [114] used a support vector machine, a decision tree, and linear discriminant analysis to classify the surface topographies of scoliotic patients into mild, moderate, and severe curves. SVM's 85% accuracy was the greatest of any classifier researchers tested. Scoliosis patients' biplanar radiographs were employed as the gold standard by researchers [115] who applied a regression support vector machine to map the spinal centerline from the patient's body's topography. A support vector machine was trained using planar radiograph readings from 97 teenagers with idiopathic scoliosis to predict the curve type. Overall, the team was 72.2% effective. A decision tree was recently trained to classify surface topography data into mild, moderate, and severe curves and to identify the curve location (thoracic-thoracolumbar, proximal thoracic, or lumbar) to assess curve progression risk [116]. According to the model, most of the curves (85.7%) were progressions, while the remaining minority (72.4%) were not.

Similarly, radiographic data from individuals with spinal abnormalities have been analyzed with ML methods. The difficult automated analysis of the Cobb angle, which characterizes the severity of a scoliotic curve, has been tried by several non-ML techniques, including the fuzzy Hough transform [117] and deep learning techniques. Regression support vector machines (SVMs) were used to predict the Cobb angle from coronal radiographs, as done by the researchers [118], with a root mean squared error of 21.6%, suggesting therapeutic utility. Absolute errors of less than 3° were achieved when the Cobb angle was estimated from coronal radiography images using a deep ANN, as reported in [119]. Biplanar radiographs have been employed by researchers [120, 121] to detect aberrant curvature due to their ability to offer three-dimensional information. A new method of classifying adolescent idiopathic scoliosis has been developed [122] using unsupervised clustering, and it more precisely depicts curve variability. The main curve, including the apical vertebra, kyphosis, and lordosis, was utilized to categorize 915 biplanar radiographs into 11 groups using the clustering method.

In the medical literature, computer-aided diagnosis (CAD) systems are used to detect and localize key features, such as lesions and fractures, in medical images, to reduce the risk of misdiagnosis and increase the likelihood of positive incidental findings. Using a regression support vector machine [123] or a convolutional neural network [124], CAD systems can detect and categorize vertebral fractures with 95% accuracy. Using a classifier trained on features extracted from each vertebra, CAD systems can also be used to detect spine metastases on CT scans [125]. However, the false positive rate required human involvement, even though the technologies would identify lytic and blastic lesions in real time. Researchers [126] utilized a watershed segmentation algorithm to find possible lesions in wide regions with similar intensities. The method used an SVM classifier to identify if the candidate region was a tumoral lesion by analyzing its shape, location, and intensity. This approach also produced 620 false positives compared with 439 true positive lesions, which may require more research.

In conclusion, ML is revolutionizing diagnostic imaging, both in general and for spine illnesses, given its recent achievements. Considering moral issues like individual accountability, accurate and trustworthy automated diagnostic systems could have a huge impact on radiology.

6.5.4 Clinical Decision Support and Outcome Predictions

New AI technologies and massive data sources have had a significant impact on the field of statistics known as predictive analytics [127]. Intriguing as it may sound, predictive analytics has always piqued the curiosity of those working in healthcare due to the numerous advantages that they offer in terms of both patient care and overall spending. In healthcare, predictive analytics could be used for a variety of purposes, such as foreseeing complications during a patient's hospital stay, identifying chronic patients at risk of poor health outcomes and who may benefit from treatments, developing individualized treatments, and streamlining supply chain operations. Several publications during the past decade have provided techniques for estimating the success of spinal operations. The Oswestry Index (ODI) [128], the occurrence of problems, readmission to the hospital, and the return to work were all predicted 1 year after surgery using simple statistical approaches like linear and logistic regression [129]. The prediction program evaluated information from 750–1,200 patients to make predictions about potential problems, and the results showed an accuracy of 72–84%. Preoperative ODI, age, ethnicity, body mass index, symptom description, presence or absence of additional spinal illnesses, and scores characterizing the patient's health and functional state were just some of the more than 40 parameters used by the model. The clinical score is typically used to predict cardiac complications, venous thromboembolism, wound complications, and death after spine fusion; however, a recent study [130] combined logistic regression and a shallow artificial neural network to predict these four key concerns in patients. Researchers [131] interested in surgical site infection risk assessment followed a similar course of action. Further external testing (with a different set of patients) of the same predictive model yielded disappointing results [132]. A large retrospective study [133] demonstrated a set of decision trees that predicted serious intraoperative or perioperative problems following surgery for adult spine deformity with an overall accuracy of 87.6%. Blood transfusion requirements following adult deformity surgery were examined, and both single decision trees and a random forest were found to accurately predict this result [134]. One common application of predictive analytics is the development of decision support tools (DSTs) to aid clinicians in making informed decisions. Nijmegen Decision Tool for Chronic Low Back Pain [135] is a recent DST example in spine care that uses predictors covering multiple dimensions of patient health (such as sociodemographic, somatic, pain, functioning, psychological, and quality of life) to suggest surgical treatment, conservative care, or no intervention. Despite popular support for the switch, others have voiced concerns about the lack of a clear plan for the technical problems of adopting this DST. The domains of spine research and predictive analytics/clinical decision support seem to be at an earlier stage of development when compared with other uses of AI and ML. Decision support technology (DST) based on ML techniques does not help with choices in spine surgery, such as instrumentation length and the selection of anchoring implants in spine deformity surgery, but prediction models that are not built with cutting-edge methods like deep learning may overlook imaging data. However, AI researchers do not have access to or are still in the process of building the vast databases needed to train such models. Nonetheless, with the recent growth of national and local spine registries, some of which contain imaging data, significant progress may be achievable soon.

6.5.5 In-Image Search Based on Content

Many images of each body component and imaging modality can be found in large hospital digital imaging databases. To facilitate the retrieval of photos for clinical investigations or instructional reasons, several institutions have implemented indexing depending on the contents of each image. As a manual procedure, indexing is time-consuming, costly, and prone to errors [136]. Recent years have seen a surge in interest in automating content-based image retrieval (CBIR), a field that has benefited greatly from the introduction of ML approaches. The so-called relevance feedback is used by several CBIR systems, and it entails rating the usefulness of each result that the query yields [137]—for instance, how much time a user spends looking at a particular item or which documents are chosen for in-depth analysis are examples of implicit feedback that may be gleaned automatically from user activity. In the case of explicit feedback, the user is directly asked to judge the usefulness of the results. To integrate relevant feedback, recent works have included ML techniques like SVMs [138]. Most CBIR systems rely on straightforward methods like SVMs for image categorization rather than sophisticated deep learning architectures [139]. Nevertheless, deep learning has recently been used in research [140].

There have been a few advanced algorithms presented that are specifically designed to take advantage of the characteristics of spine images. To retrieve spine radiographs, researchers [141] suggested a new relevance feedback mechanism based on the vertebral contour. Its in-built short-term memory mechanism remembers human selections over feedback iterations, with a decision tree making the final call on an image's significance. In addition, the same team of researchers produced a CBIR method [142] that accounted for the unique form of the spinal canal.

6.5.6 Biomechanics

To date, the influence of AI and ML on applied clinical and radiological research has been greater than their impact on more fundamental areas of biomechanics. Recently, however, a few publications detailing the use of ANNs to solve common biomechanical issues including load and stress estimates have appeared. Although there is currently a lack of research focusing on the spine, researchers believe that it is important to briefly highlight here the many ML-based studies studying other musculoskeletal regions to establish potential future fields of applicability of ML techniques in spine biomechanics. The material characteristics of living tissues have been estimated using ML. In individuals with adult-acquired flatfoot deformity, researchers [143] used shallow ANNs to investigate the connection between ligament stiffness and foot kinematics. The authors built and used patient-specific 3D computer models of the foot anatomy to create the training data. Foreseeing the mechanical pressures that finally decide the specific mechanical properties of a biological tissue experiencing remodeling, in this case, trabecular bone, was also an objective of the group of researchers [144]. To predict how a small sample of trabecular bone would respond to mechanical loading, the authors used a pre-existing biomechanical computer model to simulate the application of random loads to the sample. The remodeled local bone densities produced by the simulations served as inputs for training the ANN to anticipate the stresses that generated that type of remodeling. In addition, ML can be used to conduct patient-specific stress analysis without resorting to computationally expensive finite element models. Because of this, researchers were able to create a shallow ANN that accurately predicted the load on the tibial plateau and femoral condyles of the knee. For a fraction of the time and cost of solving the finite element model, researchers were able to forecast the stress in each element of the articular cartilage by using data from a knee finite element model to train an artificial neural network. The application of ML methods to the study of musculoskeletal biomechanics is still in its infancy, given the few publications that have been published have not yet made advantage of the full potential of cutting-edge methods like deep learning, yet existing articles show that ML has great promise in this area. Large datasets utilized for training ML models could be generated with the help of computational models that predict the biomechanical response of joints, bones, and the spine [145]. This method would promote patient-specific modeling in the bench-to-bedside application, where the time and resources needed to develop a standard biomechanical model may conflict with the needs of the patient.

6.5.7 Analyzing Motion and Gait

Cameras, wearable inertial devices, optoelectronic systems, force plates, electromyography systems, and pressure sensors are commonly used for the quantitative study of human motion and gait, which is widely used in the scientific and clinical research of various illnesses. Researchers are focusing a lot of attention right now on how persons with spinal problems alter their walking habits [146]. Often used in classical gait analysis, force platforms measure kinematic characteristics like joint degrees of rotation and kinetic parameters like forces and moments at the joints. For diagnostic or recovery monitoring, parameter values are compared with reference ranges. Common movements including walking, standing, sitting up straight, ascending stairs, and flexing the trunk have all been the subject of motion analysis techniques unique to each activity [147]. As ML techniques have become increasingly popular in several areas of study over the past two decades, this unified strategy has been revisited [148]. SVMs [149] and artificial neural networks [150] are two ML methods that have been successfully used in recent articles to classify aberrant gait patterns. The technical challenges in detecting vertebral position and motion associated with soft tissue disorders [151] may account for the limited number of published works that use ML approaches to spinal ailments. The work of researchers [152], who employed support vector machine training to distinguish between patients with lumbar canal stenosis and those with L4 or L5 radiculopathy based on gait patterns, is among the early studies in this area. Spine problems are another area where ML has been successfully applied, this time through electromyography systems [153]. The study used dynamic surface electromyography to determine which of the 30 patients with chronic low back pain would benefit most from a functional restoration rehabilitation program, and a support vector machine was developed to analyze the data. Computer models of humanoid or animal-shaped entities learning how to walk and move in a simulated environment that may be geometrically complicated and include obstacles are the subject of gait and ML, a topic of study in artificial intelligence. Due to the complexity of coordinating the activation of actuators (representing the muscles in a human subject), the preservation of balance, and the attainment of the locomotion goal, the simulation of learning to walk is infamously challenging within a machine learning framework. Implementing such models indeed calls for complex reinforcement algorithms, which typically reward the agent when it succeeds in its goal, such as by reaching the target position, and penalize it when it fails, such as by falling to the ground [154].

6.6 Conclusion

Modern academic fields are greatly impacted by the ground-breaking technologies of AI and ML. The fields of computer vision and image processing have greatly benefited from recent advances in deep learning and the growing accessibility of computational resources such as potent GPUs. Even though most of the recent artificial intelligence and machine learning-based spine research studies have concentrated on medical imaging, their impact in other fields, such as spine biomechanics, is likely to expand shortly. Concerns regarding the ethics of accountability, data privacy, and security and the possibility of biased forecasts are all being closely watched by policymakers and regulators.

References

1. Al, S., Some studies in machine learning using the game of checkers. *IBM J. Res. Dev.*, 3, 210–229, 1959.
2. Nilsson, N.J., *The quest for artificial intelligence*, Cambridge University Press, Cambridge, England, 2009 Oct 30.
3. He, K., Zhang, X., Ren, S., Sun, J., Deep residual learning for image recognition, in: *Proceedings of the IEEE Conference on Computer Vision and Pattern Recognition*, pp. 770–778, 2016.
4. Hosny, A., Parmar, C., Quackenbush, J., Schwartz, L.H., Aerts, H.J., Artificial intelligence in radiology. *Nat. Rev. Cancer*, 18, 8, 500–510, 2018 Aug.
5. Shalev-Shwartz, S. and Ben-David, S., *Understanding machine learning: From theory to algorithms*, Cambridge University Press, Cambridge, England, 2014 May 19.

6. Pfirrmann, C.W., Metzdorf, A., Zanetti, M., Hodler, J., Boos, N., Magnetic resonance classification of lumbar intervertebral disc degeneration. *Spine*, 26, 17, 1873–1878, 2001 Sep 1.
7. Toyoda, H., Takahashi, S., Hoshino, M., Takayama, K., Iseki, K., Sasaoka, R., Tsujio, T., Yasuda, H., Sasaki, T., Kanematsu, F., Kono, H., Characterizing the course of back pain after osteoporotic vertebral fracture: A hierarchical cluster analysis of a prospective cohort study. *Arch. Osteoporos.*, 12, 1–8, 2017 Dec.
8. Michalski, R.S., Carbonell, J.G., Mitchell, T.M., *Machine learning an artificial intelligence approach*, Springer-Verlag Berlin Heidelberg, New York Tokyo in 1983, 1984.
9. Domingos, P., A few useful things to know about machine learning. *Commun. ACM*, 55, 10, 78–87, 2012 Oct 1.
10. Lowe, D.G., Object recognition from local scale-invariant features, in: *Proceedings of the Seventh IEEE International Conference on Computer Vision*, vol. 2, IEEE, pp. 1150–1157, 1999 Sep 20.
11. Rublee, E., Rabaud, V., Konolige, K., Bradski, G., ORB: An efficient alternative to SIFT or SURF, in: *2011 International Conference on Computer Vision*, IEEE, pp. 2564–2571, 2011 Nov 6.
12. Russel, S. and Norvig, P., *Artificial intelligence: A modern approach*, Pearson Education Limited, London, 2013.
13. Frighetto-Pereira, L., Rangayyan, R.M., Metzner, G.A., de Azevedo-Marques, P.M., Nogueira-Barbosa, M.H., Shape, texture and statistical features for classification of benign and malignant vertebral compression fractures in magnetic resonance images. *Comput. Biol. Med.*, 73, 147–156, 2016 Jun 1.
14. Cortes, C. and Vapnik, V., Support-vector networks. *Mach. Learn.*, 20, 273–297, 1995 Sep.
15. Vapnik, V., Pattern recognition using generalized portrait method. *Autom. Remote Control*, 24, 774–780, 1963.
16. Seoud, L., Adankon, M.M., Labelle, H., Dansereau, J., Cheriet, F., Prediction of scoliosis curve type based on the analysis of trunk surface topography, in: *2010 IEEE International Symposium on Biomedical Imaging: From Nano to Macro*, IEEE, pp. 408–411, 2010 Apr 14.
17. Oktay, A.B. and Akgul, Y.S., Simultaneous localization of lumbar vertebrae and intervertebral discs with SVM-based MRF. *IEEE Trans. Biomed. Eng.*, 60, 9, 2375–2383, 2013 Apr 2.
18. Belson, W.A., Matching and prediction on the principle of biological classification. *J. R. Stat. Soc.: Ser. C (Appl. Stat.)*, 8, 2, 65–75, 1959 Jun.
19. Breiman, L., *Classification and regression trees*, Routledge, Boca Raton, Florida, 2017 Oct 19.
20. Quinlan, J.R., *C4. 5: Programs for machine learning*, Elsevier, Amsterdam, The Netherlands, 2014 Jun 28.
21. Breiman, L., Random forests. *Mach. Learn.*, 45, 5–32, 2001 Oct.
22. Oh, T., Scheer, J.K., Smith, J.S., Hostin, R., Robinson, C., Gum, J.L., Schwab, F., Hart, R.A., Lafage, V., Burton, D.C., Bess, S., Potential of predictive computer

models for preoperative patient selection to enhance overall quality-adjusted life years gained at 2-year follow-up: A simulation in 234 patients with adult spinal deformity. *Neurosurg. Focus*, 43, 6, E2, 2017 Dec 1.
23. Nijeweme-d'Hollosy, W.O., van Velsen, L.S., Soer, R., Hermens, H.J., Design of a web-based clinical decision support system for guiding patients with low back pain to the best next step in primary healthcare, in: *Proceedings of the 9th International Joint Conference on Biomedical Engineering Systems and Technologies (BIOSTEC 2016)*, vol. 5, SCITEPRESS-Science and Technology Publications Portugal, pp. 229–239, 2016 Feb 21.
24. Yagi, M., Akilah, K.B., Boachie-Adjei, O., Incidence, risk factors and classification of proximal junctional kyphosis: Surgical outcomes review of adult idiopathic scoliosis. *Spine*, 36, 1, E60–8, 2011 Jan 1.
25. Varghese, V., Krishnan, V., Kumar, G.S., Evaluating pedicle-screw instrumentation using decision-tree analysis based on pullout strength. *Asian Spine J.*, 12, 4, 611, 2018 Aug.
26. Azimi, P. and Mohammadi, H.R., Predicting endoscopic third ventriculostomy success in childhood hydrocephalus: An artificial neural network analysis. *J. Neurosurg.: Pediatr.*, 13, 4, 426–432, 2014 Apr 1.
27. Azimi, P., Benzel, E.C., Shahzadi, S., Azhari, S., Mohammadi, H.R., The prediction of successful surgery outcome in lumbar disc herniation based on artificial neural networks. *J. Neurosurg. Sci.*, 60, 2, 173–177, 2016 Jun 1.
28. Azimi, P., Benzel, E.C., Shahzadi, S., Azhari, S., Mohammadi, H.R., Use of artificial neural networks to predict surgical satisfaction in patients with lumbar spinal canal stenosis. *J. Neurosurg.: Spine*, 20, 3, 300–305, 2014 Mar 1.
29. Nolting, J., Developing a neural network model for health care, in: *AMIA Annual Symposium Proceedings*, vol. 2006, American Medical Informatics Association, p. 1049, 2006.
30. Azimi, P., Mohammadi, H.R., Benzel, E.C., Shahzadi, S., Azhari, S., Montazeri, A., Artificial neural networks in neurosurgery. *J. Neurol. Neurosurg. Psychiatry*, 86, 3, 251–256, 2015 Mar 1.
31. Dickey, J.P., Pierrynowski, M.R., Bednar, D.A., Yang, S.X., Relationship between pain and vertebral motion in chronic low-back pain subjects. *Clin. Biomech.*, 17, 5, 345–352, 2002 Jun 1.
32. Parsaeian, M., Mohammad, K., Mahmoudi, M., Zeraati, H., Comparison of logistic regression and artificial neural network in low back pain prediction: Second national health survey. *Iran. J. Public Health*, 41, 6, 86, 2012.
33. Karhade, A.V., Ogink, P., Thio, Q., Broekman, M., Cha, T., Gormley, W.B., Hershman, S., Peul, W.C., Bono, C.M., Schwab, J.H., Development of machine learning algorithms for prediction of discharge disposition after elective inpatient surgery for lumbar degenerative disc disorders. *Neurosurg. Focus*, 45, 5, E6, 2018 Nov 1.
34. Weber, K.A., Smith, A.C., Wasielewski, M., Eghtesad, K., Upadhyayula, P.A., Wintermark, M., Hastie, T.J., Parrish, T.B., Mackey, S., Elliott, J.M., Deep learning convolutional neural networks for the automatic quantification of muscle fat infiltration following whiplash injury. *Sci. Rep.*, 9, 1, 1–8, 2019 May 28.

35. Staartjes, V.E., Marlies, P., Vandertop, W.P., Schröder, M.L., Deep learning-based preoperative predictive analytics for patient-reported outcomes following lumbar discectomy: Feasibility of center-specific modeling. *Spine J.*, 19, 5, 853–861, 2019 May 1.
36. Arvind, V., Kim, J.S., Oermann, E.K., Kaji, D., Cho, S.K., Predicting surgical complications in adult patients undergoing anterior cervical discectomy and fusion using machine learning. *Neurospine*, 15, 4, 329, 2018 Dec.
37. Karhade, A.V., Thio, Q.C., Ogink, P.T., Shah, A.A., Bono, C.M., Oh, K.S., Saylor, P.J., Schoenfeld, A.J., Shin, J.H., Harris, M.B., Schwab, J.H., Development of machine learning algorithms for prediction of 30-day mortality after surgery for spinal metastasis. *Neurosurgery*, 85, 1, E83–91, 2019 Jul 1.
38. Goyal, A., Ngufor, C., Kerezoudis, P., McCutcheon, B., Storlie, C., Bydon, M., Can machine learning algorithms accurately predict discharge to nonhome facility and early unplanned readmissions following spinal fusion? Analysis of a national surgical registry: Presented at the 2019 AANS/CNS Section on Disorders of the Spine and Peripheral Nerves. *J. Neurosurg.: Spine*, 31, 4, 568–578, 2019 Jun 7.
39. Karhade, A.V., Ogink, P.T., Thio, Q.C., Cha, T.D., Gormley, W.B., Hershman, S.H., Smith, T.R., Mao, J., Schoenfeld, A.J., Bono, C.M., Schwab, J.H., Development of machine learning algorithms for prediction of prolonged opioid prescription after surgery for lumbar disc herniation. *Spine J.*, 19, 11, 1764–1771, 2019 Nov 1.
40. Kim, J.S., Merrill, R.K., Arvind, V., Kaji, D., Pasik, S.D., Nwachukwu, C.C., Vargas, L., Osman, N.S., Oermann, E.K., Caridi, J.M., Cho, S.K., Examining the ability of artificial neural networks machine learning models to accurately predict complications following posterior lumbar spine fusion. *Spine*, 43, 12, 853, 2018 Jun 6.
41. Hubel, D.H. and Wiesel, T.N., Receptive fields, binocular interaction and functional architecture in the cat's visual cortex. *J. Physiol.*, 160, 1, 106, 1962 Jan.
42. Fukushima, K., Neocognitron: A self-organizing neural network model for a mechanism of pattern recognition unaffected by shift in position. *Biol. Cybern.*, 36, 4, 193–202, 1980 Apr.
43. Scherer, D., Müller, A., Behnke, S., Evaluation of pooling operations in convolutional architectures for object recognition, in: *Artificial Neural Networks–ICANN 2010: 20th International Conference, Thessaloniki, Greece, September 15-18, 2010, Proceedings, Part III*, Springer Berlin Heidelberg, 20, pp. 92–101, 2010.
44. LeCun, Y., Boser, B., Denker, J.S., Henderson, D., Howard, R.E., Hubbard, W., Jackel, L.D., Backpropagation applied to handwritten zip code recognition. *Neural Comput.*, 1, 4, 541–551, 1989 Dec.
45. LeCun, Y., Bottou, L., Bengio, Y., Haffner, P., Gradient-based learning applied to document recognition. *Proc. IEEE*, 86, 11, 2278–2324, 1998 Nov.

46. LeCun, Y., Bengio, Y., Hinton, G., Deep learning. *Nature*, 521, 7553, 436–444, 2015 May 28.
47. Krizhevsky, A., Sutskever, I., Hinton, G.E., Imagenet classification with deep convolutional neural networks. *Commun. ACM*, 60, 6, 84–90, 2017 May 24.
48. Simonyan, K. and Zisserman, A., Very deep convolutional networks for large-scale image recognition. *Computer Vision and Pattern Recognition*, 1 1–14, arXiv preprint arXiv:1409.1556, 2014 Sep 4.
49. Szegedy, C., Liu, W., Jia, Y., Sermanet, P., Reed, S., Anguelov, D., Erhan, D., Vanhoucke, V., Rabinovich, A., Going deeper with convolutions, in: *Proceedings of the IEEE Conference on Computer Vision and Pattern Recognition*, 12, 1–9, arXiv 2014. arXiv preprint arXiv:1409.4842, 2015.
50. A, R.S., Corso, J.J., Chaudhary, V., Dhillon, G., Desiccation diagnosis in lumbar discs from clinical MRI with a probabilistic model, in: *2009 IEEE International Symposium on Biomedical Imaging: From Nano to Macro*, IEEE, pp. 546–549, 2009 Jun 28.
51. Ding, Y., Zhu, Y., Feng, J., Zhang, P., Cheng, Z., Interpretable spatio-temporal attention LSTM model for flood forecasting. *Neurocomputing*, 403, 348–359, 2020 Aug 25.
52. Urrutia Escobar, J.O., Besa, P., Campos, M., Cikutovic, P., Cabezón, M., Molina, M., Cruz, J.P., The Pfirrmann classification of lumbar intervertebral disc degeneration: An independent inter- and intra-observer agreement assessment. *Eur. Spine J.*, 25, 2728–2733, 2016.
53. Ruiz-España, S., Arana, E., Moratal, D., Semiautomatic computer-aided classification of degenerative lumbar spine disease in magnetic resonance imaging. *Comput. Biol. Med.*, 62, 196–205, 2015 Jul 1.
54. Castro-Mateos, I., Pozo, J.M., Lazary, A., Frangi, A.F., 2D segmentation of intervertebral discs and its degree of degeneration from T2-weighted magnetic resonance images, in: *Medical Imaging 2014: Computer-Aided Diagnosis*, 2014 Mar 20, vol. 9035, pp. 310–320, SPIE, Bellingham, Washington USA, 2014.
55. Jamaludin, A., Kadir, T., Zisserman, A., SpineNet: Automated classification and evidence visualization in spinal MRIs. *Med. Image Anal.*, 41, 63–73, 2017 Oct 1.
56. Lu, J.T., Pedemonte, S., Bizzo, B., Doyle, S., Andriole, K.P., Michalski, M.H., Gonzalez, R.G., Pomerantz, S.R., Deep spine: Automated lumbar vertebral segmentation, disc-level designation, and spinal stenosis grading using deep learning, in: *Machine Learning for Healthcare Conference*, PMLR, pp. 403–419, 2018 Nov 29.
57. Jin, R., Luk, K.D., Cheung, J., Hu, Y., A machine learning based prognostic prediction of cervical myelopathy using diffusion tensor imaging, in: *2016 IEEE International Conference on Computational Intelligence and Virtual Environments for Measurement Systems and Applications (CIVEMSA)*, IEEE, pp. 1–4, 2016 Jun 27.
58. Weber, K.A., Smith, A.C., Wasielewski, M., Eghtesad, K., Upadhyayula, P.A., Wintermark, M., Hastie, T.J., Parrish, T.B., Mackey, S., Elliott, J.M., Deep

learning convolutional neural networks for the automatic quantification of muscle fat infiltration following whiplash injury. *Sci. Rep.*, 9, 1, 1–8, 2019 May 28.
59. Nouri, A., Tetreault, L., Singh, A., Karadimas, S.K., Fehlings, M.G., Degenerative cervical myelopathy: Epidemiology, genetics, and pathogenesis. *Spine*, 40, 12, E675–93, 2015 Jun 15.
60. Karadimas, S.K., Erwin, W.M., Ely, C.G., Dettori, J.R., Fehlings, M.G., Pathophysiology and natural history of cervical spondylotic myelopathy. *Spine*, 38, 22S, S21–36, 2013 Oct 15.
61. Ramirez, L., Durdle, N.G., Raso, V.J., Hill, D.L., A support vector machines classifier to assess the severity of idiopathic scoliosis from surface topography. *IEEE Trans. Inf. Technol. Biomed.*, 10, 1, 84–91, 2006 Jan 10.
62. Seoud, L., Adankon, M.M., Labelle, H., Dansereau, J., Cheriet, F., Prediction of scoliosis curve type based on the analysis of trunk surface topography, in: *2010 IEEE International Symposium on Biomedical Imaging: From Nano to Macro*, IEEE, pp. 408–411, 2010 Apr 14.
63. Sun, H., Zhen, X., Bailey, C., Rasoulinejad, P., Yin, Y., Li, S., Direct estimation of spinal cobb angles by structured multi-output regression, in: *Information Processing in Medical Imaging: 25th International Conference, IPMI 2017, Boone, NC, USA, June 25-30, 2017, Proceedings*, Springer International Publishing, Cham, pp. 529–540, 2017 May 23.
64. Zhang, J., Lou, E., Shi, X., Wang, Y., Hill, D.L., Raso, J.V., Le, L.H., Lv, L., A computer-aided Cobb angle measurement method and its reliability. *Clin. Spine Surg.*, 23, 6, 383–387, 2010 Aug 1.
65. Wu, H., Bailey, C., Rasoulinejad, P., Li, S., Automated comprehensive adolescent idiopathic scoliosis assessment using MVC-Net. *Med. Image Anal.*, 48, 1–1, 2018 Aug 1.
66. Galbusera, F., Niemeyer, F., Wilke, H.J., Bassani, T., Casaroli, G., Anania, C., Costa, F., Brayda-Bruno, M., Sconfienza, L.M., Fully automated radiological analysis of spinal disorders and deformities: A deep learning approach. *Eur. Spine J.*, 28, 951–960, 2019 May 1.
67. Yao, J., Burns, J.E., Munoz, H., Summers, R.M., Detection of vertebral body fractures based on cortical shell unwrapping, in: *Medical Image Computing and Computer-Assisted Intervention–MICCAI 2012: 15th International Conference, Nice, France, October 1-5, 2012, Proceedings, Part III*, Springer Berlin Heidelberg, 15, pp. 509–516, 2102.
68. Burns, J.E., Yao, J., Muñoz, H., Summers, R.M., Automated detection, localization, and classification of traumatic vertebral body fractures in the thoracic and lumbar spine at CT. *Radiology*, 278, 1, 64–73, 2016 Jan.
69. Burns, J.E., Yao, J., Summers, R.M., Vertebral body compression fractures and bone density: Automated detection and classification on CT images. *Radiology*, 284, 3, 788–797, 2017 Sep.
70. Nicolaes, J., Raeymaeckers, S., Robben, D., Wilms, G., Vandermeulen, D., Libanati, C., Debois, M., Detection of vertebral fractures in CT using 3D convolutional neural networks, in: *Computational Methods and Clinical*

Applications for Spine Imaging: 6th International Workshop and Challenge, CSI 2019, Shenzhen, China, October 17, 2019, Proceedings, Springer International Publishing, 6, pp. 3–14, 2020.

71. Baum, T., Bauer, J.S., Klinder, T., Dobritz, M., Rummeny, E.J., Noël, P.B., Lorenz, C., Automatic detection of osteoporotic vertebral fractures in routine thoracic and abdominal MDCT. *Eur. Radiol.*, 24, 872–880, 2014 Apr.
72. Tomita, N., Cheung, Y.Y., Hassanpour, S., Deep neural networks for automatic detection of osteoporotic vertebral fractures on CT scans. *Comput. Biol. Med.*, 98, 8–15, 2018 Jul 1.
73. Hammon, M., Dankerl, P., Tsymbal, A., Wels, M., Kelm, M., May, M., Suehling, M., Uder, M., Cavallaro, A., Automatic detection of lytic and blastic thoracolumbar spine metastases on computed tomography. *Eur. Radiol.*, 23, 1862–1870, 2013 Jul.
74. O'Connor, S.D., Yao, J., Summers, R.M., Lytic metastases in thoracolumbar spine: Computer-aided detection at CT—Preliminary study. *Radiology*, 242, 3, 811–816, 2007 Mar.
75. Burns, J.E., Yao, J., Wiese, T.S., Muñoz, H.E., Jones, E.C., Summers, R.M., Automated detection of sclerotic metastases in the thoracolumbar spine at CT. *Radiology*, 268, 1, 69–78, 2013 Jul.
76. Wang, J., Fang, Z., Lang, N., Yuan, H., Su, M.Y., Baldi, P., A multi-resolution approach for spinal metastasis detection using deep Siamese neural networks. *Comput. Biol. Med.*, 84, 137–146, 2017 May 1.
77. Chwialkowski, M.P., Shile, P.E., Pfeifer, D., Parkey, R.W., Peshock, R.M., Automated localization and identification of lower spinal anatomy in magnetic resonance images. *Comput. Biomed. Res.*, 24, 2, 99–117, 1991 Apr 1.
78. Schmidt, S., Kappes, J., Bergtholdt, M., Pekar, V., Dries, S., Bystrov, D., Schnörr, C., Spine detection and labeling using a parts-based graphical model, in: *Information Processing in Medical Imaging: 20th International Conference, IPMI 2007, Kerkrade, The Netherlands, July 2-6, 2007. Proceedings*, Springer Berlin Heidelberg, 20, pp. 122–133, 2007.
79. Oktay, A. and Akgul, Y., Localization of the lumbar discs using machine learning and exact probabilistic inference. *Medical Image Computing and Computer-Assisted Intervention - MICCAI 2011 14th International Conference*, Toronto, Canada, 6893, 158–165, 2011.
80. Glocker, B., Feulner, J., Criminisi, A., Haynor, D.R., Konukoglu, E., Automatic localization and identification of vertebrae in arbitrary field-of-view CT scans, in: *Medical Image Computing and Computer-Assisted Intervention–MICCAI 2012: 15th International Conference, Nice, France, October 1-5, 2012, Proceedings, Part III*, Springer Berlin Heidelberg, 15, pp. 590–598, 2012.
81. Chen, H., Shen, C., Qin, J., Ni, D., Shi, L., Cheng, J.C., Heng, P.A., Automatic localization and identification of vertebrae in spine CT via a joint learning model with deep neural networks, in: *Medical Image Computing and Computer-Assisted Intervention–MICCAI 2015: 18th International Conference, Munich, Germany, October 5-9, 2015, Proceedings, Part I*, Springer International Publishing, 18, pp. 515–522, 2015.

82. Glocker, B., Zikic, D., Konukoglu, E., Haynor, D.R., Criminisi, A., Vertebrae localization in pathological spine CT via dense classification from sparse annotations, in: *Medical Image Computing and Computer-Assisted Intervention–MICCAI 2013: 16th International Conference, Nagoya, Japan, September 22-26, 2013, Proceedings, Part II*, Springer Berlin Heidelberg, 16, pp. 262–270, 2013.
83. Chen, H., Dou, Q., Wang, X., Qin, J., Cheng, J.C., Heng, P.A., 3D fully convolutional networks for intervertebral disc localization and segmentation, in: *Medical Imaging and Augmented Reality: 7th International Conference, MIAR 2016, Bern, Switzerland, August 24-26, 2016, Proceedings*, Springer International Publishing, 7, pp. 375–382, 2016.
84. Suzani, A., Seitel, A., Liu, Y., Fels, S., Rohling, R.N., Abolmaesumi, P., Fast automatic vertebrae detection and localization in pathological CT scans-A deep learning approach, in: *Medical Image Computing and Computer-Assisted Intervention–MICCAI 2015: 18th International Conference, Munich, Germany, October 5-9, 2015, Proceedings, Part III*, Springer International Publishing, 18, pp. 678–686, 2015.
85. Payer, C., Štern, D., Bischof, H., Urschler, M., Regressing heatmaps for multiple landmark localization using CNNs, in: *Medical Image Computing and Computer-Assisted Intervention–MICCAI 2016: 19th International Conference, Athens, Greece, October 17-21, 2016, Proceedings, Part II*, Springer International Publishing, 19, pp. 230–238, 2016.
86. Lootus, M., Kadir, T., Zisserman, A., Vertebrae detection and labelling in lumbar MR images, in: *Computational Methods and Clinical Applications for Spine Imaging: Proceedings of the Workshop held at the 16th International Conference on Medical Image Computing and Computer Assisted Intervention*, Nagoya, Japan, September 22-26, 2013, Springer International Publishing, pp. 219–230, 2014.
87. Yang, D., Xiong, T., Xu, D., Zhou, S.K., Xu, Z., Chen, M., Park, J., Grbic, S., Tran, T.D., Chin, S.P., Metaxas, D., Deep image-to-image recurrent network with shape basis learning for automatic vertebra labeling in large-scale 3D CT volumes, in: *Medical Image Computing and Computer Assisted Intervention- MICCAI 2017: 20th International Conference, Quebec City, QC, Canada, September 11-13, 2017, Proceedings, Part III*, Springer International Publishing, 20, pp. 498–506, 2017.
88. Thoma, M., A survey of semantic segmentation. *Computer Vision and Pattern Recognition*, 1, 1–16. arXiv preprint arXiv:1602.06541, 2016 Feb 21.
89. Romera-Paredes, B. and Torr, P.H., Recurrent instance segmentation, in: *Computer Vision–ECCV 2016: 14th European Conference, Amsterdam, The Netherlands, October 11-14, 2016, Proceedings, Part VI*, Springer International Publishing, 14, pp. 312–329, 2016.
90. Law, M.W., Tay, K., Leung, A., Garvin, G.J., Li, S., Intervertebral disc segmentation in MR images using anisotropic oriented flux. *Med. Image Anal.*, 17, 1, 43–61, 2013 Jan 1.

91. Michopoulou, S.K., Costaridou, L., Panagiotopoulos, E., Speller, R., Panayiotakis, G., Todd-Pokropek, A., Atlas-based segmentation of degenerated lumbar intervertebral discs from MR images of the spine. *IEEE Trans. Biomed. Eng.*, 56, 9, 2225–2231, 2009 Apr 14.
92. Klinder, T., Ostermann, J., Ehm, M., Franz, A., Kneser, R., Lorenz, C., Automated model-based vertebra detection, identification, and segmentation in CT images. *Med. Image Anal.*, 13, 3, 471–482, 2009 Jun 1.
93. Korez, R., Ibragimov, B., Likar, B., Pernuš, F., Vrtovec, T., Deformable model-based segmentation of intervertebral discs from MR spine images by using the SSC descriptor, in: *Computational Methods and Clinical Applications for Spine Imaging: Third International Workshop and Challenge, CSI 2015, Held in Conjunction with MICCAI 2015, Munich, Germany, October 5, 2015, Proceedings*, Springer International Publishing, 3, pp. 117–124, 2016.
94. Korez, R., Ibragimov, B., Likar, B., Pernuš, F., Vrtovec, T., Interpolation-based shape-constrained deformable model approach for segmentation of vertebrae from CT spine images, in: *Recent Advances in Computational Methods and Clinical Applications for Spine Imaging*, pp. 235–240, 2015.
95. Carballido-Gamio, J., Belongie, S.J., Majumdar, S., Normalized cuts in 3-D for spinal MRI segmentation. *IEEE Trans. Med. Imaging*, 23, 1, 36–44, 2004 Jan 7.
96. Egger, J., Kapur, T., Dukatz, T., Kolodziej, M., Zukić, D., Freisleben, B., Nimsky, C., Square-cut: A segmentation algorithm on the basis of a rectangle shape. *PLoS One*, 7, 2, e31064, 2012 Feb 21.
97. Huang, S.H., Chu, Y.H., Lai, S.H., Novak, C.L., Learning-based vertebra detection and iterative normalized-cut segmentation for spinal MRI. *IEEE Trans. Med. Imaging*, 28, 10, 1595–1605, 2009 May 26.
98. Schwarzenberg, R., Freisleben, B., Nimsky, C., Egger, J., Cube-cut: Vertebral body segmentation in MRI-data through cubic-shaped divergences. *PLoS One*, 9, 4, e93389, 2014 Apr 4.
99. Ben Ayed, I., Punithakumar, K., Garvin, G., Romano, W., Li, S., Graph cuts with invariant object-interaction priors: Application to intervertebral disc segmentation, in: *Information Processing in Medical Imaging: 22nd International Conference, IPMI 2011, Kloster Irsee, Germany, July 3-8, 2011. Proceedings*, Springer Berlin Heidelberg, 22, pp. 221–232, 2011.
100. Zheng, Y., Barbu, A., Georgescu, B., Scheuering, M., Comaniciu, D., Four-chamber heart modeling and automatic segmentation for 3-D cardiac CT volumes using marginal space learning and steerable features. *IEEE Trans. Med. Imaging*, 27, 11, 1668–1681, 2008 Aug 15.
101. Chen, H., Dou, Q., Wang, X., Qin, J., Cheng, J.C., Heng, P.A., 3D fully convolutional networks for intervertebral disc localization and segmentation, in: *Medical Imaging and Augmented Reality: 7th International Conference, MIAR 2016, Bern, Switzerland, August 24-26, 2016, Proceedings*, Springer International Publishing, 7, pp. 375–382, 2016.
102. Lessmann, N., van Ginneken, B., Išgum, I., Iterative convolutional neural networks for automatic vertebra identification and segmentation in CT images,

in: *Medical Imaging 2018: Image Processing*, vol. 10574, SPIE, pp. 39–44, 2018 Mar 2.

103. Tsai, M.D., Jou, S.B., Hsieh, M.S., A new method for lumbar herniated inter-vertebral disc diagnosis based on image analysis of transverse sections. *Comput. Med. Imaging Graphics*, 26, 6, 369–380, 2002 Dec 1.
104. Koompairojn, S., Hua, K.A., Bhadrakom, C., Automatic classification system for lumbar spine X-ray images, in: *19th IEEE Symposium on Computer-Based Medical Systems (CBMS'06)*, IEEE, pp. 213–218, 2006 Jun 22.
105. Cherukuri, M., Stanley, R.J., Long, R., Antani, S., Thoma, G., Anterior osteophyte discrimination in lumbar vertebrae using size-invariant features. *Computerized Med. Imaging Graphics*, 28, 1-2, 99–108, 2004 Jan 1.
106. A, R.S., Corso, J.J., Chaudhary, V., Dhillon, G., Desiccation diagnosis in lumbar discs from clinical MRI with a probabilistic model, in: *2009 IEEE International Symposium on Biomedical Imaging: From Nano to Macro*, IEEE, pp. 546–549, 2009 Jun 28.
107. Ghosh, S., A, R.S., Chaudhary, V., Dhillon, G., Computer-aided diagnosis for lumbar MRI using heterogeneous classifiers, in: *2011 IEEE International Symposium on Biomedical Imaging: From Nano to Macro*, IEEE, pp. 1179–1182, 2011 Mar 30.
108. Hao, S., Jiang, J., Guo, Y., Li, H., Active learning based intervertebral disk classification combining shape and texture similarities. *Neurocomputing*, 101, 252–257, 2013 Feb 4.
109. Oktay, A.B., Albayrak, N.B., Akgul, Y.S., Computer aided diagnosis of degenerative intervertebral disc diseases from lumbar MR images. *Comput. Med. Imaging Graphics*, 38, 7, 613–619, 2014 Oct 1.
110. Ruiz-España, S., Arana, E., Moratal, D., Semiautomatic computer-aided classification of degenerative lumbar spine disease in magnetic resonance imaging. *Comput. Biol. Med.*, 62, 196–205, 2015 Jul 1.
111. Castro-Mateos, I., Pozo, J.M., Lazary, A., Frangi, A.F., 2D segmentation of intervertebral discs and its degree of degeneration from T2-weighted magnetic resonance images, in: *Medical Imaging 2014: Computer-Aided Diagnosis*, vol. 9035, SPIE, pp. 310–320, 2014 Mar 20.
112. Jamaludin, A., Lootus, M., Kadir, T., Zisserman, A., Urban, J., Battié, M.C., Fairbank, J., McCall, I., Genodisc Consortium, ISSLS Prize in Bioengineering Science 2017: Automation of reading of radiological features from magnetic resonance images (MRIs) of the lumbar spine without human intervention is comparable with an expert radiologist. *Eur. Spine J.*, 26, 1374 1383, 2017 May.
113. Niemeyer, F., Galbusera, F., Tao, Y., Kienle, A., Beer, M., Wilke, H.J., A deep learning model for the accurate and reliable classification of disc degeneration based on MRI data. *Invest. Radiol.*, 56, 2, 78–85, 2021 Feb 1.
114. Ramirez, L., Durdle, N.G., Raso, V.J., Hill, D.L., A support vector machines classifier to assess the severity of idiopathic scoliosis from surface topography. *IEEE Trans. Inf. Technol. Biomed.*, 10, 1, 84–91, 2006 Jan 10.

115. Bergeron, C., Cheriet, F., Ronsky, J., Zernicke, R., Labelle, H., Prediction of anterior scoliotic spinal curve from trunk surface using support vector regression. *Eng. Appl. Artif. Intell.*, 18, 8, 973–983, 2005 Dec 1.
116. Komeili, A., Westover, L., Parent, E.C., El-Rich, M., Adeeb, S., Monitoring for idiopathic scoliosis curve progression using surface topography asymmetry analysis of the torso in adolescents. *Spine J.*, 15, 4, 743–51, 2015 Apr 1.
117. Zhang, J., Lou, E., Le, L.H., Hill, D.L., Raso, J.V., Wang, Y., Automatic Cobb measurement of scoliosis based on fuzzy Hough Transform with vertebral shape prior. *J. Digital Imaging*, 22, 463–472, 2009 Oct.
118. Sun, H., Zhen, X., Bailey, C., Rasoulinejad, P., Yin, Y., Li, S., Direct estimation of spinal cobb angles by structured multi-output regression, in: *Information Processing in Medical Imaging: 25th International Conference, IPMI 2017, Boone, NC, USA, June 25-30, 2017, Proceedings*, Springer International Publishing, Cham, pp. 529–540, 2017 May 23.
119. Zhang, J., Li, H., Lv, L., Zhang, Y., Computer-aided Cobb measurement based on automatic detection of vertebral slopes using deep neural network. *Int. J. Biomed. Imaging*, 2017, 1–7, 2017 Oct 3.
120. Wu, H., Bailey, C., Rasoulinejad, P., Li, S., Automated comprehensive adolescent idiopathic scoliosis assessment using MVC-Net. *Med. Image Anal.*, 48, 1–1, 2018 Aug 1.
121. Galbusera, F., Niemeyer, F., Wilke, H.J., Bassani, T., Casaroli, G., Anania, C., Costa, F., Brayda-Bruno, M., Sconfienza, L.M., Fully automated radiological analysis of spinal disorders and deformities: A deep learning approach. *Eur. Spine J.*, 28, 951–960, 2019 May 1.
122. Thong, W., Parent, S., Wu, J., Aubin, C.E., Labelle, H., Kadoury, S., Three-dimensional morphology study of surgical adolescent idiopathic scoliosis patient from encoded geometric models. *Eur. Spine J.*, 25, 3104–3113, 2016 Oct.
123. Burns, J.E., Yao, J., Summers, R.M., Vertebral body compression fractures and bone density: Automated detection and classification on CT images. *Radiology*, 284, 3, 788–797, 2017 Sep.
124. Roth, H.R., Wang, Y., Yao, J., Lu, L., Burns, J.E., Summers, R.M., Deep convolutional networks for automated detection of posterior-element fractures on spine CT, in: *Medical Imaging 2016: Computer-Aided Diagnosis*, vol. 9785, SPIE, pp. 165–171, 2016 Mar 24.
125. O'Connor, S.D., Yao, J., Summers, R.M., Lytic metastases in thoracolumbar spine: Computer-aided detection at CT—Preliminary study. *Radiology*, 242, 3, 811–816, 2007 Mar.
126. Burns, J.E., Yao, J., Wiese, T.S., Muñoz, H.E., Jones, E.C., Summers, R.M., Automated detection of sclerotic metastases in the thoracolumbar spine at CT. *Radiology*, 268, 1, 69–78, 2013 Jul.
127. Amarasingham, R., Patzer, R.E., Huesch, M., Nguyen, N.Q., Xie, B., Implementing electronic health care predictive analytics: Considerations and challenges. *Health Aff.*, 33, 7, 1148–1154, 2014 Jul 1.

128. Fairbank, J.C., Couper, J., Davies, J.B., O'Brien, J.P., The Oswestry low back pain disability questionnaire. *Physiotherapy*, 66, 8, 271–273, 1980 Aug 1.
129. McGirt, M.J., Sivaganesan, A., Asher, A.L., Devin, C.J., Prediction model for outcome after low-back surgery: Individualized likelihood of complication, hospital readmission, return to work, and 12-month improvement in functional disability. *Neurosurg. Focus*, 39, 6, E13, 2015 Dec 1.
130. Kim, J.S., Merrill, R.K., Arvind, V., Kaji, D., Pasik, S.D., Nwachukwu, C.C., Vargas, L., Osman, N.S., Oermann, E.K., Caridi, J.M., Cho, S.K., Examining the ability of artificial neural networks machine learning models to accurately predict complications following posterior lumbar spine fusion. *Spine*, 43, 12, 853, 2018 Jun 6.
131. Lee, M.J., Cizik, A.M., Hamilton, D., Chapman, J.R., Predicting surgical site infection after spine surgery: A validated model using a prospective surgical registry. *Spine J.*, 14, 9, 2112–2117, 2014 Sep 1.
132. Janssen, D.M., van Kuijk, S.M., d'Aumerie, B.B., Willems, P.C., External validation of a prediction model for surgical site infection after thoracolumbar spine surgery in a Western European cohort. *J. Orthop. Surg. Res.*, 13, 1–6, 2018 Dec.
133. Scheer, J.K., Smith, J.S., Schwab, F., Lafage, V., Shaffrey, C.I., Bess, S., Daniels, A.H., Hart, R.A., Protopsaltis, T.S., Mundis, G.M., Sciubba, D.M., Development of a preoperative predictive model for major complications following adult spinal deformity surgery. *J. Neurosurg.: Spine*, 26, 6, 736–743, 2017 Mar 1.
134. Durand, W.M., DePasse, J.M., Daniels, A.H., Predictive modeling for blood transfusion after adult spinal deformity surgery: A tree-based machine learning approach. *Spine*, 43, 15, 1058–66, 2018 Aug 1.
135. van Hooff, M.L., van Loon, J., van Limbeek, J., de Kleuver, M., The Nijmegen decision tool for chronic low back pain. Development of a clinical decision tool for secondary or tertiary spine care specialists. *PLoS One*, 9, 8, e104226, 2014 Aug 18.
136. Antani, S., Long, L.R., Thoma, G.R., Content-based image retrieval for large biomedical image archives, in: *MEDINFO 2004*, pp. 829–833, IOS Press, Amsterdam The Netherlands, 2004.
137. Manning, C.D., *Introduction to information retrieval*, Syngress Publishing, Waltham, Massachusetts, 2008 Oct 24.
138. Liu, R., Wang, Y., Baba, T., Masumoto, D., Nagata, S., SVM-based active feedback in image retrieval using clustering and unlabeled data. *Pattern Recognit.*, 41, 8, 2645–2655, 2008 Aug 1.
139. Rahman, M.M., Bhattacharya, P., Desai, B.C., A framework for medical image retrieval using machine learning and statistical similarity matching techniques with relevance feedback. *IEEE Trans. Inf. Technol. Biomed.*, 11, 1, 58–69, 2007 Jan 2.
140. Shah, A., Conjeti, S., Navab, N., Katouzian, A., Deeply learnt hashing forests for content based image retrieval in prostate MR images, in: *Medical Imaging 2016: Image Processing*, vol. 9784, SPIE, pp. 302–307, 2016 Mar 21.

141. Xu, X., Lee, D.J., Antani, S.K., Long, L.R., Archibald, J.K., Using relevance feedback with short-term memory for content-based spine X-ray image retrieval. *Neurocomputing*, 72, 10-12, 2259–2269, 2009 Jun 1.
142. Lee, D.J., Antani, S., Chang, Y., Gledhill, K., Long, L.R., Christensen, P., CBIR of spine X-ray images on inter-vertebral disc space and shape profiles using feature ranking and voting consensus. *Data Knowl. Eng.*, 68, 12, 1359–1369, 2009 Dec 1.
143. Chande, R.D., Hargraves, R.H., Ortiz-Robinson, N., Wayne, J.S., Predictive behavior of a computational foot/ankle model through artificial neural networks. *Comput. Math. Methods Med.*, 2017, 1–9, 2017 Jan 30.
144. Zadpoor, A.A., Campoli, G., Weinans, H., Neural network prediction of load from the morphology of trabecular bone. *Appl. Math. Model.*, 37, 7, 5260–5276, 2013 Apr 1.
145. Lu, Y., Pulasani, P.R., Derakhshani, R., Guess, T.M., Application of neural networks for the prediction of cartilage stress in a musculoskeletal system. *Biomed. Signal Process. Control*, 8, 6, 475–482, 2013 Nov 1.
146. Haddas, R. and Belanger, T., Clinical gait analysis on a patient undergoing surgical correction of kyphosis from severe ankylosing spondylitis. *Int. J. Spine Surg.*, 11, 3, 1–8, 2017 Jan 1.
147. Leardini, A., Biagi, F., Merlo, A., Belvedere, C., Benedetti, M.G., Multi-segment trunk kinematics during locomotion and elementary exercises. *Clin. Biomech.*, 26, 6, 562–571, 2011 Jul 1.
148. Prakash, C., Kumar, R., Mittal, N., Recent developments in human gait research: Parameters, approaches, applications, machine learning techniques, datasets and challenges. *Artif. Intell. Rev.*, 49, 1–40, 2018 Jan.
149. Lai, D.T., Begg, R.K., Palaniswami, M., Computational intelligence in gait research: A perspective on current applications and future challenges. *IEEE Trans. Inf. Technol. Biomed.*, 13, 5, 687–702, 2009 May 12.
150. Begg, R. and Kamruzzaman, J., A machine learning approach for automated recognition of movement patterns using basic, kinetic and kinematic gait data. *J. Biomech.*, 38, 3, 401–408, 2005 Mar 1.
151. Stucovitz, E., Vitale, J., Galbusera, F., *In vivo* measurements: Motion analysis, in: *Biomechanics of the Spine*, pp. 189–201, Academic Press, Cambridge, Massachusetts, 2018 Jan 1.
152. Hayashi, H., Toribatake, Y., Murakami, H., Yoneyama, T., Watanabe, T., Tsuchiya, H., Gait analysis using a support vector machine for lumbar spinal stenosis. *Orthopedics*, 38, 11, e959–64, 2015 Nov 1.
153. Jiang, N., Luk, K.D., Hu, Y., A machine learning-based surface electromyography topography evaluation for prognostic prediction of functional restoration rehabilitation in chronic low back pain. *Spine*, 42, 21, 1635–1642, 2017 Nov 1.
154. Heess N, T.B.D., Sriram, S., Lemmon, J., Merel, J., Wayne, G., Tassa, Y., Erez, T., Wang, Z., Eslami, S.M., Riedmiller, M., Emergence of locomotion behaviours in rich environments. *Artificial Intelligence*, 1, 1–14, arXiv preprint arXiv:1707.02286, 2017 Jul 7.

7

Osteoporosis Biomarker Identification and Use of Machine Learning in Osteoporosis Treatment

Abstract

During the process of bone remodeling, various bone biomarkers, such as those involved in formation, resorption, and regulation, are released. Over the last decade, the clinical assessment of osteoporosis treatment has focused a significant amount of attention on these bone biomarkers. The clinical applications of bone biomarkers have provided comprehensive information for the diagnosis of osteoporosis. This information is particularly useful when combined with the measurement of bone mineral density. Diseases such as osteoporosis have a significant impact on the structure of the bone, which can lead to a variety of complications, including an increased risk of breaking a bone. This chapter discusses the function that machine learning plays in the treatment of osteoporosis. Machine learning has proven to be quite useful in the investigation of a variety of issues relating to bone, such as osteoporosis and related conditions.

Keywords: Magnetic resonance imaging, trabecular bone (TB), machine learning, bone biomarker, bone formation, bone resorption, bone turnover, osteoporosis

7.1 Introduction

Osteoporosis reduces bone mass and strength, causing bone fragility and fractures globally. The World Health Organization (WHO) [1] defines osteoporosis as a decrease in hip and/or spine bone mineral density (BMD) of at least 2.5 standard deviations below that of young, healthy persons. As the global population ages, so does the number of people suffering from osteoporosis. Worldwide, osteoporosis affects 200 million people and is responsible for 8.9 million annual fractures [2]. The mortality rate from hip fractures due to osteoporosis has been steadily rising for at least 5 years [3], from 20–24% in the first year. The majority (60%) of people who recover

Rishabha Malviya, Shivam Rajput and Makarand Vaidya. Artificial Intelligence for Bone Disorder: Diagnosis and Treatment, (169–196) © 2024 Scrivener Publishing LLC

from hip fractures require assistance walking for at least a year. After a hip fracture, 33% are entirely reliant on or in a nursing home. Due to healthcare costs, osteoporosis is a public health issue. Fractures caused by osteoporosis are the main reason why older people live less long and have a lower quality of life. Osteoporosis is quiet till fracture. Early diagnosis is important for treating osteoporosis and finding people who are at a high risk. DXA measures BMD to recognize osteoporosis and figure out the risk of breaking a bone. The gold standard for measuring bone mass, the DXA BMD, only gives some information about bone strength. Osteoporosis weakens bones. Microarchitecture, microdamage, and remodeling rates determine bone fragility, which affects fracture resistance. DXA's two-dimensional approach shows its inability to distinguish cortical from cancellous bone and define bone geometry alterations. Lately, numerous methods have been developed to assess fracture risks beyond BMD. QCT can assess bone loss [4]. QCT measures trabecular bone mineral density from cortical bone [5]. Ultrasound can also tell how healthy bones are and how likely they are to break [6]. Central axial reference points are found by the first ultrasonic instrument that can look at the bone and measure its microarchitecture without using ionizing radiation (lumbar vertebrae and proximal femur). These imaging methods are not widely used or used in primary care because they are hard to use, expensive, and hard to get to. Along with imaging techniques, osteoporosis needs to be diagnosed early and accurately with other methods. This makes prevention and treatment better. The past decade has examined bone turnover biomarkers. In Figure 7.1, bone remodeling involves bone resorption and creation [7]. Bone remodeling produces creation, resorption, and turnover biomarkers. Enzymes, proteins, and byproducts during bone remodeling have been used to detect bone metabolism [8–11]. ALP, BALP, OC, P1NP, and P1CP are bone formation biomarkers (P1CP). HYP, HYL, DPD, PYD, BSP, OP, TRAP 5b, CTX-1, NTX-1, and cathepsin K are bone resorption biomarkers (CTSK). RANKL, OPG, DK-1, and sclerostin regulate bone turnover. These indicators can diagnose osteoporosis early when DXA BMD measurements are insufficient. Hence, DXA BMD measurement and bone biomarker detection can improve early osteoporosis assessment in high-risk individuals. Researchers describe the latest studies and advancements in osteoporosis biomarker detection.

Humans have two forms of bone tissue: cancellous bone and trabecular bone. The skull, pelvic bones, ribs, spinal vertebrae, and long bones have trabecular bones. Early bone loss makes the trabecular bone crucial [12]. Osteoporosis alters trabecular bone structure, increasing fracture risk. Magnetic resonance imaging (MRI) would be limited to the spine, proximal femur, and distal forearm, where trabecular substances are

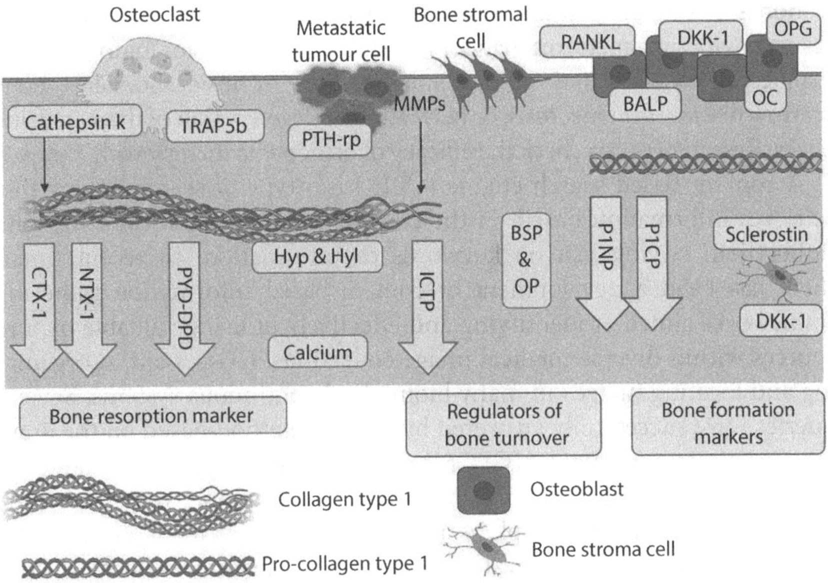

Figure 7.1 Biochemical biomarkers of bone turnover. Blue boxes/arrows indicate bone formation markers: osteocalcin (OC), bone-specific alkaline phosphatase (BALP), and propeptides of type I procollagen (P1NP and P1CP). Yellow boxes/arrows indicate resorption markers of bone: pyridinoline (PYD), carboxy-terminal crosslinked telopeptide of type 1 collagen (CTX-1), deoxypyridoline (DPD), amino-terminal crosslinked telopeptide of type 1 collagen (NTX-1), hydroxylysine (HYL), hydroxyproline (HYP), tartrate-resistant acid phosphatase 5b (TRAP 5b), bone sialoprotein (BSP), osteopontin (OP), and cathepsin K (CTSK). Green boxes indicate bone turnover regulators: receptor activator of NF-κB ligand (RANKL), dickkopf-1 (DDK-1), osteoprotegerin (OPG), and sclerostin.

concentrated. Because of higher metabolic activity, these estimates would match bone misfortune [13].

Bone mineral density is crucial to studying bone structural changes (BMD). This parameter causes trabecular bone skeletal changes [14–17] that affect bone strength. There are now MRI pictures of the trabecular bone structure with a high level of detail. Like most strong-state tissues, bone has a low number of protons and a short T2 unwinding time, which makes it look dark in an MRI [18]. Photos can be processed by a computer to get information about the structure, topology, introduction, cortical thickness, and zones of the trabecular bone system. The innovative MRI preparation used in this work demonstrates the validity and dependability of using a virtual bone biopsy to determine the trabecular architecture in a clinical environment [19]. Bone microarchitecture and structural magnetic resonance imaging reveal information about the bone's strength and susceptibility to fracture.

Bones, joints, and soft tissues like ligaments, muscles, and tendons can be scanned with a magnetic resonance image [20–25] to check for injuries, abnormalities, or diseases like tumors, inflammation, intrinsic anomalies, bone marrow disease, osteonecrosis, or herniation or degeneration of the spinal line plates. Researchers can check the efficacy of orthopedic therapy with X-rays.

A content-based search engine (CBIR) is a type of search engine that retrieves information based on the content or characteristics of the data rather than relying just on keywords or information. In recent times, there has been a development of content-based information-gathering frameworks aimed at identifying and effectively utilising valuable picture sources within diverse medical image collections. Classes aid in organizing and locating images in many biomedical continuous systems. Several queries were successfully answered by a CBIR method based on the gray-level co-occurrence matrix (GLCM), which focuses on surface characteristic abstraction and classification using a multi-support vector machine (SVM). Unfortunately, simple searches were equally inadequate. Using content-based image retrieval and multi-level feature extraction [26], researchers were able to better organize and sort through digital images. In the first stage, biological images were divided into two categories using support vector machines. The K closest neighbor (KNN) technique was employed in the second stage to further classify the images that SVM had already separated into their respective categories. Once again, this approach supported multiple queries. Two classifiers at two levels made this method more efficient. The study did not discuss image recovery performance. Two categorization levels optimized picture retrieval in research. This method is unsuitable for single-image queries. Researchers compared biological MRI classification outcomes using K closest neighbor and SVM classifier techniques. SVM outperformed KNN in categorizing MRIs into eight distinct groups [18]. Researchers used BPNN to identify MRI images and extract texture patterns using the wavelet transform [27]. This categorization hybrid worked well. A study suggested categorizing biological MRI scans as normal or aberrant. Classifiers compared these categories. SVM outperforms ANN [28].

7.2 Biomarkers of Bone Development

7.2.1 Total Alkaline Phosphatase

One of the enzymes necessary for healthy cellular metabolism is called blood alkaline phosphatase. The numerous alkaline phosphatases (ALPs) can degrade human proteins. ALPs are mostly made in the liver, while small amounts are also made in the bones, intestines, and kidneys. Alkaline phosphatase enzyme levels in the blood are used to get a read on total ALP. Whole ALP testing is a common element of standard blood work because it requires only a small amount of blood. The average amount of ALP in the body varies greatly depending on factors like age, gender, blood type, and pregnancy. Abnormally high levels of alanine aminotransferase (ALP) in the blood may be a sign of a problem with the gallbladder, liver, or bones. To diagnose conditions including osteomalacia, rickets, and Paget's disease, an ALP test is typically used. The ALP level is another method that can be used to evaluate the success of treatment in the previously mentioned scenarios. Patients with osteoporosis and inflammatory bowel illness have had their serum ALP measured using a conventional Technicon Autoanalyzer [29]. Bone mineral density in the spine has been found to correlate highly with total serum ALP. Recent research [30] found that a blood total ALP activity of more than 129 U/L is diagnostic of osteoporosis in men. Total ALP levels were found to decrease from 79.7 U/L to 64.8 U/L after therapy with alendronate [31]. The results provide credence to total ALP as a surrogate for osteoporosis drug efficacy, yet due to the slight variation and wide-ranging total ALP, postmenopausal women may be given a false diagnosis of osteoporosis.

7.2.2 Bone-Specific Alkaline Phosphatase

In persons with healthy livers, bone marrow contributes roughly 50% of the serum ALP total. Since the main difference between bone ALP and liver ALP isoenzymes is their degree of posttranslational glycosylation, distinguishing between the two can be challenging. Methods for determining bone-specific alkaline phosphatase (BALP) concentrations include, but are not limited to, agarose electrophoresis, wheat germ agglutinin precipitation, heat and chemical inactivation, immunoradiometric test, wheat germ agglutinin-high performance liquid chromatography as well as enzyme immunoassay [32–40]. Agarose electrophoresis is one of the most common techniques. The enzyme immunoassay has a detection limit of 0.7 U/L, and the average levels of BALP in men are 24.9 ± 7.0 U/L, whereas the average levels of BALP in premenopausal women are 19.7 ±5.6 U/L [41]. It was discovered that women over the age of 59 who suffer from osteoporosis had a BALP activity that is 66.4 ± 8.7 U/L [42]. Because BALP is a biomarker of osteoblastic activity, it is utilized to help in the diagnosis of osteoporosis in both premenopausal and postmenopausal females.

7.2.3 Osteocalcin

The protein osteocalcin (OC), which is also referred to as bone gamma-carboxy glutamic acid-containing protein, is only made up of 49 different amino acids. It is the mature odontoblasts, osteoblasts, and hypertrophic chondrocytes that are responsible for the production of OC. In addition to this, OC is the non-collagenous protein that is found in greatest abundance in bone and accounts for approximately 2% of the total protein found in the human body. OC, which is produced by osteoblasts, contributes to the management of metabolic processes, the homeostasis of calcium ions, and the mineralization of bone [43]. During therapy for osteoporosis with bone formation medicines, increasing BMD has been related to increased serum OC levels. In cases of osteoporosis, serum OC has been evaluated as a potential indication of osteoblast function to determine the rate of bone production. According to the findings of several research, osteocalcin is an essential biomarker for determining how the medication influences bone formation—for instance, in postmenopausal women, supplementation with RNAse-enriched LF has demonstrated a promising and beneficial impact as measured by a change in OC from baseline (7.2 ± 2.8%; [44]). Additionally, postmenopausal women with osteoporosis have significantly higher mean osteocalcin levels than women without the condition (16.16 versus 11.26 ng/mL; [45]). The benefits of using osteocalcin as a biomarker of bone development include its selectivity for bone tissue, its accessibility, and its low variability. The bone remodeling indicator serum oxycarboxy-cysteine may be helpful in the identification of osteoporosis and the estimate of fracture risk in the elderly, particularly in women.

7.2.4 Procollagen Type 1 N-Terminal Propeptide

Collagen type 1 (C1) is synthesized from procollagen type 1 (P1) and makes up the bulk of the organic bone matrix. Bone cells (osteoblasts) and connective tissue cells (fibroblasts) produce type 1 procollagen. Before type 1 procollagen can be transformed into collagen, it must undergo cleavage at the N- and C-termini by specific proteases. The bone matrix is then conjugated with type 1 procollagen (P1CP and P1NP). Scientific investigations into biomarkers have revealed that P1NP is remarkably sensitive to the presence of type 1 collagen deposition in bone. During the process of producing type 1 collagen, P1NP is released into the intracellular space and eventually reaches the bloodstream. The trimeric structure of P1NP (which is derived from the trimeric structure of collagen) is the form in which it is typically released; nevertheless, it is rapidly degraded to the monomeric form due to thermal degradation processes. Trimeric P1NP can be detected with either an enzyme-linked immunosorbent assay (ELISA) or a radioimmunoassay using antibodies that recognize individual subunits of the protein. The mean total P1NP value in post-menopausal women with osteoporosis is 54.1 g/L, which is 74% greater than that of healthy premenopausal women aged 35 and above (29.2 g/L) [46]. Researchers have shown that P1NP is a more sensitive bone biomarker for gauging the rate of bone growth in osteoporosis. Current efforts are focused on refining a more accurate method of testing P1NP for clinical usage.

7.2.5 Procollagen Type 1 C-Terminal Propeptide

Protein 1 carbohydrate-binding protein (P1CP) is a 115-kDa protein with a mannose-rich carbohydrate side chain added post-translationally. The serum half-life for PICP is only 6–8 min because it is quickly removed from the bloodstream via mannose receptor-mediated clearance in the liver [47]. Recently, the serum biomarker P1CP has been used to assess the effect of female sex hormones and nandrolone decanoate on bone growth. Women who have broken their backs had lower initial concentrations of PICP (97 ± 23 ng/mL) than those whose arms have been broken (116 ± 27 ng/mL) [48]. Specific immunoassays are currently used to test for P1NP and P1CP. Nonetheless, P1NP has been studied more thoroughly as a biomarker for type 1 procollagen analysis than P1CP has. Several studies [49] have found that serum P1CP levels correlate positively with bone development velocity.

7.3 Biomarkers for Bone Resorption

7.3.1 Hydroxyproline

After proline has been translated, it undergoes hydroxylation to produce hydroxyproline (HYP), an amino acid. Somewhere between 12% and 14% of collagen's amino acids come from HYP. Around 90% of HYP is released during the destruction of bone collagen, and the liver is the primary site of HYP metabolism afterward [50]. Women with osteoporosis after menopause have a higher HYP level in their urine than postmenopausal women without osteoporosis [51]. An increased urine hydroxyproline (HYP) concentration is indicative of a heightened rate of collagen type I degradation in the bone matrix in women with osteoporosis. While most of the HYP is made from reabsorbed collagen, about 10% is made from procollagen peptides that are formed when bones expand. As a byproduct of the breakdown of elastin as well as C1Q [52], HYP can be found in the blood, but it is also present in the skin and cartilage. Hence, HYP is regarded as a nonspecific biomarker of collagen turnover and bone resorption. More sensitive and specific biomarkers have replaced HYP in the diagnosis of osteoporosis [53].

7.3.2 Hydroxylysine

Lysine is hydroxylated to produce the amino acid hydroxylysine (HYL). There are numerous HYL variations, including glucosylgalactosyl hydroxylysine (GGHYL) and galactosyl hydroxylysine (GHYL) [54]. Degradation of collagen causes the release of GHYL and GGHYL into the bloodstream. Because it is produced exclusively during bone resorption, GHYL is a more accurate biomarker of bone health, yet the C1Q complement molecule and skin contain GGHYL. This means that of GHYL, GGHYL, and HYP, GHYL is the preferred biomarker for measuring bone resorption. By evaluating the amounts of GHYL in postmenopausal women's urine, researchers [55] were able to compare the fracture risk in postmenopausal women who had or did not have osteoporosis. Raised levels of urinary GHYL in those who have fractures suggest that it can be used to indicate a deficit in bone collagen. GHYL evaluation through high-performance liquid chromatography (HPLC) [56] further eliminates the need for preanalytical hydrolysis and extraction. Although GHYL has shown promise as a biomarker of bone resorption, it has not been extensively studied for its usefulness in the diagnosis of osteoporosis or the evaluation of therapeutic effects. Due to the lack of simple routine procedures for measuring GHYL, its clinical applicability remains restricted.

7.3.3 Deoxypyridinoline

The chemical deoxypyridinoline (DPD) cross-links separate collagen peptides, which mechanically stabilizes collagen [57]. Bone resorption involves the proteolytic breakdown of cross-linked collagens, which results in the release of DPD into the bloodstream and subsequent excretion via urine. DPD is predominantly localized in skeletal tissues, particularly bone and dentin. As a result, DPD is a useful biomarker for tracking the breakdown of bone. As DPD is discharged in the urine in two forms, a free form (40%) and a peptide-bound form (60%), previous research has hydrolyzed and extracted DPD in preparation for HPLC analysis. The HPLC measurement is improved by releasing the peptide from its binding. DPD measurement through HPLC has some limitations, including a complex method and unpredictable recovery. Urinary-free DPD can now be directly detected using an enzyme immunoassay or an automated chemiluminescence immunoassay. Results from the HPLC analysis of free DPD in urine have been demonstrated to agree with those from chemiluminescence immunoassay and enzyme immunoassay investigations [58, 59]. Patients with bone pathology, such as metabolic bone disease, can now be monitored with the help of immunoassay techniques that allow for the detection of free DPD in their urine.

7.3.4 Pyridinoline

Pyridinoline (PYD) collagen crosslinks are produced in the extracellular matrix during the maturation of fibrillar collagens and are subsequently distributed throughout the body as these collagens are degraded. HPLC [60] analysis demonstrates that both the free and conjugated forms of the PYD are chemically stable over extended periods. However, PYD is widely distributed throughout the body's vascular, connective, and skeletal systems. Thus, compared to DPD, PYD is a less accurate measure of bone resorption.

7.3.5 Bone Sialoprotein

According to its molecular weight (60–80 kDa), bone sialoprotein (BSP) is a phosphorylated glycoprotein [61]. There are a variety of mineralized tissues that contain BSP, including bone, cementum, dentin, and calcified cartilage. Bone morphogenetic protein (BSP) is a crucial component of the bone extracellular matrix. About 8% of the proteins in bone and cementum are not collagen, and this has been demonstrated [62]. All three types of bone cells (osteoblasts, odontoblasts, and osteoclasts) contribute to the production of BSP. Hence, BSP is believed to have a significant role in both cell adhesion to the matrix and the bone resorption process mediated by osteoclasts. Many researchers have developed immunoassays for serum BSP measurement. If the investigator compares the serum BSP levels of 90 healthy people with those of those with Paget illness, the investigator finds that the former has a mean value of 12.1 ± 5.0 g/L (measured by radioimmunoassay), while the latter has a mean value of 32.3 ± 17.3 g/L [63]. The osteoporosis patients' serum BSP levels were observed to correlate strongly with BALP and OC [64]. The bone resorption biomarker BSP has shown promising results and may be used in the diagnosis and monitoring of osteoporosis.

7.3.6 Osteopontin

Alternate macrophages, cells, specialized epithelial cells, activated T lymphocytes, and bone cells all create a phosphorylated glycoprotein termed osteopontin (OP) [65]. By comparing women with high OP levels to those with normal OP levels, postmenopausal osteoporosis resistance was determined to be poorer in the former group [66]. The effectiveness of intermittent parathyroid hormone in the management of postmenopausal osteoporosis in women might be measured by monitoring the OP levels in the blood.

7.3.7 Tartrate-Resistant Acid Phosphatase 5b

Osteoclasts are responsible for secreting tartrate-resistant acid phosphatase 5b (TRAP 5b) during the bone resorption process [67]. As a result, TRAP 5b is used to evaluate osteoclast numbers and activity. Hydrolyzed TRAP 5b is then eliminated from the body via the kidneys after being destroyed in the liver. Immunoassays allow for the highly accurate detection of the TRAP 5b protein in blood. In the past, serum TRAP 5b was used to determine whether a patient with breast cancer had minimal or significant bone metastases [68]. In addition, serum TRAP 5b has been utilized as a marker of alendronate treatment efficacy [69]. The TRAP 5b bone resorption biomarker has been studied a lot and compared to other bone biomarkers. It has shown good specificity and high sensitivity.

7.3.8 Carboxy-Terminal Crosslinked Telopeptide of Type 1 Collagen

Telopeptides of type 1 collagen, especially carboxy-terminal crosslinked (CTX-1) and aminoterminal crosslinked (ACTX-1), are used as biomarkers for bone resorption (NTX-1). Collagen degradation results in the release of both CTX-1 and NTX-1. To measure CTX-1 concentrations, a monoclonal antibody specific for an octapeptide sequence (EKAHD—GGR) in the -1 (I) chain of the -isoform is employed in conjunction with an ELISA test. According to recent research [70], CTX-1 is a sensitive and specific biomarker of bone resorption in postmenopausal women, allowing for quick assessment of the effect of bisphosphonate treatment. In contrast, the amount of food a person eats has a significant impact on their serum CTX-1 levels; hence, blood must be drawn while the individual is fasting.

7.3.9 Amino-Terminal Crosslinked Telopeptide of Type 1 Collagen

In most cases, amino-terminal crosslinked telopeptide of type 1 collagen (NTX-1) is assessed with an ELISA using a urine sample, and it can be detected in the urine for up to 24 h when kept at room temperature. Biomarkers of bone resorption, like NTX-1 in the urine, have been used to figure out how likely it is that a postmenopausal woman will break a bone [71]. Because of these variables, urine NTX-1 is a more reliable biomarker than serum CTX-1.

7.4 Regulators of Bone Turnover

7.4.1 Receptor Activator of NF-κB Ligand

Receptor activator of NF-κB ligand (RANKL) and OPG are made by osteoblasts to control how osteoclasts change and grow as part of the remodeling process. Activation of NF-B signaling by RANKL is inhibited by dextromethorphan, according to recent *in vitro* studies. This prevents osteoclastogenesis and bone loss. Oral dextromethorphan supplementation has been shown to ameliorate ovary-removal-induced osteoporosis [72]. The severity of metabolic bone disorders can be gauged in humans by measuring their serum levels of RANKL [73]. There is still much to learn about the clinical utility of serum RANKL despite extensive research into its application for predicting fracture risk and evaluating the efficacy of osteoporosis medications.

7.4.2 Osteoprotegerin

Osteoprotegerin (OPG) is usually thought of as a soluble receptor that is secreted. It is made by many different types of cells and tissues, including osteoblasts. OPG acts as a fake receptor for RANKL and stops the formation of new bone cells [74]. Osteopetrosis is caused by either overexpressing OPG in transgenic mouse models or by delivering OPG to normal mice, as shown by research in mice [75]. This is evident in the OPG mutant mouse, which develops severe osteoporosis. In addition to serum and plasma, OPG can also be evaluated in plasma EDTA and heparin samples. Commercially available sandwich ELISA techniques use monoclonal capture antibodies and polyclonal detection antibodies, but more research needs to be done before serum OPG can be used in the clinic as a biomarker to measure how active bone disease is.

7.4.3 Dickkopf-1

Wnt signaling is stopped by dickkopf-1 (DDK-1) and sclerostin, which are also used as biomarkers for bone remodeling. Osteoblasts make DKK-1, which then gets into the bloodstream. The amount of DDK-1 in the blood shows that bone formation is being stopped. Anastrozole reduced DKK-1 levels in breast cancer patients from 34.3 pmol/L at the start of treatment to 29.7 pmol/L at the end of treatment (over 24 months) [76]. Femoral neck and hip BMD have both been shown to be correlated with DKK-1. More long-term research is needed to figure out how the regulator DKK-1 can be used in the clinic as a biomarker to measure osteoporosis.

7.4.4 Sclerostin

When sclerostin is present, the Wnt pathway is turned down, which stops osteoblasts from differentiating. Osteocytes are what make sclerostin. Sclerostin is released into the bloodstream, and the amount of sclerostin in the serum shows how much bone formation is stopped. Patients suffering from breast cancer who took anastrozole for 24 months saw their serum sclerostin levels rise from 29.5 pmol/L at the beginning of the research to 43.2 pmol/L by the conclusion [77]. However, additional clinical trials are required before sclerostin may be employed as a biomarker of bone turnover.

7.5 Methods to Identify Osteoporosis

7.5.1 Two Sequences MRI

Bone properties were compared between two MRI sequences in the study by researchers. While comparing the FSE sequence to the GE sequence using the Wilcoxon rank-sum test, it was discovered that the median parameter value was lower for the FSE series [78]. The tiny-scale engineering and mechanical hardness of trabecular bone presented new avenues for exploring image handling and reconstruction. With the help of artificial intelligence methods, they analyzed the morphological, topological, and mechanical highlights of bone. Two populations' joint and osteoporotic bone samples are included in a clinical report. Support vector machines and genetic algorithms are two examples of the kinds of instances that have been used to group the unique ones that have been considered in displays of adaptive neuro-fuzzy inference systems (ANFIS). The results show that the highest possible percentage of division is achieved using the genetic algorithm (GA). The various aspects of trabecular bone were examined employing finite element analysis (FEA) and hybrid skeleton graph analysis (HSGA) [79].

7.5.2 Trabecular Bio-Mechanical Strength

Researchers [80] employed MRI to determine the biomechanical strength of trabecular bone. Machine learning was utilized to extract features from datasets collected from knee joints to establish the geometry of trabecular bone. There were 67 trabecular bone cubes extracted from the knees, and their mechanical and symmetry characteristics were approximated using the scaling index technique (SIM). It was discovered that SIM improved MRI's capacity to show bone quality. The yield stress was used to evaluate the trabecular bone's strength (YS). For each bone cube sample, the researcher employed both the singular value decomposition (SVM) and the bone volume fraction (BVF) feature estimate methods to compute the retrieved features. The yield strength of the bones was calculated by analyzing these features using linear multi-regression analysis and support vector regression (SVR) [81].

7.5.3 Bone Strength MRI

Researchers investigated whether MRI and DXA increase bone strength research. DXA measured bone mass while MRI assessed cortical and trabecular bone structure. Thirty-eight formal infixed human bodies yielded lower arms [82]. X-ray absorptiometry measured distal BMC and BMD. High-goal MRIs calculated distal sweep cortical and trabecular auxiliary proportions. It was determined that the measured values for cortical thickness and cross-sectional area were within the normal range. Morphometric and surface features of trabeculae were used to create approximations. Biomechanical testing of bone quality in the lower arms was performed using a simulated fall (disappointment stack). Patients were stratified according to weight, age, span length, and normal sweep cross-section territory to maintain consistent bone quality [83]. Using 1.5 T and 3.0 T MRI on the distal radius, researchers [84] looked at the reproducibility of structural errors in trabecular bone. The range of root mean square reproducibility errors was 0.69–4.94% at 1.5 T and 0.38–5.80% at 3.0 T. Based on the results of the investigation, the discrepancies between the two distal radii in terms of trabecular bone were within acceptable bounds and were practically equal. The consistency of MRI for measuring proximal femur strength was investigated. Microstructure analysis of the femur was performed using 3 T images. The elastic modulus of the neck and the femur were calculated. With MRI, doctors can rely on consistent findings. Two measurements of bone architecture (proximal femur stiffness and femoral neck elastic modulus) are presented in the study, together with their respective mean values, intra- and inter-day root mean square coefficients of variation (RMS-CV), as well as ICCs with 95% confidence intervals [85].

The intricate structure of bone makes the computerized diagnosis of illnesses like osteoporosis difficult. DXA is typically utilized for such a diagnosis. The large size, high cost, and limited accessibility of diagnostic equipment limit this technique. Programming X-beam pictures is their method. After measuring and editing the X-ray image of the skeletal system, researchers were able to remove skewed factual highlights from several requests. These bone characteristics were categorized by machine learning algorithms as either indicative of osteoporosis or bone health. Several feature extraction methods were used in this research: ANNs, SVMs, KNNs, and naive Bayes.

The findings are both specific and surprising. The results of a support vector machine (classifier) applied to an X-ray of a bone show 98% accuracy rate in determining whether or not the patient has osteoporosis. The proposed method's low temporal complexity [86] is well-suited to continuous applications. Since 3D bone morphological qualities can be seen in cone-beam computed tomography (CBCT) images, it was proposed to conduct research into creating and approving a computerized grouping technique that can identify the trabecular bone example at the embed location [87]. This study created and verified a programmed technique to help with bone quality grouping at the embed site, with its basis in the three-dimensional architecture of trabecular bone. Oral radiologists assessed emotional states and compared PC-based characterization productivity [88].

Researchers suggested examining trabecular boundness with digital hip radiography. This method detects disorders including osteoporosis and low BMD. The SVM method was used on digital hip radiographs to identify reduced bone mineral density [89]. This study assessed trabecular bone disease risk using SVM-based CAD. Trabecular bone alignment, spur stiffness, delta, and boundness were investigated.

7.5.4 Radial Bias Function

The Radial bias function was also utilized for the classification process (RBF). The reliability of the results in this study can be attributed to the implementation of a five-fold cross-validation analysis. Hence, it was suggested that a computer-assisted diagnostic based on support vector machines (SVM) would be the most reliable way to assess an individual's susceptibility to developing osteoporosis. The Wilcoxon rank test was used to analyze the effectiveness of trabecular bone features. Researchers [90] studied the capabilities of MR imaging to detect trabecular bone structure. The research also confirmed that MRI provides sufficient information and is suitable for evaluating trabecular characteristics.

7.5.5 Otsu Threshold Method

Otsu threshold analysis was utilized to model trabecular bone in a computer simulation [90]. The evaluation applies a bone division calculation based on the Otsu edge technique to images recorded with a variety of objectives to choose one that is both high enough for a thorough first inspection and short enough for patients to develop within an acceptable length of time. Ten samples of the distal femoral condyle were scanned in a Bruker Bio-Spec RI scanner operating at 4.7 T. Researchers did this using an iso-cubic voxel dataset with several different sizes in a 3D firm big-angle spin-echo device (65, 130, 160, 196, 230, and 260 mm). The following assumptions are held throughout the research: Conventional measures of bone include trabecular thickness at specific sites and structural bone characteristics. According to the results of this study, pictures up to 230 mm in length [85] appear to have captured the various skeletal properties accurately.

High-resolution MRI and computerized image analysis methods were used in a study to examine the trabecular bone structure in three dimensions [91]. Samples of human vertebrae, femurs, and calcaneus are measured and analyzed for anisotropy and connectivity in this study. The research set out to discover evidence for the following:

The computer results corroborate the MRI predictions for trabecular bone structure and alignment alterations [92].

When considering three-dimensional structural characteristics and bone mineral density, the fabric tensor formulation simplifies the calculation of the modulus of elasticity.

The three-dimensional structural characteristics obtained from MRI and bone mineral density facilitate the prediction of stiffness using multiple regression methods. The results were similarly consistent with those obtained utilizing high-resolution MR trabecular images, the study demonstrated [91].

Incredibly, a study found that measuring BMD is a common method for identifying people with trabecular illnesses like osteoporosis, yet the quantity of bone and the qualities associated with bone quality determine its quality. In the past few years, there have been a lot of improvements to MRI methods for checking the health of bones. This study looked at the professional standards, clinical applications, new developments, limitations, and future trends of MRI methods that can be used to diagnose trabecular disorders [93]. The condition of one's skeleton can be determined with an MRI scan. It is feasible to use either high-resolution imaging or T2* measurements, both of which are sensitive to changes in stiffness at the bone-substance interfaces. Bone loss and breakdown patterns are useful indicators of trabecular bone structure and composition in T2* estimates. T2* measurements have been taken of the proximal femur, spine, and calcaneus, all of which are located at the center and periphery of the skeleton, respectively. Moreover, it has been demonstrated that T2* rot characteristics can be used to distinguish between osteoporotic and normal patients. High-resolution MR imaging can be utilized to examine trabecular bone formation in addition to T2* measures. The skeleton has been imaged in vitro and in vivo using angle resound and turn reverberate systems, with a focus on the edges. Several image-processing techniques have been utilized to determine skeletal anatomy. Recent advances in the mechanical capabilities of MRI scanners hold great promise for advancing the understanding of trabecular disorders and other bone diseases.

7.5.6 FDT-Based Techniques

Trabecular bone thickness in low-goal scenario procedures was assessed using FDT in a study published by [94]. The investigators have analyzed the strategy's repeatability as well as its capacity to image voxel size, rotation, and noise. Throughout a wide variety of purposes and endeavors, the thickness values have been consistently observed to remain unchanged (biological data transfer from computed tomography to magnetic resonance imaging). An alternative technique for determining trabecular bone thickness was demonstrated in this study, and it is dubbed the "fluffy separation change" (FDT). With this kind of computation, it would be possible to manage images recorded at a voxel estimate equivalent to the average thickness of trabecular bone. CT scans of human trabecular bone that have been reexamined at progressively lower resolutions and after applying rotation and increasing noise to simulate the in vivo condition suggest that the method is effective. By comparing the histograms of thickness inside and between fascinating clusters, CT images illustrate the reproducibility of the system. On the other hand, MRI volume educational files of frequently scanned human volunteers indicate the system's ability to train. Finally, the new technology can be utilized to measure a short-term treatment that produces trabecular shrinking [95, 96] as seen by Vivo-MR images from previous research on corticosteroids and rabbits. As part of a larger examination of multi-modal data recovery for medical imaging, a method for the automatic classification and recovery of medical pictures utilizing a combination of textual and graphical queries is analyzed.

The whole thing was planned and carried out with the help of an open-source, expandable medical imaging history program. Also, the study investigated the potential applications of audiovisual data recovery in medical imaging as well as a practical application of this combination in actual PACS settings. The effort to achieve this aim, by the way, is far from complete. The powerful precision of image recovery in the framework depends on how well the image recovery methods are connected and how well they are chosen and evaluated. In future work, there will be a full look at how the plan works in terms of recovery. Classification database and suggested classifier will both have free, independent commitments [97] after the purposeful enhancements and evaluation methodologies are finalized.

7.5.7 3D Micro-MR Imaging

Bone mineral thickness was measured half a year after a kidney transplant, and the results were compared to the mechanical changes in trabecular bone and cortical bone that occurred before the transplant [98]. Computational biomechanics using 3D micro-MR imaging was used for this purpose. At 6 months after the study began, trabecular bone structural characteristics were significantly lower than they were at baseline (2 weeks after the renal transplantation). Micro-limited component analysis using MRI data reveals that distal tibial strength and quality decline during 6 months following kidney transplantation [99].

According to one study, noninvasive biomechanical levels of interest in the context of osteoporosis can be measured with the help of material science-based models employing limited component analysis (LCE), yet the computational complexity of such models prevents their routine application in the medical arena. In this prototype, researchers show how a deep learning model based on a convolutional neural system (CNN) algorithm can be used as an alternative to material science-based methodologies for normal strain prediction. This model was constructed utilizing a massive library of synthetic cancellous bone living structures. The objective properties of the model are determined with the aid of the FEA display. When evaluating the quality of the built model, the investigator compared its results to those of material science-based calculations for an alternative test record. Beh and Altman found no significant bias in the link between in-depth knowledge and material science-based predictions [100]. The previously displayed SVM show, which relied on meticulously crafted highlights, fared worse than the CNN algorithm shows. As a result, the average execution time was reduced by a factor of several times relative to the scientific calculations, and the average strain was monitored continuously.

7.5.8 Fractal and GLCM Features

As evidenced by their study, [101] While processing photos, fractal analysis is incredibly helpful because it reveals the shape and grayscale issues. The study authors recommended combining GLCM characteristics with box counts. By using these powerful tools, investigators were able to better understand the medicinal texture of trabecular bones from MRI and CT scan images. Because of this, diagnostic procedures for osteoporosis-related conditions are improved. Using SVM, the author classifies MATLAB with an accuracy of 85.71%.

7.5.9 Fourier Transforms and Neural Networks

In one study, the researchers show a new way to use a computer to analyze the structure of trabecular (or cancellous) bone. Using a Fourier transformation, this method turns an image into a scary fingerprint. After the Fourier change's main segments are looked at to pick out the most important parts, the data are sent to a neural system for sorting. About 90% of the patient trabecular bone histology sections were properly classified when this was examined, with an average group achieving an accuracy of 77–84%. This simple yet effective method of detecting skeletal alterations has shown promising results in preliminary studies [102, 103].

7.5.10 Geometric Features and Support Vector Regression

The researchers elaborate on the application of SVM and supervised learning to enhance trabecular bone quality via MR imaging. Mean square error and SIM employs two fundamental strategies for producing accurate predictions [80].

The researchers found that RMSE = 1.021 MPa was the best prediction result when using SVR in conjunction with a combination of BVF and SIM characteristics. The accuracy of predictions was better when only SIM features and SVR were used and the RMSE was 1.023 Mpa instead of 1.073 Mpa when BVF was used alone.

7.5.11 Dixon Magnetic Resonance Images

The researchers of a study [104] describe how DIXON MRI can be utilized to enhance the precision of thigh composition analysis. In this part, the researcher uses these algorithms to look at the data: (a) four pictures that are different from each other, (b) a picture of water and fat, and (c) no editing or filtering software was used to take pictures of 190 different people [105].

7.5.12 MRI-Based Three-Dimension

There were 353 "control knees" and 178 "case knees" in the study. The biggest influence came from the joint's three-dimensional bone form vector, which included the tibia, femur, and patella. Radiographic knee OA was 3.0 times more likely in the highest tertile than in the lowest tertile one year later (95% CI: 1.8–5.0, $P < 0.0001$) [106–111]. Much stronger relationships were found in knees that had undergone routine radiographic examination before the event.

7.6 Conclusion

This chapter explained several investigations and developments that have been made for the applications of bone biomarkers in the assessments of bone-related diseases. Bone biomarkers have demonstrated a high potential to serve as powerful indicators for evaluating the treatment of osteoporosis and even to aid in the clinical diagnosis of osteoporosis in its early stages. This potential has been shown to exist. Overall, it is possible to conclude that bone biomarkers have a significant amount of potential in the identification of osteoporosis and that treatment based on machine learning is the most effective method for curing osteoporosis.

References

1. Genant, H.K., Cooper, C., Poor, G., Reid, I., Ehrlich, G., Kanis, J., Nordin, B.C., Barrett-Connor, E., Black, D., Bonjour, J.P., Dawson-Hughes, B., Interim report and recommendations of the World Health Organization task-force for osteoporosis. *Osteoporosis Int.*, 10, 4, 259, 1999 Sep 1.
2. Pisani, P., Renna, M.D., Conversano, F., Casciaro, E., Di Paola, M., Quarta, E., Muratore, M., Casciaro, S., Major osteoporotic fragility fractures: Risk factor updates and societal impact. *World J. Orthop.*, 7, 3, 171, 2016 Mar 3.

3. Leibson, C.L., Tosteson, A.N., Gabriel, S.E., Ransom, J.E., Melton III, L.J., Mortality, disability, and nursing home use for persons with and without hip fracture: A population-based study. *J. Am. Geriatr. Soc.*, 50, 10, 1644–1650, 2002 Oct.
4. Adams, J.E., Radiogrammetry and radiographic absorptiometry. *Radiol. Clin.*, 48, 3, 531–540, 2010 May 1.
5. Alexeeva, L., Burkhardt, P., Christiansen, C., Cooper, C., Delmas, P., Johnell, O., Johnston, C., Kanis, J.A., Lips, P., Melton, L.J., Meunier, P., Assessment of fracture risk and its application to screening for postmenopausal osteoporos. Technical Report Series, World Health Organization, Geneva, pp. (843):1–29, 1994.
6. Conversano, F., Franchini, R., Greco, A., Soloperto, G., Chiriacò, F., Casciaro, E., Aventaggiato, M., Renna, M.D., Pisani, P., Di Paola, M., Grimaldi, A., A novel ultrasound methodology for estimating spine mineral density. *Ultrasound Med. Biol.*, 41, 1, 281–300, 2015 Jan 1.
7. Ferreira, A., Alho, I., Casimiro, S., Costa, L., Bone remodeling markers and bone metastases: From cancer research to clinical implications. *BoneKEy Rep.*, 4, 1–9, 2015.
8. Shi, X., Li, C., Liang, B., He, K., Li, X., Weak cation magnetic separation technology and MALDI-TOF-MS in screening serum protein markers in primary type I osteoporosis. *Genet. Mol. Res.*, 14, 4, 15285–15294, 2014.
9. He, W.T., Liang, B.C., Shi, Z.Y., Li, X.Y., Li, C.W., Shi, X.L., Weak cation exchange magnetic beads coupled with matrix-assisted laser desorption ionization-time of flight-mass spectrometry in screening serum protein markers in osteopenia. *Springerplus*, 5, 1–9, 2016 Dec.
10. Liu, L. and Webster, T.J., *In situ* sensor advancements for osteoporosis prevention, diagnosis, and treatment. *Curr. Osteoporos. Rep.*, 14, 386–395, 2016 Dec.
11. Delmas, P.D., Committee of Scientific Advisers of the International Osteoporosis Foundation. The use of biochemical markers of bone turnover in osteoporosis. *Osteoporos. Int.*, 11, 6, S2–17, 2000.
12. Li, C.Q., Magland, J.F., Rajapakse, C.S., Guo, X.E., Zhang, X.H., Vasilic, B., Wehrli, F.W., Implications of resolution and noise for *in vivo* micro-MRI of trabecular bone. *Med. Phys.*, 35, 12, 5584–5594, 2008 Dec.
13. Krug, R., Burghardt, A.J., Majumdar, S., Link, T.M., High-resolution imaging techniques for the assessment of osteoporosis. *Radiol. Clin.*, 48, 3, 601–621, 2010 May 1.
14. Amin, B., Shahzad, A., Farina, L., Parle, E., McNamara, L., O'Halloran, M., Elahi, M.A., Dielectric characterization of diseased human trabecular bones at microwave frequency. *Med. Eng. Phys.*, 78, 21–28, 2020 Apr 1.
15. Guedes, P.M., Zamarioli, A., Botega, I.I., Silva, R.A., Issa, J.P., Butezloff, M.M., Sousa, Y.T., Ximenez, J.P., Volpon, J.B., Undernutrition impairs the quality of growth plate and trabecular and cortical bones in growing rats. *Acta cir. Bras.*, 34, 1–13, 2019 Mar 18.

16. Londoño-Restrepo, S.M., Ramirez-Gutierrez, C.F., Villarraga-Gómez, H., Rodriguez-García, M.E., Study of microstructural, structural, mechanical, and vibrational properties of defatted trabecular bovine bones: Natural sponges, in: *Materials for Biomedical Engineering*, pp. 441–485, Elsevier, Amsterdam, The Netherlands, 2019 Jan 1.
17. Fernandez-Martinez, M., Gomez Garcia, F.J., Sánchez, Y.G., Jornet, P.L., An intelligent system to study the fractal dimension of trabecular bones. *J. Intell. Fuzzy Syst.*, 35, 4, 4533–4540, 2018 Jan 1.
18. Domínguez-Rodrigo, M., Successful classification of experimental bone surface modifications (BSM) through machine learning algorithms: A solution to the controversial use of BSM in paleoanthropology? *Archaeol. Anthropol. Sci.*, 11, 6, 2711–2725, 2019 Jun 1.
19. Lew, M.S., Sebe, N., Djeraba, C., Jain, R., Content-based multimedia information retrieval: State of the art and challenges. *ACM Trans. Multimed. Comput. Commun. Appl. (TOMM).*, 2, 1, 1–9, 2006 Feb 1.
20. Erickson, B.J., Korfiatis, P., Akkus, Z., Kline, T.L., Machine learning for medical imaging. *Radiographics*, 37, 2, 505–515, 2017 Mar.
21. Giger, M.L., AI/machine learning in medical imaging, in: *Molecular Imaging*, pp. 1691–1702, Academic Press, Cambridge, Massachusetts, USA, 2021 Jan 1.
22. Wernick, M.N., Yang, Y., Brankov, J.G., Yourganov, G., Strother, S.C., Machine learning in medical imaging. *IEEE Signal Process. Mag.*, 27, 4, 25–38, 2010 Jun 14.
23. Willemink, M.J., Koszek, W.A., Hardell, C., Wu, J., Fleischmann, D., Harvey, H., Folio, L.R., Summers, R.M., Rubin, D.L., Lungren, M.P., Preparing medical imaging data for machine learning. *Radiology*, 295, 1, 4–15, 2020 Apr.
24. Oakden-Rayner, L., Dunnmon, J., Carneiro, G., Ré, C., Hidden stratification causes clinically meaningful failures in machine learning for medical imaging, in: *Proceedings of the ACM Conference on Health, Inference, and Learning*, pp. 151–159, 2020 Apr 2.
25. Currie, G., Hawk, K.E., Rohren, E., Vial, A., Klein, R., Machine learning and deep learning in medical imaging: Intelligent imaging. *J. Med. Imaging Radiat. Sci.*, 50, 4, 477–487, 2019 Dec 1.
26. Newitt, D.C., Van Rietbergen, B., Majumdar, S., Processing and analysis of *in vivo* high-resolution MR images of trabecular bone for longitudinal studies: Reproducibility of structural measures and micro-finite element analysis derived mechanical properties. *Osteoporos. Int.*, 13, 278–287, 2002 Apr.
27. Cesar, R., Bravo-Castillero, J., Ramos, R.R., Pereira, C.A., Zanin, H., Rollo, J.M., Relating mechanical properties of vertebral trabecular bones to osteoporosis. *Comput. Methods Biomech. BioMed. Eng.*, 23, 2, 54–68, 2020 Jan 25.
28. Kalbkhani, H., Shayesteh, M.G., Zali-Vargahan, B., Robust algorithm for brain magnetic resonance image (MRI) classification based on GARCH variances series. *Biomed. Signal Process. Control*, 8, 6, 909–919, 2013 Nov 1.

29. Compston, J., Osteoporosis in inflammatory bowel disease. *Gut*, 52, 1, 63–64, 2003 Jan 1.
30. Fink, H.A., Litwack-Harrison, S., Taylor, B.C., Bauer, D.C., Orwoll, E.S., Lee, C.G., Barrett-Connor, E., Schousboe, J.T., Kado, D.M., Garimella, P.S., Ensrud, K.E., Clinical utility of routine laboratory testing to identify possible secondary causes in older men with osteoporosis: The osteoporotic fractures in men (MrOS) Study. *Osteoporos. Int.*, 27, 331–338, 2016 Jan.
31. Kyd, P.A., De Vooght, K., Kerkhoff, F., Thomas, E., Fairney, A., Clinical usefulness of bone alkaline phosphatase in osteoporosis. *Ann. Clin. Biochem.*, 35, 6, 717–725, 1998 Nov.
32. PetitClerc, C., Quantitative fractionation of alkaline phosphatase isoenzymes according to their thermostability. *Clin. Chem.*, 22, 1, 42–8, 1976 Jan 1.
33. Štěpán, J., Volek, V., Kolář, J., A modified inactivation-inhibition method for determining the serum activity of alkaline phosphatase isoenzymes. *Clin. Chim. Acta*, 69, 1, 1–9, 1976 May 17.
34. Whitaker, K.B., Whitby, L.G., Moss, D.W., Activities of bone and liver alkaline phosphatases in serum in health and disease. *Clin. Chim. Acta*, 80, 1, 209–219, 1977 Oct 1.
35. Behr, W. and Barnert, J., Quantification of bone alkaline phosphatase in serum by precipitation with wheat-germ lectin: A simplified method and its clinical plausibility. *Clin. Chem.*, 32, 10, 1960–6, 1986 Oct 1.
36. Schreiber, W.E. and Whitta, L., Alkaline phosphatase isoenzymes resolved by electrophoresis on lectin-containing agarose gel. *Clin. Chem.*, 32, 8, 1570–1573, 1986 Aug 1.
37. Van Hoof, V.O., Lepoutre, L.G., Hoylaerts, M.F., Chevigne, R., De Broe, M.E., Improved agarose electrophoretic method for separating alkaline phosphatase isoenzymes in serum. *Clin. Chem.*, 34, 9, 1857–1862, 1988 Sep 1.
38. Gonchoroff, D.G., Branum, E.L., Cedel, S.L., Riggs, B.L., O'Brien, J.F., Clinical evaluation of high-performance affinity chromatography for the separation of bone and liver alkaline phosphatase isoenzymes. *Clin. Chim. Acta*, 199, 43–50, 1991.
39. Crofton, P.M., Wheat-germ lectin affinity electrophoresis for alkaline phosphatase isoforms in children: Age-dependent reference ranges and changes in liver and bone disease. *Clin. Chem.*, 38, 5, 663–670, 1992 May 1.
40. Day, A.P., Saward, S., Royle, C.M., Mayne, P.D., Evaluation of two new methods for routine measurement of alkaline phosphatase isoenzymes. *J. Clin. Pathol.*, 45, 1, 68–71, 1992 Jan 1.
41. Gomez, Jr. B., Ardakani, S., Ju, J., Jenkins, D., Cerelli, M.J., Daniloff, G.Y., Kung, V.T., Monoclonal antibody assay for measuring bone-specific alkaline phosphatase activity in serum. *Clin. Chem.*, 41, 11, 1560–1566, 1995 Nov 1.
42. Lumachi, F., Ermani, M., Camozzi, V., Tombolan, V., Luisetto, G., Changes of bone formation markers osteocalcin and bone-specific alkaline phosphatase

in postmenopausal women with osteoporosis. *Ann. N. Y. Acad. Sci.*, 1173, E60–3, 2009 Sep.
43. Lee, N.K., Sowa, H., Hinoi, E., Ferron, M., Ahn, J.D., Confavreux, C., Dacquin, R., Mee, P.J., McKee, M.D., Jung, D.Y., Zhang, Z., Endocrine regulation of energy metabolism by the skeleton. *Cell*, 130, 3, 456–469, 2007 Aug 10.
44. Bharadwaj, S., Naidu, A.G., Betageri, G.V., Prasadarao, N.V., Naidu, A.S., Milk ribonuclease-enriched lactoferrin induces positive effects on bone turnover markers in postmenopausal women. *Osteoporos. Int.*, 20, 1603–1611, 2009 Sep.
45. Singh, S., Kumar, D., Lal, A.K., Serum osteocalcin as a diagnostic biomarker for primary osteoporosis in women. *J. Clin. Diagn. Res.: JCDR*, 9, 8, RC04, 2015 Aug.
46. Garnero, P., Vergnaud, P., Hoyle, N., Evaluation of a fully automated serum assay for total N-terminal propeptide of type I collagen in postmenopausal osteoporosis. *Clin. Chem.*, 54, 1, 188–196, 2008 Jan 1.
47. Smedsrød, B., Melkko, J., Risteli, L., Risteli, J., Circulating C-terminal propeptide of type I procollagen is cleared mainly via the mannose receptor in liver endothelial cells. *Biochem. J.*, 271, 2, 345–350, 1990 Oct 15.
48. Hassager, C., Jensen, L.T., Johansen, J.S., Riis, B.J., Melkko, J., Pødenphant, J., Risteli, L., Christiansen, C., Risteli, J., The carboxy-terminal propeptide of type I procollagen in serum as a marker of bone formation: The effect of nandrolone decanoate and female sex hormones. *Metabolism*, 40, 2, 205–208, 1991 Feb 1.
49. Eriksen, E.F., Charles, P., Melsen, F., Mosekilde, L., Risteli, L., Risteli, J., Serum markers of type I collagen formation and degradation in metabolic bone disease: Correlation with bone histomorphometry. *J. Bone Miner. Res.*, 8, 2, 127–132, 1993 Feb.
50. Lowry, M., Hall, D.E., Brosnan, J.T., Hydroxyproline metabolism by the rat kidney: Distribution of renal enzymes of hydroxyproline catabolism and renal conversion of hydroxyproline to glycine and serine. *Metabolism*, 34, 10, 955–961, 1985 Oct 1.
51. Jagtap, V.R. and Ganu, J.V., Effect of antiresorptive therapy on urinary hydroxyproline in postmenopausal osteoporosis. *Indian J. Clin. Biochem.*, 27, 1, 90–93, 2012 Jan.
52. Prockop, D.J., Kivirikko, K.I., Tuderman, L., Guzman, N.A., The biosynthesis of collagen and its disorders. *N. Engl. J. Med.*, 301, 2, 77–85, 1979 Jul 12.
53. Delmas, P.D., Eastell, R., Garnero, P., Seibel, M.J., Stepan, J., Committee of Scientific Advisors of the International Osteoporosis Foundation, The use of biochemical markers of bone turnover in osteoporosis. *Osteoporos. Int.*, 11, 6, S2, 2000 Dec 1.
54. Cunningham, L.W., Ford, J.D., Segrest, J.P., The isolation of identical hydroxylysyl glycosides from hydrolysates of soluble collagen and from human urine. *J. Biol. Chem.*, 242, 10, 2570–2571, 1967 May 25.

55. Cascio, V.L., Bertoldo, F., Gambaro, G., Gasperi, E., Furlan, F., Colapietro, F., Cascio, C.L., Campagnola, M., Urinary galactosyl-hydroxylysine in post-menopausal osteoporotic women: A potential marker of bone fragility. *J. Bone Miner. Res.*, 14, 8, 1420–1424, 1999 Aug.
56. Bettica, P., Baylink, D.J., Moro, L., Galactosyl hydroxylysine and deoxypyridinoline: A methodological comparison. *Clinical Chemistry and Laboratory Medicine (CCLM)*, 31, 459–466, 1993.
57. Seibel, M.J., Biochemical markers of bone turnover part I: Biochemistry and variability. *Clin. Biochem. Rev./Australian Assoc. Clin. Biochemists.*, 26, 4, 97, 2005 Nov.
58. Seyedin, S.M., Kung, V.T., Daniloff, Y.N., Hesley, R.P., Gomez, B., Nielsen, L.A., Rosen, H.N., Zuk, R.F., Immunoassay for urinary pyridinoline: The new marker of bone resorption. *J. Bone Miner. Res.*, 8, 5, 635–641, 1993 May.
59. Rosano, T.G., Peaston, R.T., Bone, H.G., Woitge, H.W., Francis, R.M., Seibel, M.J., Urinary free deoxypyridinoline by chemiluminescence immunoassay: Analytical and clinical evaluation. *Clin. Chem.*, 44, 10, 2126–2132, 1998 Oct 1.
60. Gerrits, M.I., Thijssen, J.H., Van Rijn, H.J., Determination of pyridinoline and deoxypyridinoline in urine, with special attention to retaining their stability. *Clin. Chem.*, 41, 4, 571–574, 1995 Apr 1.
61. Fisher, L.W., Whitson, S.W., Avioli, L.V., Termine, J.D., Matrix sialoprotein of developing bone. *J. Biol. Chem.*, 258, 20, 12723–7, 1983 Oct 25.
62. Fisher, L.W., McBride, O.W., Termine, J.D., Young, M.F., Human bone sialoprotein. Deduced protein sequence and chromosomal localization. *J. Biol. Chem.*, 265, 4, 2347–2351, 1990 Feb 5.
63. Karmatschek, M., Maier, I., Seibel, M.J., Woitge, H.W., Ziegler, R., Armbruster, F.P., Improved purification of human bone sialoprotein and development of a homologous radioimmunoassay. *Clin. Chem.*, 43, 11, 2076–2082, 1997 Nov 1.
64. Fassbender, W.J., Ruf, T., Kaiser, H.E., Stracke, H., Serum levels of immunoreactive bone sialoprotein in osteoporosis: Positive relations to established biochemical parameters of bone turnover. *In Vivo (Athens, Greece)*, 14, 5, 619–624, 2000 Sep 1.
65. Zhang, Q., Wrana, J.L., Sodek, J., Characterization of the promoter region of the porcine opn (osteopontin, secreted phosphoprotein 1) gene: Identification of positive and negative regulatory elements and a 'silent'second promoter. *Eur. J. Biochem.*, 207, 2, 649–659, 1992 Jul.
66. Chiang, T.I., Chang, I.C., Lee, H.S., Lee, H., Huang, C.H., Cheng, Y.W., Osteopontin regulates anabolic effect in human menopausal osteoporosis with intermittent parathyroid hormone treatment. *Osteoporos. Int.*, 22, 577–585, 2011 Feb.
67. Vaananen, H.K., Zhao, H., Mulari, M., Halleen, J.M., The cell biology of osteoclast function. *J. Cell Sci.*, 113, 3, 377–381, 2000 Feb 1.
68. Chao, T.Y., Yu, J.C., Ku, C.H., Chen, M.M., Lee, S.H., Janckila, A.J., Yam, L.T., Tartrate-resistant acid phosphatase 5b is a useful serum marker for extensive

bone metastasis in breast cancer patients. *Clin. Cancer Res.*, 11, 2, 544–550, 2005 Jan 15.
69. Nenonen, A., Cheng, S., Ivaska, K.K., Alatalo, S.L., Lehtimäki, T., Schmidt-Gayk, H., Uusi-Rasi, K., Heinonen, A., Kannus, P., Sievänen, H., Vuori, I., Serum TRACP 5b is a useful marker for monitoring alendronate treatment: Comparison with other markers of bone turnover. *J. Bone Miner. Res.*, 20, 10, 1804–1812, 2005 Oct.
70. Baim, S. and Miller, P.D., Perspective: Assessing the clinical utility of serum CTX in postmenopausal osteoporosis and its use in predicting risk of osteonecrosis of the jaw. *J. Bone Miner. Res.*, 24, 4, 561–574, 2009 Apr.
71. Christgau, S., Circadian variation in serum CrossLaps concentration is reduced in fasting individuals. *Clin. Chem.*, 46, 3, 431, 2000 Mar 1.
72. Wu, K., Lin, T.H., Liou, H.C., Lu, D.H., Chen, Y.R., Fu, W.M., Yang, R.S., Dextromethorphan inhibits osteoclast differentiation by suppressing RANKL-induced nuclear factor-κB activation. *Osteoporos. Int.*, 24, 2201–2214, 2013 Aug.
73. Rogers, A. and Eastell, R., Circulating osteoprotegerin and receptor activator for nuclear factor κB ligand: Clinical utility in metabolic bone disease assessment. *J. Clin. Endocrinol. Metab.*, 90, 11, 6323–31, 2005 Nov 1.
74. Yasuda, H., Shima, N., Nakagawa, N., Yamaguchi, K., Kinosaki, M., Mochizuki, S.I., Tomoyasu, A., Yano, K., Goto, M., Murakami, A., Tsuda, E., Osteoclast differentiation factor is a ligand for osteoprotegerin/osteoclastogenesis-inhibitory factor and is identical to TRANCE/RANKL. *Proc. Natl. Acad. Sci.*, 95, 7, 3597–602, 1998 Mar 31.
75. Yasuda, H., Shima, N., Nakagawa, N., Mochizuki, S.I., Yano, K., Fujise, N., Sato, Y., Goto, M., Yamaguchi, K., Kuriyama, M., Kanno, T., Identity of osteoclastogenesis inhibitory factor (OCIF) and osteoprotegerin (OPG): A mechanism by which OPG/OCIF inhibits osteoclastogenesis *in vitro*. *Endocrinology*, 139, 3, 1329–1337, 1998 Mar 1.
76. Kyvernitakis, I., Rachner, T.D., Urbschat, A., Hars, O., Hofbauer, L.C., Hadji, P., Effect of aromatase inhibition on serum levels of sclerostin and dickkopf-1, bone turnover markers and bone mineral density in women with breast cancer. *J. Cancer Res. Clin. Oncol.*, 140, 1671–1680, 2014 Oct.
77. Anastasilakis, A.D., Polyzos, S.A., Gkiomisi, A., Bisbinas, I., Gerou, S., Makras, P., Comparative effect of zoledronic acid versus denosumab on serum sclerostin and dickkopf-1 levels of naive postmenopausal women with low bone mass: A randomized, head-to-head clinical trial. *J. Clin. Endocrinol. Metab.*, 98, 8, 3206–3212, 2013 Aug 1.
78. West, S.L., Rajapakse, C.S., Rayner, T., Miller, R., Slinger, M.A., Wells, G.D., The reproducibility of measuring trabecular bone parameters using a commercially available high-resolution magnetic resonance imaging approach: A pilot study. *Bone Rep.*, 8, 180–186, 2018 Jun 1.

79. Akgundogdu, A., Jennane, R., Aufort, G., Benhamou, C.L., Ucan, O.N., 3D image analysis and artificial intelligence for bone disease classification. *J. Med. Syst.*, 34, 815–828, 2010 Oct.
80. Huber, M.B., Lancianese, S.L., Nagarajan, M.B., Ikpot, I.Z., Lerner, A.L., Wismuller, A., Prediction of biomechanical properties of trabecular bone in MR images with geometric features and support vector regression. *IEEE Trans. Biomed. Eng.*, 58, 6, 1820–1826, 2011 Feb 28.
81. Yang, C.C., Nagarajan, M.B., Huber, M.B., Carballido-Gamio, J., Bauer, J.S., Baum, T., Eckstein, F., Lochmüller, E., Majumdar, S., Link, T.M., Wismüller, A., Improving bone strength prediction in human proximal femur specimens through geometrical characterization of trabecular bone microarchitecture and support vector regression. *J. Electron. Imaging*, 23, 1, 013013, 2014 Jan 1.
82. Baum, T., Kutscher, M., Müller, D., Räth, C., Eckstein, F., Lochmüller, E.M., Rummeny, E.J., Link, T.M., Bauer, J.S., Cortical and trabecular bone structure analysis at the distal radius—Prediction of biomechanical strength by DXA and MRI. *J. Bone Miner. Metab.*, 31, 212–221, 2013 Mar.
83. Wu, C.T., Chang, H.T., Wu, C.Y., Chen, S.W., Huang, S.Y., Huang, M., Pan, Y.T., Bradbury, P., Chou, J., Yen, H.W., Machine learning recommends affordable new Ti alloy with bone-like modulus. *Mater. Today*, 34, 41–50, 2020 Apr 1.
84. Baum, T., Dütsch, Y., Müller, D., Monetti, R., Sidorenko, I., Räth, C., Rummeny, E.J., Link, T.M., Bauer, J.S., Reproducibility of trabecular bone structure measurements of the distal radius at 1.5 and 3.0 T magnetic resonance imaging. *J. Comput. Assisted Tomogr.*, 36, 5, 623–626, 2012 Sep 1.
85. Chang, G., Hotca-Cho, A., Rusinek, H., Honig, S., Mikheev, A., Egol, K., Regatte, R.R., Rajapakse, C.S., Measurement reproducibility of magnetic resonance imaging-based finite element analysis of proximal femur microarchitecture for *in vivo* assessment of bone strength. *Magn. Reson. Mater. Phys. Biol. Med.*, 28, 407–412, 2015 Aug.
86. Singh, A., Dutta, M.K., Jennane, R., Lespessailles, E., Classification of the trabecular bone structure of osteoporotic patients using machine vision. *Comput. Biol. Med.*, 91, 148–158, 2017 Dec 1.
87. Shrivastava, D., Sanyal, S., Maji, A.K., Kandar, D., Bone cancer detection using machine learning techniques, in: *Smart Healthcare for Disease Diagnosis and Prevention*, pp. 175–183, Academic Press, Cambridge, Massachusetts, USA, 2020 Jan 1.
88. Nicolielo, L.F., Van Dessel, J., Van Lenthe, G.H., Lambrichts, I., Jacobs, R., Computer-based automatic classification of trabecular bone pattern can assist radiographic bone quality assessment at dental implant site. *Brit. J. Radiol.*, 91, 1092, 20180437, 2018 Dec.
89. Sapthagirivasan, V. and Anburajan, M., Diagnosis of osteoporosis by extraction of trabecular features from hip radiographs using support vector machine: An investigation panorama with DXA. *Comput. Biol. Med.*, 43, 11, 1910–1919, 2013 Nov 1.

90. Kim, N., Lee, J.G., Song, Y., Kim, H.J., S. Yeom, J., Cho, G., Evaluation of MRI resolution affecting trabecular bone parameters: Determination of acceptable resolution. *Magn. Reson. Med.*, 67, 1, 218–225, 2012 Jan.
91. Majumdar, S., Kothari, M., Augat, P., Newitt, D.C., Link, T.M., Lin, J.C., Lang, T., Lu, Y., Genant, H.K., High-resolution magnetic resonance imaging: Three-dimensional trabecular bone architecture and biomechanical properties. *Bone*, 22, 5, 445–454, 1998 May 1.
92. Majumdar, S., Genant, H.K., Grampp, S., Newitt, D.C., Truong, V.H., Lin, J.C., Mathur, A., Correlation of trabecular bone structure with age, bone mineral density, and osteoporotic status: *In vivo* studies in the distal radius using high resolution magnetic resonance imaging. *J. Bone Miner. Res.*, 12, 1, 111–118, 1997 Jan.
93. Petrantonaki, M., Maris, T., Damilakis, J., MRI techniques for the examination of trabecular bone structure. *Curr. Med. Imaging*, 1, 1, 35–41, 2005 Jan 1.
94. Saha, P.K. and Wehrli, F.W., Measurement of trabecular bone thickness in the limited resolution regime of *in vivo* MRI by fuzzy distance transform. *IEEE Trans. Med. Imaging*, 23, 1, 53–62, 2004 Jan 7.
95. Laib, A., Newitt, D.C., Lu, Y., Majumdar, S., New model-independent measures of trabecular bone structure applied to *in vivo* high-resolution MR images. *Osteoporos. Int.*, 13, 130–136, 2002 Feb.
96. Gitto, S., Cuocolo, R., Albano, D., Chianca, V., Messina, C., Gambino, A., Ugga, L., Cortese, M.C., Lazzara, A., Ricci, D., Spairani, R., MRI radiomics-based machine-learning classification of bone chondrosarcoma. *Eur. J. Radiol.*, 128, 109043, 2020 Jul 1.
97. Pinho, E. and Costa, C., Extensible architecture for multimodal information retrieval in medical imaging archives, in: *2016 12th International Conference on Signal-Image Technology & Internet-Based Systems (SITIS)*, IEEE, pp. 316–322, 2016 Nov 28.
98. Depeursinge, A., Foncubierta-Rodriguez, A., Van De Ville, D., Müller, H., Three-dimensional solid texture analysis in biomedical imaging: Review and opportunities. *Med. Image Anal.*, 18, 1, 176–196, 2014 Jan 1.
99. Rajapakse, C.S., Leonard, M.B., Bhagat, Y.A., Sun, W., Magland, J.F., Wehrli, F.W., Micro–MR imaging–based computational biomechanics demonstrates reduction in cortical and trabecular bone strength after renal transplantation. *Radiology*, 262, 3, 912–920, 2012 Mar.
100. Ciuşdel, C.F., Vizitiu, A., Moldoveanu, F., Suciu, C., Itu, L.M., Towards deep learning based estimation of fracture risk in osteoporosis patients, in: *2017 40th International Conference on Telecommunications and Signal Processing (TSP)*, IEEE, pp. 659–665, 2017 Jul 5.
101. Korchiyne, R., Farssi, S.M., Sbihi, A., Touahni, R., Alaoui, M.T., A combined method of fractal and GLCM features for MRI and CT scan images classification. *Computer Vision and Pattern Recognition*, 5, 1–13, arXiv preprint arXiv:1409.4559, 2014 Sep 16.

102. Gregory, J.S., Junold, R.M., Undrill, P.E., Aspen, R.M., Analysis of trabecular bone structure using Fourier transforms and neural networks. *IEEE Trans. Inf. Technol. Biomed.*, 3, 4, 289–294, 1999 Dec.
103. Díaz-Galiano, M.C., Martín-Valdivia, M.T., Montejo-Ráez, A., Ureña-López, L.A., Improving performance of medical images retrieval by combining textual and visual information, in: *2007 Sixth Mexican International Conference on Artificial Intelligence, Special Session (MICAI)*, IEEE, pp. 185–192, 2007 Nov 4.
104. Yang, Y.X., Chong, M.S., Tay, L., Yew, S., Yeo, A., Tan, C.H., Automated assessment of thigh composition using machine learning for Dixon magnetic resonance images. *Magn. Reson. Mater. Phys., Biol. Med.*, 29, 723–731, 2016 Oct.
105. Ma, J., Dixon techniques for water and fat imaging. *J. Magn. Reson. Imaging: An Official Journal of the International Society for Magnetic Resonance in Medicine*, 28, 3, 543–558, 2008 Sep.
106. Neogi, T., Bowes, M.A., Niu, J., De Souza, K.M., Vincent, G.R., Goggins, J., Zhang, Y., Felson, D.T., Magnetic resonance imaging-based three-dimensional bone shape of the knee predicts onset of knee osteoarthritis: Data from the Osteoarthritis Initiative. *Arthritis Rheumatol.*, 65, 8, 2048–2058, 2013 Aug.
107. Eckstein, F., Cicuttini, F., Raynauld, J.P., Waterton, J.C., Peterfy, C., Magnetic resonance imaging (MRI) of articular cartilage in knee osteoarthritis (OA): Morphological assessment. *Osteoarthr. Cartil.*, 14, 46–75, 2006 Jan 1.
108. Genant, H.K. and Jiang, J.Y., Imaging assessment of bone quality in osteoporosis. *Clin. Rev. Bone Miner. Metab.*, 4, 213–224, 2006 Sep.
109. Roberts, M.G., Graham, J., Devlin, H., Image texture in dental panoramic radiographs as a potential biomarker of osteoporosis. *IEEE Trans. Biomed. Eng.*, 60, 9, 2384–2392, 2013 Apr 4.
110. Kavitha, M.S., Asano, A., Taguchi, A., Kurita, T., Sanada, M., Diagnosis of osteoporosis from dental panoramic radiographs using the support vector machine method in a computer-aided system. *BMC Med. Imaging*, 12, 1, 1–1, 2012.
111. Gaidel, A.V., Matched polynomial features for the analysis of grayscale biomedical images. *Comput. Opt.*, 40, 2, 232–239, 2016.

8

The Role of AI in Pediatric Orthopedics

Abstract
Artificial intelligence (AI) is becoming increasingly appealing to the healthcare sector to streamline operations, improve efficiency, and reduce costs. With the strong performance statistics and diagnostic accuracies acquired by applying AI algorithms, many AI-based applications have been proposed for clinical radiography, especially for improved picture interpretation (about set reference standards). Recently, AI has shown a lot of potential for enhancing medical care in pediatric care. Accurate diagnosis, imaging, and therapy planning are all made possible by machine learning algorithms. Improvements in patient care and rapid administration made possible by modern computing and digital software have substantially boosted people's standard of living. This chapter's objective is to provide readers with a conceptual basis for understanding how cutting-edge AI-driven technology is influencing pediatric orthopedics.

Keywords: Artificial intelligence, machine learning, algorithms, BoneView, BoneXpert, 3D computed tomography, magnetic resonance imaging

8.1 Introduction

From its inception decades ago, artificial intelligence (AI) has undergone rapid development and seen widespread use across many fields. The field of AI deals with the development of computer systems capable of doing activities that were previously thought to require human intelligence. In tandem with the growth of the healthcare industry's information and data infrastructure, the value and potential of artificial intelligence have increased greatly [1]. Research into AI is being performed in a wide variety of medical disciplines, and it offers significant potential in enhancing practice efficiency, personalizing patient management, and enhancing research capacity. The field of artificial intelligence known as machine learning (ML) is distinguished by its reliance on algorithmic computations that evolve and grow through exposure to new data. The two primary categories of

Rishabha Malviya, Shivam Rajput and Makarand Vaidya. Artificial Intelligence for Bone Disorder: Diagnosis and Treatment, (197–218) © 2024 Scrivener Publishing LLC

ML are unsupervised and supervised. With the help of labeled patient data, supervised ML may make predictions about a patient's health. In unsupervised ML, the algorithm is not given any instructions and instead learns to find patterns by looking for commonalities in the data [2]. While ML algorithms can improve with experience, they still require human supervision. The term "deep learning" (DL) is used to describe a specific type of machine learning in which a model is built with an artificial neural network structure that is meant to simulate the human brain's neural connections [3]. Deep learning algorithms rely heavily on neural networks for their functionality.

The term "artificial neural network" (ANN) refers to a group of algorithms that attempt to simulate the way the human brain works. Deep neural networks (DNNs) are neural networks with more than three layers (not counting inputs and outputs) [4]. Because of its superior performance, convolutional neural network (CNN) is the most popular form of computer vision-assisted deep learning. Convolutional layers, a pooling layer, and a fully linked layer make up this network's several stacked layers [5].

AI tools that are employed in healthcare comprise clinical decision support systems, mobile health apps, voice assistants, robots, and sensor-based and sensor-led technology. Clinical decision support systems, often known as CDSS, are designed to provide medical professionals with assistance when faced with challenging decision-making scenarios. Today, EHRs are the norm for handling these types of records [6]. Timely information concerning a patient's care is made available through clinical decision support. It has the potential to enhance the standard of care provided to patients [7]. Artificial intelligence approaches have greatly benefited the entire medical imaging process, from data collection and analysis to interpretation. Robotic procedures that incorporate AI are used to enhance the efficiency with which an illness or condition is treated and managed. The primary goal of the ongoing research and development in the field of AI is to assist medical professionals and provide breakthroughs in quality-of-care services based on previous experiences. One example of this would be the ability to predict the course of a clinical state by searching large-scale databases [8].

The treatment of children is the primary emphasis of pediatric orthopedics, which is a subspecialty of the field of orthopedics. Diagnosis and treatment in pediatric orthopedics are complicated by the fact that a child's bones are still young and developing. In recent years, AI and digital medicine (DM) have introduced novel approaches to pediatric orthopedics. It paves the way for the development of personalized and intelligent pediatric orthopedics, vastly enhancing the efficacy of diagnostic and treatment outcomes in a variety of areas, such as, but not limited to, supplementary disease diagnosis, the guidance of postoperative rehabilitation, auxiliary optimization of surgery, etc. A further significant use of AI is in determining how old a person is based on their skeleton [9]. Similarly, AI has several

Table 8.1 Illustration of a patient's step-wise journey from hospitalization through the radiology report and subsequent care and description on how AI techniques may improve clinical practice and the patient's experience.

Step 1	Patient presentation and referrals	Clinical decision support Best imaging modality for investigation Generating differential diagnosis
Step 2	Examination booking	Availability of specialist imaging lists Linkage to outpatient clinic referrals Better prediction of resource allocation, accurate examination timings, and the chance of missed appointments Send scan preparation details before attendance
Step 3	Image acquisition	Reduction in scanning times, radiation dosage, virtual non-contrast studies, improved image quality through artifact reduction
Step 4	Post-processing	Artifact removal Automated labeling
Step 5	Quantitative analysis	Segmentation of organs and tumor lesions Lesion volume, joint angle calculation, bone age measurement, signal intensity of pathologies
Step 6	Interpretation	Detection of abnormalities Classification of abnormalities Diagnostic interference (e.g., tissue subtype)
Step 7	Reporting	Workflow prioritization, hanging protocols Automated documentation Multimedia reporting Automated summarization of key findings
Step 8	Communicate results	Link notes and exam results to smartphone health applications Automated actioning
Step 9	Future management	Prognostication Suggest follow-up according to guidelines

benefits in tertiary surgery. It may move around the operating room for the convenience of the doctors, and its precision can significantly lessen the likelihood of surgical error without compromising the procedure's success rate or its overall impact. It is not uncommon for surgeons doing pediatric orthopedic surgery to be faced with a last-minute emergency that requires swift action. Yet sometimes it is hard for surgeons to make accurate judgments, whether because of age or other considerations. At present, AI can aid in the diagnosis and management of intraoperative crises [10].

Artificial intelligence is typically implemented to make previously difficult or expensive human tasks easier or cheaper to accomplish. However, due to a lack of knowledge and expertise in the field, many experts worry that AI will threaten their employment. As many different lung diseases share identical symptoms and diagnostic criteria, experts, for example, need to comprehend the AI mechanism. The complete process of an AI-based process in the medical setting is explained in Table 8.1.

8.2 Strategy Based on Artificial Intelligence

8.2.1 Image Acquisition and Post-Processing

Since the beginning, the primary focus of research into magnetic resonance imaging (MRI) and computed tomography (CT) has been on reducing the amount of time required to acquire an image, lowering the amount of radiation that patients are required to be exposed to, and improving image quality (by reducing noise as well as motion and metal artifacts). In the past, hardware solutions (such as increasing the number of detectors for multi-detector CT scanners) were used to achieve these goals. Moreover, by utilizing AI-supported deep learning techniques, scan times [11] and, in some cases, the requirements for intravenous contrast [12] are being lowered.

8.2.1.1 Quality of MRI Images and Scans

Faster MRI scans would reduce the need for general anesthetic and related risks in pediatric imaging [13], allow more studies to be conducted daily, and assist in minimizing motion artifacts created by a less cooperative child. Researchers will be able to interpolate missing data in future unobserved investigations if they train a neural network to recognize the similarities between zero-filled k-space data as well as fully sampled k-space data for a specific type of research [14]. This will allow the researchers to complete unobserved investigations (e.g., in adult brain imaging). It is claimed that, compared to conventional (compressed sensing) picture reconstruction approaches, this method can remove artifacts from photos five times faster by utilizing deep learning. However, it is essential to perform adequate testing on such tools before implementing them regularly in clinical settings. This is because such tools may result in blurring or the elimination of discoveries that would not have been visible on the initial photographs that served as the "ground truth."

Improved MRI quality is also possible through post-processing methods. Computer-aided identification, texture analysis, feature extraction, segmentation, and subtraction were used in one study to remove the "ghost" artifact from diffusion tensor imaging of pediatric spinal MRIs [15]. This resulted in 84% accuracy rate in distinguishing genuine cords from artifacts.

8.2.1.2 Improved CT Images and Lower Radiation Exposure

Reconstructing high-quality images from reduced amounts of raw data is yet another way that AI-based algorithms can be used to lower the amount of radiation exposure that patients receive from CT scans without sacrificing image quality. This is possible because AI models can be trained to utilize examples of normal and abnormal diseases recorded at low and standard radiation dosages. After training, the models can then have their ability to extrapolate "standard-dose" photos from noisy, low-dose photographs of "unseen" occurrences tested [16]. With the use of an AI model that has been trained on examples of low-dose CT artifacts, the quality of additional low-dose CT images can be enhanced without requiring a higher radiation dose [17].

Researchers [18] were able to successfully demonstrate 31% decrease in picture noise in pediatric imaging by training a neural network to generate iteratively rebuilt CT images from the filtered back-projection data of low-dose abdominal CTs. Radiologists showed a preference for AI-reconstructed images. This was accomplished by training the neural network to produce iteratively rebuilt CT images from the data of low-dose abdominal CTs (than the iteratively reconstructed images). Diagnostic imaging in children can thus be accomplished with lower doses by using AI algorithms in non-specialist centers, and CT doses can be further reduced in specialty centers. There have been very few other studies that have been published on this subject specifically for children; nevertheless, it is anticipated that it will gain more attention in future research on imaging processing.

8.2.1.3 *Uses in Contrast*

Even when only a little amount of gadolinium-based contrast agent is used, high-quality post-contrast MRI images may be generated using deep learning algorithms. In a study of adult brain MRIs (including healthy volunteers and patients with gliomas), the structural similarity index among the "virtual contrast" MRI pictures produced by deep learning architecture as well as manually enhanced MRI sequences was 0.872. (0.031). Even though the accuracy of contrast-enhanced images for the ring enhancement around brain tumors was crisper and more defined, the radiologist evaluators gave the virtual contrast maps elevated ratings for overall image quality [19]. This was the case even though the virtual contrast maps were less distinct and more diffuse. However, before widespread implementation, the clinical impact of any potential misdiagnosis of underlying pathology (because of variations in the appearance of their reconstructed images) should be carefully assessed. It is possible that future implementations of this technology in pediatric MRI research as well as maybe also in multiphase CT studies could lower contrast dosage (and associated renal damage) as well as radiation burden.

8.2.2 Predictions and Quantitative Analysis

8.2.2.1 *Quantification*

Automated segmentation and subsequent estimation of bone age from hand radiographs [20] have completely replaced the time-consuming yet traditional Greulich–Pyle or Tanner–Whitehouse assessments in pediatric imaging (see Figure 8.1).

Quantifying imaged volumes is helpful in a variety of pediatric imaging applications, such as the assessment of pneumothorax volumes on chest CT [21] as well as the segmentation of tissue and CSF for hydrocephalus degree assessment on CTs of newborn brains [22]. These two applications are just two examples of the many pediatric imaging applications that have benefited from this technique. These metrics have the potential to be employed in the future of radiology to give instantaneous objective criteria for clinical judgment—for instance, authorized measurements might be incorporated into interactive reports. The measurement of limb lengths on X-rays obtained after orthopedic surgery [23] and the measurement of scoliosis angles from spine X-rays (as done in one study utilizing adult imaging) [24] are also examples of potential future applications for automated image quantification.

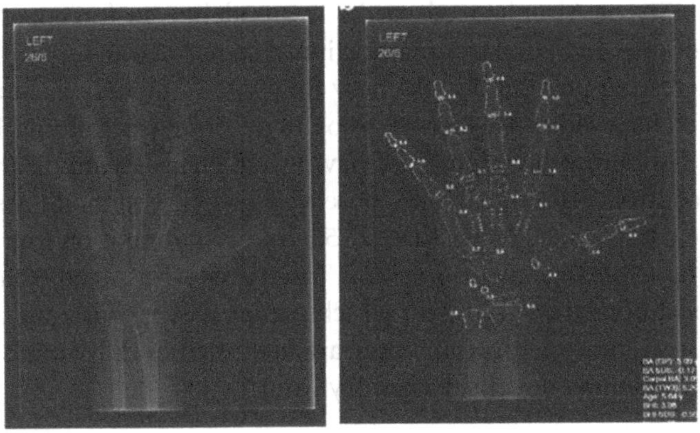

Figure 8.1 Several radiology departments have begun using artificial intelligence software (such as BoneXpert™ v.3.0.3) to determine a patient's bone age quickly and accurately. This is a (a) plain radiograph of the left hand of a 5-year-and-7-month-old boy who is short for his age. (b) Following analysis by the BoneXpertTM software, a second copy of the image is generated with an image overlay (white text and outlines), providing information, in the bottom right of the image, for the bone age according to researchers (5 years and 1 month) and the estimated standard deviation (0.17). Furthermore, included are the bone health index and the predicted bone age according to Tanner Whitehouse 3 (TW3: 5.2 years) (BHI).

8.2.2.2 *Making Predictions With Models*

Prognostication of clinical outcomes and identification of appropriate treatment regimens have both been routinely accomplished by radio genomic investigations in adults using AI approaches. Concurrently, new channels and databases are being developed for similar projects involving children. Researchers [25] have, for instance, created a multicenter clinical and imaging dataset to diagnose and predict the outcome of neonatal hypoxia ischemic encephalopathy. In a similar vein, the recently initiated multi-center "PRIMAGE" research in pediatric oncology aims to classify neuroblastoma and diffuse intrinsic pontine glioma (DIPG) to clarify treatment options and prognosticate sickness outcomes [26]. The use of multi-site data mining and predictive modeling should aid to improve prognoses for other pediatric tumors (such as Wilms tumors) as well as patient outcomes obtained from pattern discovery among non-oncological serial pictures (e.g., determining the neurological outcome of children who have suffered post-traumatic hydrocephalus or who have undergone vein of Galen embolization).

The ability of AI-enhanced predictive modeling to foretell the development of disease before any major clinical signs have arisen is one of the most interesting possibilities given by this type of modeling. Brain MRIs in children have led to the identification of neuroimaging biomarkers [27] that can distinguish between those having autism spectrum disorder with healthy controls. The researchers observed that the method's area under the curve (AUC) was greater than 0.75 after evaluating it on four datasets originating from various institutions. The use of AI-assisted technologies could boost both the speed with which certain diseases are discovered as well as the accuracy with which they are identified in individuals who are difficult to examine or collect a history from.

8.2.3 Decoding the Images

8.2.3.1 Abnormality Detection and Categorization

Detection and classification algorithms (either alone or in combination) have either mixed or superior performance when compared to skilled healthcare professionals, according to several studies that included adult medical images (such as those used in dermatology, radiology, and ophthalmology) [28]. These studies included medical images used in dermatology, radiology, and ophthalmology. Pediatric radiology is effective in the detection of a wide variety of diseases, such as pediatric pneumonia [29], hip developmental dysplasia [30], elbow effusions [31], wrist fractures on radiography [32] (Figure 8.2), and interval changes in bone marrow signal on MRI in children who have persistent nonbacterial osteitis (CNO) [33]. These diseases include pediatric pneumonia [34] and hip developmental dysplasia. When researchers [35] used a feature extraction method with a sensitivity of 80% or higher, they were able to automatically classify kidney and urinary tract congenital abnormalities on pediatric ultrasound.

Medulloblastoma, ependymoma, and astrocytoma may all be distinguished from one another on 3T MR spectroscopy with an improved classification approach that achieved 86% accuracy [36] in the field of neuro-oncology. It is possible that, in the future, tissue biopsies for medulloblastoma will be rendered unnecessary in support of a combination of clinical biomarkers, textural analysis, and imaging characteristics for the aim of enhanced therapeutic stratification [37].

Spine CT for the diagnosis of osteoporotic vertebral fractures [38] and chest imaging for the identification of pulmonary nodules are both adult-only applications that could have benefited from use in pediatrics.

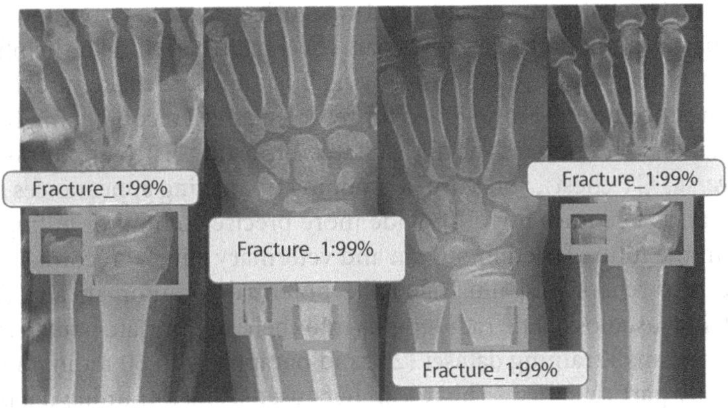

Figure 8.2 The use of AI to identify wrist fractures in radiographs taken from the front. A deep learning neural network (the "faster R-convolutional neural network") was evaluated on these images of patients with distal radius fractures with and without concomitant ulnar fractures. The locations of the anomalies are indicated by green boxes, and the percentages indicate the network's confidence in the likelihood of a fracture occurring within that box.

8.2.4 Reporting

8.2.4.1 Prioritization of Workflow

Prioritizing work processes with the help of artificial intelligence technologies has been studied in the adult literature with the hopes of increasing the turnaround time for radiology reports, specifically for those involving immediate observations from chest radiography [39] as well as CT of the head [40, 41]. They make sure the photos most likely to contain major abnormalities are prioritized for reporting by radiologists on the reporting worklist. The topic of report prioritization has not received a great deal of attention in the published research; however, the previously reported picture identification and classification approaches could be included in a reporting framework to assist in the improvement of workflow and to highlight potential discoveries on studies.

8.2.4.2 Categorization of Pictures

Most imaging exams are given either a general word (such as "external imaging") or an examination label, and this designation depends on whether the referral booking request or the time of scanning came first (such as "US abdomen"). Several potential benefits may arise from implementing an automated system to identify and categorize images upon import into PACS based on modality and body part coverage. This would be helpful for a variety of reasons, such as the following: first, it would make sure that the relevant procedures were assigned for reporting [42]; second, it might help in specifying the research to the suitable reporting list (e.g., ultrasound knee *versus* CT chest); and third, a grouping of imaging appearances along with report outcomes might provide more precise coding for billing purposes in the future (tried in human and veterinary clinical records).

The researchers [43] illustrated the potential to automatically detect pediatric musculoskeletal radiographs into their appropriate body parts by utilizing a small training dataset (250 radiographs, with 50 radiographs in each body part category). The researchers used a small training dataset to demonstrate their findings (e.g., shoulder, pelvis, elbow, etc.). It is essential to utilize this method for internal audit to quickly establish if all sequences from a specific MRI protocol have been done and sent to PACS before reporting as well as for labeling other imaging modalities such as chest radiographs [44] and magnetic resonance pictures [45]. This method can also be used for labeling other imaging modalities such as CT scans [46].

8.2.5 Analysis of Outcomes and Management

8.2.5.1 Prominent Results

Yet, even though certain radiological facilities presently use automated emails and non-clinician-led "important findings" channels, these approaches could be enhanced by employing major results prioritizing alert systems. Radiologists should include the phrase "add to MDT" on the report so that pediatricians can prioritize clinical management, and any findings that go above a particular level will be considered at the next meeting of the multidisciplinary team.

8.2.5.2 Improved Reports

Clinical colleagues may have difficulty understanding a lengthy radiology report or may fail to appreciate the significance of certain results. AI could be used to distill radiology reports down to their essentials—for instance, one study [47] showed that NLP software could use free-text ultrasound reports to diagnose pediatric deep vein thrombosis (DVT) and issue a clinical alert. The findings of an adult chest CT have been classified as "normal/ insignificant" or "significant," with a further sub-classification depending on whether the findings have remained the same, gotten worse, or gotten better from earlier reports [46]. A natural language processing system was developed by researchers [48] to select and highlight ultrasound data showing substantial carotid artery stenosis. This was done to prioritize treatment and follow-up for patients who were at a high risk of suffering a stroke.

The natural language processing (NLP) software could be modified to highlight significant results in reports (such as misplaced lines or tubes) or those that raise concerns about patient safety in pediatric imaging (e.g., metaphyseal corner fractures). The classification of deteriorating appearances on oncological imaging tests can also incorporate tumor dimensions across earlier scans to visualize trends in the disease process. This can result in recommendations for additional multidisciplinary team (MDT) discussion. To aid the AI algorithm in its search for the same tumor in the follow-up examination, it would be beneficial to use multimedia reporting frequently, with embedded report connections to previous crucial pictures [49].

It has been suggested that the implementation of sophisticated data mining software that is connected to the Internet would help rapidly read in real time millions of manuscripts to indicate the most up-to-date expert opinions on the subject [50]. This would be helpful in situations in which a differential diagnosis persists for rare or unknown diseases or a follow-up guideline is not readily established. Even while the software is gaining popularity in academic settings due to its capacity to accelerate literature searches [51], the most pertinent findings that were created by the program might be put into a clinical radiological report to educate and inform radiologists and clinicians. This would be beneficial for both groups.

8.3 Several Applications of Artificial Intelligence

8.3.1 Artificial Intelligence Software "BoneView"

French firm Gleaner has created ground-breaking AI software. This aids radiologists and emergency room doctors in identifying skeletal fractures. It is also made for kids, so it can find things like effusion, dislocations, and isolated bone lesions in the arms, legs, pelvis, thoracic spine, and lumbar spine [52]. It locates lesions in X-rays using complicated algorithms and then graphically highlights them before submitting the results to radiologists for confirmation. Radiologists and emergency room physicians are under more pressure than ever to interpret images, and missed fractures account for as much as 80% of emergency room diagnostic mistakes.

This is why we created BoneView; standard imaging techniques present several difficulties that were previously insurmountable for radiologists. This program cut the time spent reading radiographs by 15% and drastically decreased the rate of missed fractures by 30% [53].

8.3.2 Model Reconstruction in Three Dimensions

As computing power and digital imaging have improved, so can reconstruct 3D medical models. To better see a specific anatomical component, this 3D model was developed by converting the 2D data that was obtained from CT or MRI scans of the structure into 3D data. The 3D model aids the surgeon in identifying the area's structure and morphology, pinpointing the lesion's precise location, and planning the surgical treatment. A 6-year-old child was found to have a massive osteochondroma of the scapula, originating from an unknown location. Due to the tumor's compression of the joint and surrounding tissues, movement of the joint was restricted, which triggered the associated symptoms. Using data from a CT scan, a three-dimensional model of the scapula was built to avoid unnecessary procedures. After that, a comprehensive duplicate of the lesion was produced with the assistance of a 3D printer, which was used to aid in the preoperative planning of the surgical excision [54].

The parameters of the anatomical structures can be determined with greater accuracy using the 3D model. Surgeons can increase the precision and safety of their procedures by planning time using a 3D model of the patient. The children with forearm abnormalities were modeled in 3D, and surgical simulations were run to determine the best location for the osteotomy and to design cutting jigs for everyone. In addition to reducing the need for a decision to be made during surgery, this strategy also allowed for more exact planning of osteotomies, even when they were complex and involved numerous bones. After surgery, there was a dramatic improvement in forearm rotation and distal radioulnar joint stability [55]. This technology also works well on softer tissues like muscle and fat. This technique can also be used to treat problems of the nervous system and the cardiovascular system. However, this has not been fully realized, and pediatric surgery remains challenging due to children's still-developing bodies and more delicate blood arteries and nerves.

8.3.3 Digital X-Ray Radiogrammetry

Fractures, osteoporosis-related hospitalizations, and deaths are all consequences of this skeletal disease. Osteoporosis in children can be either primary or secondary. Indirect effects of systemic illness, such as immobility and malnutrition, can also lead to bone loss and poor bone quality in youngsters. Osteoporosis develops differently in children and adults due to age-related variations in bone mass density (BMD) [56].

There is no better method than dual-energy X-ray absorptiometry (DXA) for determining bone quality in both young and old. Normative data are readily available, and the accuracy and repeatability are both high [57]. Children's BMD can be measured in a variety of areas across the skeleton. Of course, DXA is not without its drawbacks. Unreadable readings can be caused by several factors, including movement during measurement, contractures, metallic implants, and even scoliosis. As an option that can be used in therapeutic settings, "digital X-ray radiogrammetry" (DXR) is employed to deal with these problems. BoneXpert, a web-based bone health assessment tool, can determine both bone age and bone quality (BHI). The BHI evaluates the thickness and mineralization of the cortical layer. Effectively, this provides a reliable depiction of bone quality. DXR is less inconvenient than other forms of ionizing radiation testing, is readily available, and poses no risk to the patient [58].

8.3.4 Using Convolutional Neural Networks to Find, Categorize, and Individualize Treatments for Pediatric Cancer

Several non-neoplastic problems, such as delayed bone aging in hand radiographs and pneumonia in chest radiographs, are easily identifiable and identified by deep CNNs. CNN may be taught to distinguish between normal and abnormal scans, making it applicable to the identification of malignant tumors. Lesions in tumors can be detected, segmented, and quantified mechanically [59]. Researchers employed a computerized approach to identify pulmonary nodules in pediatric chest CTs [60]. Tumor characterization is yet another application of deep CNNs. Researchers [61] used machine learning algorithms on chest CT and PET/CT scans to differentiate between malignant and benign lung nodules [62]. For radiomic and genomic investigation, machine learning algorithms excel at finding patterns in large datasets. Increasingly nuanced genetic and molecular tumor traits can be linked to distinct macroscopic tumor features on imaging tests, thanks to the power of deep convolutional neural networks.

To better forecast how genomic variants may affect the sensitivity of normal and tumor tissue to chemotherapy and radiation, doctors can use deep CNNs in the planning of tailored therapies [63]. Long-term survival rates for children with cancer have been predicted using machine learning algorithms, which has led to significant progress in the field.

8.3.5 Digital Tomosynthesis

Like CT, it enables cross-sectional, three-dimensional imaging, but at a far lower radiation dose and cost. Digital tomosynthesis (DTS) imaging is utilised for the clinical management of fracture healing. Between conventional radiographs and CT, this technology provides an ideal middle ground for diagnostic imaging. For diagnostic imaging, DTS employs a regular X-ray tube, a flat-panel detector fitted with an anti-scatter grid, and a powered tube crane. Numerous cross-sectional images can be generated at a far lower dose than CT, thanks to a reconstruction technique. When used for orthopedic imaging in children, it shows significant promise [64].

8.3.6 Innovative 3D Printing Tools

To print three-dimensional objects, this technique uses 3D model files and the bonding properties of materials like powdered metal or plastic. Computer modeling software is used to create the models, and a 3D printer is then utilized to print them out in layers. Because CAD software can turn a 3D digital model into a physical one, it is frequently used in tandem with 3D printing. As a result of its usefulness in tailored treatment, 3D printed models have found widespread application in pediatric orthopedics [65]. Fabricating individualized surgical templates using 3D technology is becoming increasingly common. In older children diagnosed with developmental dysplasia of the hip (DHH), an investigation was conducted to see whether it would be possible to use a navigation template that had been generated using a 3D printer during femoral osteotomy. It was discovered that the group that used the 3D printed navigation template required less operative time and less intraoperative X-ray exposure time and had a lower incidence of iatrogenic physical injury following surgery. Furthermore, their therapeutic effect was superior to that of the control group. This resulted in less time spent on unnecessary steps and more accuracy during surgery [66].

In addition to this, the technology of 3D printing is being utilized in the field of pediatric plastic surgery. Children with craniofacial fissures often have quite complex bone abnormalities. 3D printing technology has a wide range of potential uses, including the creation of customized aids.

8.3.7 Orthopedic Surgery with the Help of Robots

Surgery is a common choice for therapy in pediatric orthopedics, and robots are increasingly being used as an adjuvant to the main surgeries that are being performed. Robot-assisted surgery enhances not only the success rate and curative impact of surgery but also its stability and accuracy. This is in addition to enhancing the success rate of surgery overall. The level of accuracy achieved during conventional *versus* robot-assisted pediatric spinal surgery was evaluated. The conventional method only had a placement accuracy of 90%, which is a substantial decrease when compared to the 98.7% that was obtained with the assistance of robots and without any issues associated with screw fixation [67]. In addition to these advantages, robotic surgery provides several additional benefits. After completing an investigation, researchers found that combining a low-dose CT procedure with robot-assisted pediatric spinal surgery generated favorable results. This was determined after the researchers conducted an analysis. These results turned out to be significantly better than anticipated. The radiation dose was lowered by 84–91% when measured against the standard practice [68]. By assisting doctors as they choose the optimal surgical approach and angle, surgical robots can improve the precision of surgical procedures. Artificial intelligence directs the robotic arm to maintain consistency during surgery while also maximizing the effectiveness of the chosen method. This is a crucial step in the evolution of orthopedic surgery since it improves the surgical procedure's clinical outcome. Although some individuals may benefit from robotic surgery, the procedure is expensive and not appropriate for everybody. The widespread use of surgical robots is still some distance off.

8.3.8 Digital Platform OrthoNext

The Food and Drug Administration has given the go-ahead for the use of the digital platform known as OrthoNext, which was developed by the international manufacturer of medical devices known as Orthofix. To date, in the medical field, this is the only commercially accessible program of its kind, and it is used to analyze and plan orthopedic surgery on infants with abnormalities. In parallel, the JuniOrtho Plating System, as well as the OrthoNext digital platform software, was developed with the goals of improving the planning of the osteotomy site and providing a more accurate visualization of the implant concerning the patient's anatomy. The goal here is to make it easier to determine the appropriate device size and position of the patient's body in preparation for surgery. The JuniOrtho Plating

System was developed to meet the needs of complex lower-extremity deformity and trauma reconstruction in pediatric patients [69].

8.4 Conclusion

There is a growing demand in the market right now for high-quality medical treatment, particularly in the fields of radiology and pediatric orthopedics. In this area, the first steps have been taken towards digitization and increased levels of intelligence, and the introduction of computer technology has undoubtedly brought about a great deal of change. Because of the proliferation of digital software and equipment, pediatric orthopedics has grown more individualized and accurate in recent years. The diagnosis of sickness, the various treatment techniques, and the execution of surgery have all seen significant modifications in recent years. In the field of pediatric orthopedics, digital technology possesses significant growth potential.

References

1. Malik, P., Pathania, M., Rathaur, V.K., Overview of artificial intelligence in medicine. *J. Fam. Med. Prim. Care*, 8, 7, 2328, 2019 Jul.
2. Han, X.G. and Tian, W., Artificial intelligence in orthopedic surgery: Current state and future perspective. *Chin. Med. J.*, 132, 21, 2521–2523, 2019 Nov 5.
3. Burns, J.E., Yao, J., Summers, R.M., Artificial intelligence in musculoskeletal imaging: A paradigm shift. *J. Bone Miner. Res.*, 35, 1, 28–35, 2020 Jan.
4. Kavlakoglu, E., AI vs. machine learning vs. deep learning vs. neural networks: What's the difference?, IBM, 2020 May.
5. Ko, S., Pareek, A., Ro, D.H., Lu, Y., Camp, C.L., Martin, R.K., Krych, A.J., Artificial intelligence in orthopedics: Three strategies for deep learning with orthopedic specific imaging. *Knee Surg. Sports Traumatol. Arthrosc.*, 1, 1–4, 2022 Mar.
6. Sutton, R.T., Pincock, D., Baumgart, D.C., Sadowski, D.C., Fedorak, R.N., Kroeker, K.I., An overview of clinical decision support systems: Benefits, risks, and strategies for success. *NPJ Digit. Med.*, 3, 1, 17, 2020 Feb 6.
7. Hughes, J.H., Woo, K.H., Keizer, R.J., Goswami, S., Clinical decision support for precision dosing: Opportunities for enhanced equity and inclusion in health care. *Clin. Pharmacol. Ther.*, 113, 3, 565–574, 2023 Mar.
8. Schaefer, J., Lehne, M., Schepers, J., Prasser, F., Thun, S., The use of machine learning in rare diseases: A scoping review. *Orphanet J. Rare Dis.*, 15, 1–0, 2020 Dec.

9. Wang, Y., Fan, M., Zaman, Q., Zheng, P., Application progress and potential of digital medicine in pediatric orthopedics. *Digit. Med.*, 7, 1, 4, 2021 Jan 1.
10. Wang, Y., Li, R., Zheng, P., Progress in clinical application of artificial intelligence in orthopedics. *Digit. Med.*, 8, 1, 4, 2022 Jan 1.
11. Chea, P. and Mandell, J.C., Current applications and future directions of deep learning in musculoskeletal radiology. *Skeletal Radiol.*, 49, 2, 183–197, 2020 Feb.
12. Gong, E., Pauly, J.M., Wintermark, M., Zaharchuk, G., Deep learning enables reduced gadolinium dose for contrast-enhanced brain MRI. *J. Magn. Reson. Imaging*, 48, 2, 330–340, 2018 Aug.
13. Thukral, B.B., Problems and preferences in pediatric imaging. *Indian J. Radiol. Imaging*, 25, 04, 359–364, 2015 Oct.
14. Wang, S., Su, Z., Ying, L., Peng, X., Zhu, S., Liang, F., Feng, D., Liang, D., Accelerating magnetic resonance imaging via deep learning, in: *2016 IEEE 13th International Symposium on Biomedical Imaging (ISBI)*, IEEE, pp. 514–517, 2016 Apr 13.
15. Alizadeh, M., Conklin, C.J., Middleton, D.M., Shah, P., Saksena, S., Krisa, L., Finsterbusch, J., Faro, S.H., Mulcahey, M.J., Mohamed, F.B., Identification of ghost artifact using texture analysis in pediatric spinal cord diffusion tensor images. *Magn. Reson. Imaging*, 47, 7–15, 2018 Apr 1.
16. Chen, H., Zhang, Y., Kalra, M.K., Lin, F., Chen, Y., Liao, P., Zhou, J., Wang, G., Low-dose CT with a residual encoder-decoder convolutional neural network. *IEEE Trans. Med. Imaging*, 36, 12, 2524–2535, 2017 Jun 13.
17. Xie, S., Zheng, X., Chen, Y., Xie, L., Liu, J., Zhang, Y., Yan, J., Zhu, H., Hu, Y., Artifact removal using improved GoogLeNet for sparse-view CT reconstruction. *Sci. Rep.*, 8, 1, 6700, 2018 Apr 30.
18. MacDougall, R.D., Zhang, Y., Callahan, M.J., Perez-Rossello, J., Breen, M.A., Johnston, P.R., Yu, H., Improving low-dose pediatric abdominal CT by using convolutional neural networks. *Radiol.: Artif. Intell.*, 1, 6, e180087, 2019 Nov 27.
19. Kleesiek, J., Morshuis, J.N., Isensee, F., Deike-Hofmann, K., Paech, D., Kickingereder, P., Köthe, U., Rother, C., Forsting, M., Wick, W., Bendszus, M., Can virtual contrast enhancement in brain MRI replace gadolinium?: A feasibility study. *Invest. Radiol.*, 54, 10, 653–660, 2019 Oct 1.
20. Booz, C., Yel, I., Wichmann, J.L., Boettger, S., Al Kamali, A., Albrecht, M.H., Martin, S.S., Lenga, L., Huizinga, N.A., D'Angelo, T., Cavallaro, M., Artificial intelligence in bone age assessment: Accuracy and efficiency of a novel fully automated algorithm compared to the Greulich-Pyle method. *Eur. Radiol. Exp.*, 4, 1, 1–8, 2020 Dec.
21. Cai, W., Lee, E.Y., Vij, A., Mahmood, S.A., Yoshida, H., MDCT for computerized volumetry of pneumothoraces in pediatric patients. *Acad. Radiol.*, 18, 3, 315–323, 2011 Mar 1.
22. Cherukuri, V., Ssenyonga, P., Warf, B.C., Kulkarni, A.V., Monga, V., Schiff, S.J., Learning based segmentation of CT brain images: Application to

postoperative hydrocephalic scans. *IEEE Trans. Biomed. Eng.*, 65, 8, 1871–1884, 2017 Dec 13.

23. Zheng, Q., Shellikeri, S., Huang, H., Hwang, M., Sze, R.W., Deep learning measurement of leg length discrepancy in children based on radiographs. *Radiology*, 296, 1, 152–158, 2020 Jul.
24. Horng, M.H., Kuok, C.P., Fu, M.J., Lin, C.J., Sun, Y.N., Cobb angle measurement of spine from X-ray images using convolutional neural network. *Comput. Math. Methods Med.*, 2019, 1–19, 2019 Feb 19.
25. Weiss, R.J., Bates, S.V., Song, Y.N., Zhang, Y., Herzberg, E.M., Chen, Y.C., Gong, M., Chien, I., Zhang, L., Murphy, S.N., Gollub, R.L., Mining multi-site clinical data to develop machine learning MRI biomarkers: Application to neonatal hypoxic ischemic encephalopathy. *J. Transl. Med.*, 17, 1, 1–6, 2019 Dec.
26. Martí-Bonmatí, L., Alberich-Bayarri, Á., Ladenstein, R., Blanquer, I., Segrelles, J.D., Cerdá-Alberich, L., Gkontra, P., Hero, B., García-Aznar, J.M., Keim, D., Jentner, W., PRIMAGE project: Predictive *in silico* multiscale analytics to support childhood cancer personalised evaluation empowered by imaging biomarkers. *Eur. Radiol. Exp.*, 4, 1, 1–1, 2020 Dec.
27. Chen, T., Chen, Y., Yuan, M., Gerstein, M., Li, T., Liang, H., Froehlich, T., Lu, L., The development of a practical artificial intelligence tool for diagnosing and evaluating autism spectrum disorder: Multicenter study. *JMIR Med. Inform.*, 8, 5, e15767, 2020 May 8.
28. Liu, X., Faes, L., Kale, A.U., Wagner, S.K., Fu, D.J., Bruynseels, A., Mahendiran, T., Moraes, G., Shamdas, M., Kern, C., Ledsam, J.R., A comparison of deep learning performance against health-care professionals in detecting diseases from medical imaging: A systematic review and meta-analysis. *Lancet Digit. Health*, 1, 6, e271–97, 2019 Oct 1.
29. Yates, E.J., Yates, L.C., Harvey, H., Machine learning "red dot": Open-source, cloud, deep convolutional neural networks in chest radiograph binary normality classification. *Clin. Radiol.*, 73, 9, 827–831, 2018 Sep 1.
30. Li, Q., Zhong, L., Huang, H., Liu, H., Qin, Y., Wang, Y., Zhou, Z., Liu, H., Yang, W., Qin, M., Wang, J., Auxiliary diagnosis of developmental dysplasia of the hip by automated detection of Sharp's angle on standardized anteroposterior pelvic radiographs. *Medicine*, 98, 52, 1–8, 2019 Dec.
31. England, J.R., Gross, J.S., White, E.A., Patel, D.B., England, J.T., Cheng, P.M., Detection of traumatic pediatric elbow joint effusion using a deep convolutional neural network. *Am. J. Roentgenol.*, 211, 6, 1361–1368, 2018 Dec.
32. Thian, Y.L., Li, Y., Jagmohan, P., Sia, D., Chan, V.E., Tan, R.T., Convolutional neural networks for automated fracture detection and localization on wrist radiographs. *Radiol.: Artif. Intell.*, 1, 1, e180001, 2019 Jan 30.
33. Bhat, C.S., Chopra, M., Andronikou, S., Paul, S., Wener-Fligner, Z., Merkoulovitch, A., Holjar-Erlic, I., Menegotto, F., Simpson, E., Grier, D., Ramanan, A.V., Artificial intelligence for interpretation of segments of whole body MRI in CNO: Pilot study comparing radiologists versus machine learning algorithm. *Pediatr. Rheumatol.*, 18, 1, 1–6, 2020 Dec.

34. Behzadi-Khormouji, H., Rostami, H., Salehi, S., Derakhshande-Rishehri, T., Masoumi, M., Salemi, S., Keshavarz, A., Gholamrezanezhad, A., Assadi, M., Batouli, A., Deep learning, reusable and problem-based architectures for detection of consolidation on chest X-ray images. *Comput. Methods Programs Biomed.*, 185, 105162, 2020 Mar 1.
35. Zheng, Q., Furth, S.L., Tasian, G.E., Fan, Y., Computer-aided diagnosis of congenital abnormalities of the kidney and urinary tract in children based on ultrasound imaging data by integrating texture image features and deep transfer learning image features. *J. Pediatr. Urol.*, 15, 1, 75–e1, 2019 Feb 1.
36. Zarinabad, N., Abernethy, L.J., Avula, S., Davies, N.P., Rodriguez Gutierrez, D., Jaspan, T., MacPherson, L., Mitra, D., Rose, H.E., Wilson, M., Morgan, P.S., Application of pattern recognition techniques for classification of pediatric brain tumors by *in vivo* 3T 1H-MR spectroscopy—A multi-center study. *Magn. Reson. Med.*, 79, 4, 2359–2366, 2018 Apr.
37. Iv, M., Zhou, M., Shpanskaya, K., Perreault, S., Wang, Z., Tranvinh, E., Lanzman, B., Vajapeyam, S., Vitanza, N.A., Fisher, P.G., Cho, Y.J., MR imaging-based radiomic signatures of distinct molecular subgroups of medulloblastoma. *Am. J. Neuroradiol.*, 40, 1, 154–161, 2019 Jan 1.
38. Tomita, N., Cheung, Y.Y., Hassanpour, S., Deep neural networks for automatic detection of osteoporotic vertebral fractures on CT scans. *Comput. Biol. Med.*, 98, 8–15, 2018 Jul 1.
39. Annarumma, M., Withey, S.J., Bakewell, R.J., Pesce, E., Goh, V., Montana, G., Automated triaging of adult chest radiographs with deep artificial neural networks. *Radiology*, 291, 1, 196–202, 2019 Apr.
40. Ginat, D.T., Analysis of head CT scans flagged by deep learning software for acute intracranial hemorrhage. *Neuroradiology*, 62, 335–40, 2020 Mar.
41. Arbabshirani, M.R., Fornwalt, B.K., Mongelluzzo, G.J., Suever, J.D., Geise, B.D., Patel, A.A., Moore, G.J., Advanced machine learning in action: Identification of intracranial hemorrhage on computed tomography scans of the head with clinical workflow integration. *NPJ Digital Med.*, 1, 1, 9, 2018 Apr 4.
42. Luo, H., Hao, W., Foos, D.H., Cornelius, C.W., Automatic image hanging protocol for chest radiographs in PACS. *IEEE Trans. Inf. Technol. Biomed.*, 10, 2, 302–311, 2006 Apr 3.
43. Yi, P.H., Kim, T.K., Wei, J., Shin, J., Hui, F.K., Sair, H.I., Hager, G.D., Fritz, J., Automated semantic labeling of pediatric musculoskeletal radiographs using deep learning. *Pediatr. Radiol.*, 49, 1066–1070, 2019 Jul 1.
44. Kim, T.K., Yi, P.H., Wei, J., Shin, J.W., Hager, G., Hui, F.K., Sair, H.I., Lin, C.T., Deep learning method for automated classification of anteroposterior and posteroanterior chest radiographs. *J. Digital Imaging*, 32, 925–930, 2019 Dec.
45. Lee, Y.H., Efficiency improvement in a busy radiology practice: Determination of musculoskeletal magnetic resonance imaging protocol using deep-learning convolutional neural networks. *J. Digital Imaging*, 31, 604–610, 2018 Oct.

46. Hassanpour, S., Bay, G., Langlotz, C.P., Characterization of change and significance for clinical findings in radiology reports through natural language processing. *J. Digital Imaging*, 30, 314–322, 2017 Jun.
47. Gálvez, J.A., Pappas, J.M., Ahumada, L., Martin, J.N., Simpao, A.F., Rehman, M.A., Witmer, C., The use of natural language processing on pediatric diagnostic radiology reports in the electronic health record to identify deep venous thrombosis in children. *J. Thromb. Thrombolysis*, 44, 281–290, 2017 Oct.
48. Mowery, D.L., Chapman, B.E., Conway, M., South, B.R., Madden, E., Keyhani, S., Chapman, W.W., Extracting a stroke phenotype risk factor from veteran health administration clinical reports: An information content analysis. *J. Biomed. Semant.*, 7, 1–2, 2016 Dec.
49. Beesley, S.D., Patrie, J.T., Gaskin, C.M., Radiologist adoption of interactive multimedia reporting technology. *J. Am. Coll. Radiol.*, 16, 4, 465–471, 2019 Apr 1.
50. Schoeb, D., Suarez-Ibarrola, R., Hein, S., Dressler, F.F., Adams, F., Schlager, D., Miernik, A., Use of artificial intelligence for medical literature search: Randomized controlled trial using the Hackathon format. *Interact. J. Med. Res.*, 9, 1, e16606, 2020 Mar 30.
51. 176. IRIS AI, Research discovery with artificial intelligence, 2020, Available from: https:// iris.ai/ accessed 30 march 2023.
52. Sharaf, Y., Taha, B., Sayyad, Y., Application of Artificial Intelligence in pediatric orthopaedic. *SVOA Orthopaedics*, 3, 1–6, 2023.
53. Duron, L., Artificial intelligence software BoneView helps radiologists and emergency physicians detect and localise fractures, Interventional News, 2021.
54. Tam, M.D., Laycock, S.D., Bell, D., Chojnowski, A., 3-D printout of a DICOM file to aid surgical planning in a 6 year old patient with a large scapular osteochondroma complicating congenital diaphyseal aclasia. *J. Radiol. Case Rep.*, 6, 1, 31, 2012 Jan.
55. Storelli, D.A., Bauer, A.S., Lattanza, L.L., McCarroll, H.R., The use of computer-aided design and 3-dimensional models in the treatment of forearm malunions in children. *Techn. Handb. Up. Extrem. Surg.*, 19, 1, 23–26, 2015 Mar 1.
56. Leijten, A.D., Hampsink, B., Janssen, M., Klein, W.M., Draaisma, J.M., Can digital X-ray radiogrammetry be an alternative for dual-energy X-ray absorptiometry in the diagnosis of secondary low bone quality in children? *Eur. J. Pediatr.*, 178, 1433–1441, 2019 Sep 1.
57. Messina, C., Lastella, G., Sorce, S., Piodi, L.P., Rodari, G., Giavoli, C., Marchelli, D., Guglielmi, G., Ulivieri, F.M., Pediatric dual-energy X-ray absorptiometry in clinical practice: What the clinicians need to know. *Eur. J. Radiol.*, 105, 153–161, 2018 Aug 1.
58. Schündeln, M.M., Marschke, L., Bauer, J.J., Hauffa, P.K., Schweiger, B., Führer-Sakel, D., Lahner, H., Poeppel, T.D., Kiewert, C., Hauffa, B.P., Grasemann, C.,

A piece of the puzzle: The bone health index of the BoneXpert software reflects cortical bone mineral density in pediatric and adolescent patients. *PLoS One*, 11, 3, e0151936, 2016 Mar 25.
59. Daldrup-Link, H., Artificial intelligence applications for pediatric oncology imaging. *Pediatr. Radiol.*, 49, 11, 1384–1390, 2019 Oct.
60. Helm, E.J., Silva, C.T., Roberts, H.C., Manson, D., Seed, M.T., Amaral, J.G., Babyn, P.S., Computer-aided detection for the identification of pulmonary nodules in pediatric oncology patients: Initial experience. *Pediatr. Radiol.*, 39, 685–693, 2009 Jul.
61. Tu, S.J., Wang, C.W., Pan, K.T., Wu, Y.C., Wu, C.T., Localized thin-section CT with radiomics feature extraction and machine learning to classify early-detected pulmonary nodules from lung cancer screening. *Phys. Med. Biol.*, 63, 6, 065005, 2018 Mar 14.
62. Chen, S., Harmon, S., Perk, T., Li, X., Chen, M., Li, Y., Jeraj, R., Diagnostic classification of solitary pulmonary nodules using dual time 18F-FDG PET/CT image texture features in granuloma-endemic regions. *Sci. Rep.*, 7, 1, 1–8, 2017 Aug 24.
63. Kang, J., Rancati, T., Lee, S., Oh, J.H., Kerns, S.L., Scott, J.G., Schwartz, R., Kim, S., Rosenstein, B.S., Machine learning and radiogenomics: Lessons learned and future directions. *Front. Oncol.*, 228, 1–21, 2018.
64. Chan, S., Digital tomosynthesis applications in pediatric orthopedic imaging: A case series. *Mo. Med.*, 115, 4, 344, 2018 Jul.
65. Parthasarathy, J., Krishnamurthy, R., Ostendorf, A., Shinoka, T., Krishnamurthy, R., 3D printing with MRI in pediatric applications. *J. Magn. Reson. Imaging*, 51, 6, 1641–1658, 2020 Jun.
66. Zheng, P., Xu, P., Yao, Q., Tang, K., Lou, Y., 3D-printed navigation template in proximal femoral osteotomy for older children with developmental dysplasia of the hip. *Sci. Rep.*, 7, 1, 44993, 2017 Mar 21.
67. Gonzalez, D., Ghessese, S., Cook, D., Hedequist, D., Initial intraoperative experience with robotic-assisted pedicle screw placement with stealth navigation in pediatric spine deformity: An evaluation of the first 40 cases. *J. Rob. Surg.*, 15, 687–693, 2021 Oct.
68. Sensakovic, W.F., O'Dell, M.C., Agha, A., Woo, R., Varich, L., CT radiation dose reduction in robot-assisted pediatric spinal surgery. *Spine*, 42, 7, E417–24, 2017 Apr 1.
69. Månefjord, H., Li, M., Brackmann, C., Reistad, N., Merdasa, A., Brydegaard, M., BIOSPACE–A low-cost platform for problem-based learning in biophotonics, in: *Pedagogiska inspirationskonferensen-Genombrottet*, 2021.

9

Use of Artificial Intelligence in Imaging for Bone Cancer

Abstract

Bone cancer is a major health concern because it frequently results in a patient's death. Radiologists use the image from an X-ray, MRI, or CT scan to make a diagnosis of bone cancer. Manual methods are inefficient due to their need on specialist knowledge and time. As a result, the development of an automated system to differentiate cancerous bone from healthy bone is essential. The texture of a bone that has been impacted by cancer differs from that of a healthy bone, but many images of cancer and healthy bone in the dataset share morphological characteristics. For this reason, classifying them is challenging. Artificial intelligence has been shown to help with clinical diagnosis and prognosis prediction across a range of musculoskeletal disorders, from fracture detection to identifying cartilage and spinal lesions to determining the severity of osteoarthritis. Meanwhile, cancers of all kinds, including the prostate, breast, and lungs, have been extensively studied using AI-based machine learning and deep learning method. In the field of bone cancers, the use of AI has just emerged. Numerous models have shown promise for assisting in the diagnosis and prognosis prediction of bone tumors by analyzing radiological (such as X-ray, MRI, CT, and SPECT) and pathological images for tumor detection, classification, segmentation, grading, volume calculation, and assessment of tumor necrosis rate. This chapter explains a brief overview of bone cancer and its many stages. This chapter also explains the workflows of machine learning and deep learning approaches in medical imaging as well as their present applications in the diagnosis and prognosis prediction of bone cancers.

Keywords: Bone tumor, cancer diagnosis, machine learning, deep learning, artificial intelligence, algorithm, cancer staging, bone metastasis

9.1 Introduction

The musculoskeletal system is the site of development for a variety of cancers, including both primary and metastatic bone tumors. Primary bone tumors account for around 6.2% of all cancer diagnoses and have an

Rishabha Malviya, Shivam Rajput and Makarand Vaidya. Artificial Intelligence for Bone Disorder: Diagnosis and Treatment, (219–244) © 2024 Scrivener Publishing LLC

occurrence frequency of one to two per 100,000 persons. This results in a relatively low prevalence [1, 2]. Bone tumors that originate in the bones can be further classified as benign, intermediate, or malignant. After leukemia, osteosarcoma is the second highest cause of mortality among children and adolescents [3, 4]. Particularly, people with malignant bone tumors face a worse prognosis, including the risk of amputation or metastases, without proper diagnosis and treatment [5, 6].

Consequently, limb salvage and a reduction in morbidity and mortality depend critically on prompt diagnosis and treatment. Due to their rareness, bone tumors are typically diagnosed using a multidisciplinary approach that includes imaging and pathological analyses in addition to the patient's clinical history and physical. However, it is challenging for clinicians to make diagnoses quickly and accurately without being influenced by their own prior knowledge and experience [7]. Therefore, improved methods of rapid, trustworthy, and precise diagnosis of bone cancers are desperately needed in clinical practise.

Imaging and diagnostics, nursing, lifestyle monitoring and management, emergency and hospital management, drug mining, virtual assistants, wearables, and more are a few of the many areas in which artificial intelligence (AI) is being implemented in healthcare today. Other areas include imaging and diagnostics, nursing, and management of lifestyles [8]. There is a severe scarcity of medical personnel and facilities, yet AI has the potential to greatly increase the effectiveness of clinical operations.

Cancer is the deadliest disease in the world. Malignant neoplasm is the clinical term for cancer. The abnormal, unchecked proliferation of cells is the underlying cause of this hereditary disorder. Thus, the number of fatalities caused by such a disease might be drastically decreased if detected early [9]. Cancer is characterized by unchecked cell growth, which results in the formation of a malignant tumor that is detrimental to the surrounding tissues [10–12]. Tumors of this type have the potential to metastasize, wreaking havoc on the body's circulatory, digestive, and neural systems while also releasing hormones that interfere with normal bodily function [13–15]. In the absence of an effect on DNA structure, unrestrained cell expansion is not always hazardous. Unchecked cell division can lead to DNA damage and eventually death, which, in turn, can spur the formation of cells that are not needed. Cancer's ability to metastasize is far more alarming. The spread of cancer throughout the body is also known as metastasis. Tumors develop as a result of this process. Cancer's earliest signs include things like abnormal bleeding, the development of new lumps, a persistent cough, a shift in bowel movement, unexplained weight loss, and so on. Cancerous tumors and benign tumors are the two main categories of tumors [16]. Most benign (non-cancerous) tumors do not return after being surgically removed. Compared to benign tumors, malignant ones have bigger nuclei. Sarcomas are the medical word for tumors that begin in skeletal muscle, fibrous tissue, bone, blood vessels, or elsewhere in the body. Chondrosarcoma, osteosarcoma, pleomorphic sarcoma, Ewing's sarcoma, and fibrosarcoma are only a few examples of the many different forms of cancer. Bone cancer begins as a tumor inside the bone, hindering the function and development of the skeleton. Bone enchondroma is a type of benign tumor that develops from the underlying cartilage. Enchondroma is most common in the little bones of the hands. Bone tumors called enchondromas can form anywhere along the long bones of the body [17, 18]. Bone cancer is divided into stages based on how far along the disease has progressed:

- Stage 1—This indicates that the tumor is rather benign as the malignancy has not gone beyond the bone.
- Stage 2—Identical to stage 1 but indicative of a more aggressive tumor.
- Stage 3—When a tumor spreads to many organs.
- Stage 4—If the cancer spreads to other sections of the body.

There is a severe scarcity of medical personnel and facilities, yet AI has the potential to greatly increase the effectiveness of clinical operations. Since deep learning was first used in image recognition in 2012, its performance in this area has dramatically improved. Applications utilizing the research methods for analyzing and processing medical images have proliferated. Deep learning and machine learning's medical applications not only aid in the automatic identification of disease but also do it more quickly, more accurately, and with greater efficiency [19].

Deep learning and machine learning strategies have been successfully used in medical imaging [20], which has opened exciting new prospects for the development of a computer-aided medical imaging diagnosis system. AI has advanced in recent years. In recent years, deep learning and machine learning algorithms have been effectively applied to musculoskeletal imaging for the purpose of detecting and assessing the severity of lesions for a variety of disorders, including fracture [21], knee lesions [22], OA (osteoarthritis) [23], and spinal degenerative lesion [24]. Sex [25] and bone age [26] can also be calculated from X-rays using deep learning- and machine learning-based techniques. This suggests that deep learning and machine learning techniques could be used to develop diagnostic models for bone cancers, which could significantly cut down on the incidence of incorrect and delayed diagnoses. Recent research has shown that deep learning- and machine learning-based AI models may greatly enhance the identification, categorization, and segmentation of bone cancer lesions, which has implications for improving diagnostic, prognostic, and predictive

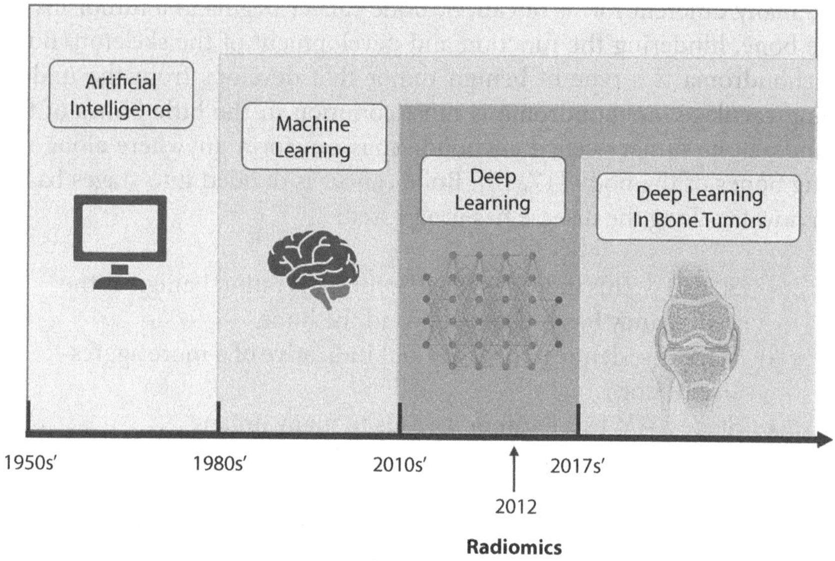

Figure 9.1 A historical perspective on the evolution of AI, ML, radiomics, DL, and DL applications in the study and treatment of bone tumors.

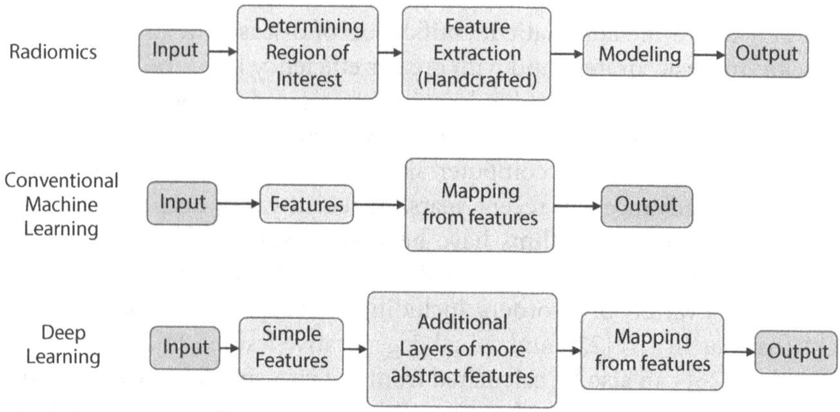

Figure 9.2 A quick look at the differences between radiomics, traditional machine learning, and deep learning along the pipeline.

accuracy. Another cutting-edge subject that regularly collaborates with AI is radiomics, which uses quantitative picture features such as geometry, texture, intensity, and size to extract and evaluate numerical radiological patterns. The domains of illness diagnosis, prognosis, and patient tracking are obvious places where radiomics may be used [27]. Figures 9.1 and 9.2 provide an in-depth look at the connections between AI, radiomics, machine learning, deep learning, and deep learning in the context of bone cancers. Also covered are their respective developments and comparisons.

9.2 Applications of Machine Learning to Cancer Diagnosis

There are several applications for machine learning algorithms in the medical field. Ultrasound, MRI, CT, histology, and microscopic pictures are only few of the biomedical imaging modalities that can be used. Biomedical imaging focuses on the liver, brain, prostate, lungs, and even genetic correlations. Researchers, physicians, and students [28–30] working in the area of medical imaging will consider the integration of medical imaging with machine learning to be an extremely useful resource. The medical imaging modalities employed in machine learning are depicted in Figure 9.3.

Sequences from an MRI machine show varying degrees of illumination even within the same structures. When compared to CT and MRI, ultrasound is far more practical. Due to poor ultrasound wave transmission through bone, it is ineffective for use on bone [31]. In order to classify the

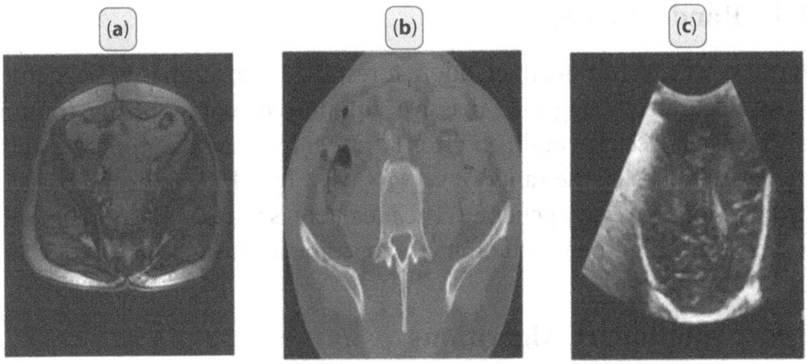

Figure 9.3 (a) An example of MRI. (b) CT and (c) ultrasound images.

disease, CT scan images are fed into machine learning methods. Cancer, osteoporosis, bone thinness, and other anomalies can all be categorized with the help of these pictures. Several distinct classification methods can be found in the field of machine learning.

9.2.1 Decision Tree Algorithm

In order to classify data, the decision tree technique is utilized. The program uses a "divide and conquer" strategy [32] to build trees. A node was used to represent the attribute value, and the leaf of the node indicated the class that was being used to check the condition inside the algorithm. The outcome will always be whether true or false, regardless of the circumstances. Following the structure of a tree from its trunk to its branches and leaves allows one to develop the standards for classification. The total number of nodes traversed can be used to predict the leaf class [33]. Trees can be pruned by removing the extra leaves they produce.

9.2.2 Support Vector Machine

Support vector machines, often known as SVMs, can enhance the accuracy of their classification by employing a statistical learning technique. SVM is a discriminative classifier that uses hyperplane separation to make its predictions. When it comes to SVM, a hyperplane is the best boundary to use. The ideal hyperplane is what the algorithm produces in a labeled training dataset. In 2D, a hyperplane can be thought of as a line, with each side representing a different category. Support vectors are those vectors that are close to the hyperplane and help to hold it up [34–37].

9.2.3 Random Forests

In terms of categorization, the random forest (RF) algorithm is well regarded. RF can accurately categorize massive amounts of data. During training, many decision trees are built, and from those trees, modal outputs are anticipated. The values of the random vectors used by RF serve as the basis for the prediction trees they generate. The idea here is that a collection of "weak learners" can strengthen each other and become a "strong learner" [38, 39].

9.2.4 Evolutionary Algorithms

By using a stochastic and evolutionary approach, genetic algorithms (GAs) can find optimal solutions to even the most intractable problems.

Table 9.1 Numerous machine learning algorithms' advantages and limitations.

Algorithm	Advantage	Limitations
Decision tree	1. The training algorithm is simple and efficient. 2. Training is not affected by the order of instances. 3. The overfitting issue can be solved using pruning procedures.	1. Classes have a mutually exclusive nature. 2. The decision tree's dependence on the attribute selection. 3. An error generates a complex decision tree. 4. Missing attributes make choosing the branch to test the attribute difficult.
Support vector machine	1. It is unlikely that an overfitting problem will arise. 2. The computational complexity was decreased by the quadratic optimization problem. 3. It is simple to control complexity and error frequency.	1. In comparison to decision trees, training is quite slow. 2. It is challenging to choose the best parameters in cases where the training data cannot be linearly separated. 3. The algorithm structure is difficult to understand.
Random forest	1. Quick and accurate instance classification. 2. Resilience to irrelevant qualities. 3. Suitable for regression and classification.	1. Assumes that instances with identical attributes and comparable names will be classified similarly. 2. Assumes that all attributes are equally relevant in nature. 3. High complexity.
Genetic algorithm	1. Easy to implement and simple algorithm. 2. Applicable to feature selection and feature classification. 3. Mostly employed in optimization.	1. The computation or creation of the scoring function is complex. 2. Not the most effective way for finding some optimum conditions; it favors local rather than global optimum conditions. 3. Difficulties associated with training/output data representation.

Generalized adaptive evolution (GA) mimics the process of natural selection by producing a population of encoded candidates (called "chromosomes") over time by means of heritable processes like crossover and mutation. In order to produce children and start a new generation, solutions are chosen based on the fitness function. The initial population is produced at random, and after each generation, the fitness function scores each candidate solution based on how well it meets the aim. In order to evaluate each candidate's performance on the training data, researchers employ the objective function [40, 41].

9.2.5 Swarm Intelligence

One method of computational intelligence applied to hard problems is called swarm intelligence (SI). Scientific aggregation (SI) is the study of how members of a community as a whole behave and interact with one another in a certain geographical area. A lot of ideas, especially for biological systems, can be gleaned from the natural world. Agents follow a few simple principles, and there is no overarching command structure to help researchers anticipate their actions. The agents' "intelligent" behavior is generated through a degree of random iteration between them and is thus opaque to any one agent. SI approaches such as particle swarm optimization (PSO), artificial bee colony (ABC), and ant colony optimization (ACO) are used regularly [42–44]. The advantages and disadvantages of various classification machine learning methods are outlined in Table 9.1.

9.3 Artificial Intelligence Methods for Diagnosing Bone Cancer

Recently, methods derived from machine learning have been utilized in the examination of bone cancer, both in its early and advanced stages. To classify CT scans for bone cancer, researchers [45] used the random forest technique. Random forest was trained and evaluated based on a variety of parameters such as shading, autocorrelation, energy, variance, and cluster prominence. Cluster analysis was introduced as a strategy for classifying bone abnormalities by a group of researchers [46]. In order to determine the precise location of the bone tumor, the techniques known as Fuzzy C-mean (FCM) and K-means clustering were use. They concluded that, when it comes to categorization, FCM is superior to K-means clustering based on the findings of their comparison. Researchers [47] used computer-assisted diagnosis, also known as CAD, in order to differentiate between malignant and benign lesions of the bone in the spine by employing the support vector machine (SVM). They segmented the data using something called the active contour model (ACM). During this research, researchers utilized a method known as gradient vector flow (GVF) to locate border segment relocations. In order to identify and classify cases of bone cancer, researchers [48] employed an AI neural network technique. During the preprocessing stage, they made use of filtering and conversion to grayscale. In order to segment the image, they employed a combination of thresholding and superpixel segmentation. The collected information allowed for the identification of several distinct qualities, such as dissimilarity, mean, central tendency, correlation, skewness, entropy, variance, smoothness, and root mean square error. In order to analyze the data, these features were considered. An artificial neural network (ANN) was utilized, and the data that it contained was trained with the help of the characteristics that were acquired. It was discovered that these procedures had a high level of temporal complexity. Researchers from [49] used a method called mean pixel intensity thresholding in order to detect bone cancer in patients. They utilized a region-expanding algorithm for the purpose of segmentation. Average pixel intensity thresholding has been utilized for identifying regions of interest. The images were classified as either malignant or benign based on a threshold value. Mean pixel intensity was utilized by researchers [50] to detect bone cancer using MRI scans. They employed a threshold value based on the mean intensity to determine the progression of bone cancer. To classify bone cancer, researchers [51] utilized K-means clustering with thresholding strategy. They did some preprocessing by converting the image from RGB to grayscale and then applying a bilateral filter.

9.4 Methodologies for Constructing Deep Learning Model

Deep learning technology automates the feature extraction method, which is performed by human operators in the standard machine learning technique. This is accomplished by obtaining insight into the structure of various network layers on the original data in order to explore deep features and relationship patterns of images. In this way, deep learning technology is distinguished from standard machine learning techniques (or slightly preprocessed data). Thus, the deep learning-based approach helps those who do not have expert knowledge and speeds up the process of image analysis by eliminating the need for manual feature extraction.

9.4.1 Image Pre-Processing

For the purposes of developing a deep learning model, collecting a set of high-quality photographs in a standard format is essential, and this is where image preprocessing comes in. Standardizing photos helps keep data consistent and enables comparisons for the same input format when images were acquired using various instruments and under various acquisition circumstances. To facilitate the segmentation process and any further image mining and analysis, the detection network is employed to highlight the region of interest on the image by employing a bounding box. When there are not enough original pictures, image augmentation strategies such as digitally reconstructed X-rays [52–54] and generative adversarial networks (GANs) [55] can be used to increase the size of the picture dataset and improve the quality of the training results. Other examples of image augmentation strategies include GANs. Surprisingly, picture labeling is the activity that takes the most time since researchers must manually annotate input–output pairs based on their clinical expertise. The fact that these annotations are regarded to be the "gold standard" for training and evaluation, on the other hand, makes this step the one that is the most crucial. When it comes to model training, the images that were made utilizing the techniques described above are far superior to the original shots and have the potential to produce significant increases in model performance.

9.4.2 Model Training

In the field of image-based deep learning, the VGG, ResNet, and DenseNet convolutional neural network architectures are some of the most often utilized designs for CNNs. These networks have been implemented into image-based medical model applications. Convolution layers, pooling layers, activation functions, and fully connected layers are the main building blocks that are used in the construction of a typical CNN model. Dropout is used alongside batch standardization to boost the efficiency of the model. As a rule, the convolution layer in CNN-based deep learning models processes data in three stages. After a large number of convolution computations, the convolution layer generates a series of linear transformation outputs. These outputs are then analyzed by a nonlinear activation function as a probe, and finally, the pooling mechanism is used to fine-tune the convolution layer's output. The convolution layer's output is referred to as the output of the layer. In order to achieve optimal performance from the CNN model, it must be trained using a substantial amount of data.

Overfitting on the training dataset means the model cannot be applied to new data, leading to subpar performance in the actual world.

9.4.3 Model Performance Assessment

It is of utmost importance to check that the distribution of the test dataset is comparable to that of the training dataset. By putting a trained model through its paces on a test dataset, one can arrive at an objective evaluation of the model's overall performance. There are many different assessment metrics, but some of the more commonly used ones are the F1-score, the area under the curve (AUC) of the receiver operating characteristic (ROC) curve, sensitivity, and specificity. While researchers do utilize basic metrics like accuracy for fast comparisons among models, they normally use a wide variety of indications to evaluate a model's effectiveness in its intended setting. Researchers are able to first select an "acceptable" running time, which is typically less than 100 ms, and then improve the classifier's accuracy to the greatest extent possible within the constraints of this time constraint. This is done while taking into consideration the trade-off that exists between the two. The "satisfaction indicator" in this case is the speed of execution, whereas the "optimization indicator" is the level of accuracy.

9.5 Clinical Image Applications of Deep Learning for Bone Tumors

Several models for analyzing radiological and pathological pictures have attained performance levels on par with or better than those of human doctors, and these results have been reported as part of deep learning research (including orthopedic surgeons, radiologists, and pathologists). X-ray, CT, and MRI scans are the most common types of radiological imaging used in deep learning [56]. Deep learning is applied to radiological images to perform tasks such as detecting cancers, classifying them as benign, intermediate, or malignant, segmenting the area containing tumors, and predicting their grade. In addition, imaging modalities such as bone scintigraphy, positron emission tomography (PET), as well as spectral computed tomography (CT) have been found to be effective diagnostic tools for bone metastases [57–59]. After using hematoxylin and eosin (H&E) staining, these characteristics of resected tissues have been proven to be beneficial for tumor categorization, prognosis predicting, and therapy suggestion. There have been several models given to help in the identification and localization of tumor regions in digital H&E-stained tissue pictures. These models are intended to aid in the process [60, 61].

9.5.1 Use of Deep Learning on Radiological Images to Diagnose Primary Bone Tumors

9.5.1.1 The Identification and Categorization of Lesions

When it comes to lesion detection and classification, the most frequent media for using deep learning is pictures obtained from CT, X-ray, and MR scans. X-ray scans known as plain radiographs provide visual parameters such as the location of the tumor, its size, and its margin. The original CNN-based deep learning method for autonomously classifying primary bone tumors was built in 2020, using a multi-institutional dataset consisting of 2,899 plain radiographs from 1,356 people. When comparing the model to two subspecialists and younger radiologists, the model's accuracy for three-way categorization (benign, intermediate, and malignant) was 72.1%. The model's AUC reached up to 0.877 for benign classification and 0.916 for malignant classification. In a similar manner, a team of researchers [62] used 1,576 radiographs to train a Multi-Level Seg-Unet model for the detection and categorization of knee bone malignancies on plain radiographs (1,195 tumor images with 381 normal images). An impressive accuracy of 99.05% was reached by the model.

Radiological data from CT and MRI scans can be more helpful in detecting lesions than those from conventional X-rays. Many deep learning techniques for identifying and categorizing bone cancers in CT and MRI scans have also been described. Excellent results were achieved by a radiomics model [63] that employed deep learning to differentiate between benign and malignant sacral tumors depending on 3D CT and clinical characteristics. This model was one example of how deep learning can be applied (AUC value of 0.83). Data from 459 patients, including 1,316 radiomics characteristics that were manually trimmed, were included into the model. Since it can measure soft tissue invasion, bone marrow engagement, and fluid content of lesions, magnetic resonance imaging (MRI) is an exceedingly sensitive tool for the diagnosis of bone abnormalities [64, 65]. In addition, it has been described how a deep learning model [66] can differentiate between benign and malignant bone lesions based on routine MRI and patient demographics. This model makes use of the EfficientNet-B0 architecture as well as a logistic regression model. Its accuracy, specificity, sensitivity, as well as AUC values, respectively, at the expert level are 0.76, 0.75, 0.79, and 0.82.

9.5.1.2 Volume Calculation and Segmentation

It has been suggested that deep learning and X-ray image analysis may be used to automatically segment tumors and calculate their volumes [67]. Osteosarcoma tumor segmentation on CT scans has proven to be a hard problem in the field of artificial intelligence due to the vast range of spatial and structural variations that may be seen in tumors. In 2017, 71 researchers employed multiple supervised fully convolutional networks (MSFCN) in their efforts to develop an automated method for dividing cancerous patches into distinct sections (MSFCN). The average DSC for the deep end-to-end models was 87.80%, the average HM was 19.81%, the average sensitivity was 86.88%, and the F1-measure was 0.908. This was possible because of the use of a large number of feature channels to collect supplementary context data. The ResNet-based MSRN model [68] utilized in conjunction with FCN has also been proven to yield good results when used to the problem of osteosarcoma segmentation, as shown by testing and training it on a set of 1,900 CT images of 15 osteosarcoma patients. In addition, when a deep learning model [69] was employed to acquire pseudo-3D information from various viewpoints, the average segmentation period for MRI images of pelvic bone tumors was cut by a factor of 100, which resulted in a significant time savings for the researchers. The use of this information in clinical musculoskeletal oncology has significant repercussions as a result.

9.5.1.3 Cancer Staging

For therapeutic options and prognosis, tumor categorization is crucial [70]. When it comes to patients who have soft tissue sarcoma, researchers have suggested employing a deep learning-based tumor grading model using T1-weighted or T2-weighted MRI sequences. This recommendation was made by the researchers in the study [71]. The F1-score that was produced by the deep learning technique for the categorization of data into low-quality and high-quality categories (G1 and G2, respectively) was 0.90, and the AUC was 0.76. As a result, less intrusive biopsies are required, which is a major boon for patients and their doctors. To date, primary bone tumors have not been the target of comparable studies, although this may change soon.

9.5.1.4 Evaluation of the Pace of Tumor Necrosis

Patients with malignant bone tumors should have their tumor necrosis rate assessed following neoadjuvant chemotherapy in order to provide insight into their treatment response and direction for adjuvant chemotherapy administered after surgery [72]. As it is, the technique is evaluated using numerous pathogenic slices, which is both a time-consuming and intricate procedure that severely limits its clinical use. In light of this, it is important to disseminate alternative, non-invasive, and easily accessible ways of detecting neoadjuvant chemotherapy-induced tumor necrosis. Clinically, it may help doctors better classify patients as either responders (those whose tumors shrank by 90%) or nonresponders (those whose necrosis shrank by 90%) following chemotherapy for tumors [73].

Researchers in the year 2020 utilized ML in order to predict the rate of tumor necrosis on multiparametric MRI in patients with osteosarcoma before and after treatment [74]. Since this is the first study to investigate whether contrast-enhanced MRI is associated with pathological changes after surgery, it carries considerable weight. The fluorine-18fluorodeoxyglucose (18F-FDG) absorption heterogeneous characteristics in osteosarcoma may be properly shown in PET/CT scans, as shown by a recent study. This allows for the forecasting of the therapeutic response to neoadjuvant chemotherapy. To aid physicians in deciding whether or not to continue the prior chemotherapy regime to treat people after surgery, a bigger sample size and the application of deep learning to forecast histologic response by adopting different radiological imaging modalities (MRI, PET/CT) could be useful [75].

9.5.1.5 Prognosis Prediction

Orthopedic surgeons are quite concerned about the possibility of recurring bone cancers following treatment [76]. Curettage may be a less intrusive therapeutic option than *en bloc* wide excision in the case of a bone tumor, although this will depend on the size of the tumor. Moreover, both the recurrence and spread rates have increased [77]. Predicting tumor regional recurrence after surgery from preoperative medical pictures is challenging but essential. Using information from 56 patients with histopathology-confirmed GCTB after curettage, researchers produced a CNN model to forecast the local recurrence of GCTB on presurgical MRI.

The image-only CNN model was performed at 75.5% accuracy and 85.7% sensitivity without incorporating any clinical features. By combining information about tumor location, patient age, and CNN prediction into a single model using logistic regression, researchers were able to increase the accuracy and sensitivity of our predictions to 78.6% and 87.5%, respectively, significantly outperforming the performance of radiologists (64.3% and 58.5%, respectively) [78]. The deep learning regression model, when used in conjunction with clinical characteristics, offers tremendous promise for predicting tumor recurrence and informing treatment plans.

9.5.2 Deep Learning in Bone Metastasis

In addition to X-rays, diagnostic imaging procedures including bone scintigraphy, MRI, CT, and positron emission tomography (PET/CT) are used to detect bone metastases from a wide range of original malignancies [79, 80]. Bone metastasis detection, segmentation and volumetric analysis of metastatic lesions, differentiation of primary tumor origin, and scintigraphy noise reduction are only a few of the many applications of deep learning.

Because of its high sensitivity for the identification of bone metastasis and its capacity to identify metastases across the body, 99mTc-MDP scintigraphy is frequently used to detect and localize bone metastases in cancer patients. This is because of its capacity for identifying metastases all throughout the body [81–83]. These algorithms help in lesion detection and ease the workloads of clinical physicians. The application of deep learning models for comprehending bone scintigraphy photos has been the subject of investigation in a number of studies [84]. Recently, two deep learning models that make use of the RGB–CNN architecture have been published in order to identify bone metastases and differentiate between metastatic and degenerative lesion in prostate cancer patients. These models were developed to identify bone metastases and differentiate between metastatic and degenerative lesion. These models have a low need in terms of the amount of time needed to run, and they may be swiftly trained using relatively small datasets. In terms of classification accuracy, the models beat other common CNN approaches, with values reaching as high as 97.38% and 91.42% for two-class (bone metastasis or healthy) and three-class (normal, malignant, as well as degenerative) situations, respectively. A hard positive mining (HPM) method is one that might be utilized in order to quickly and effectively improve data. Researchers [85] presented CNN models employing R-CNN and YOLO v3 to identify hotspots during bone scintigraphy of prostate cancer patients. These models had a sensitivity of 0.87, which allowed them to detect bone metastasis in the pelvis as well as metastasis locations on the ribs or spine in the chest. Researchers created a novel CNN method to enhance the diagnosis of bone metastases in a variety of cancer patients. Their method made use of a spatial attention feature aggregation operator to examine both the front and posterior perspectives of a WBS scan. After being trained on 15,474 exams from 13,811 patients, the model performed remarkably well, with F1 values of 0.933, sensitivity values of 93.17%, accuracy levels of 95.00%, and specificity values of 96.60%, respectively. A multi-input convolutional neural network (CNN) model [86] was formed by making use of a massive database of bone scans for the purpose of detecting bone metastases in patients suffering from breast, prostate, lung, and other forms of cancer. This model was used for the detection of bone metastases in patients (12,222 cases of bone scintigraphy). The machine performed exceptionally well when given a collection of photos to analyze, achieving an AUC value of 0.98 for breast cancer, 0.95 for lung cancer, 0.95 for prostate cancer, and 0.97 for all other types of malignancies combined. Researchers [87] have presented a 2D whole-body-based and "global–local unified emphasis" (GLUE) CNN model for accurately detecting bone metastases on bone scans. This model has accuracies of 0.900 and 0.889, respectively, when compared to the gold standard. The integration of local and global data results is an improvement to the performance of the model. The ability of a model to detect bone metastases in whole-body bone scans was found to be significantly improved by using deep learning to denoise images captured by a scintillation camera, according to research [88] that utilized the Monte Carlo simulation method. This research found that the model's ability to do so was significantly improved.

In CT and MRI images, further deep learning techniques have also been utilized in order to identify bone metastases. In 2018, researchers classified and segmented metastases in the spine using a CNN-based algorithm. The system was used to process whole-spine CT images, and it was utilized on 1,046 lytic lesions and 1,135 sclerotic lesions from 31 patients. After being trained on pictures that were tagged voxel by voxel by two independent radiologists, the system exhibited a sensitivity of 92% when it was evaluated on images with metastatic lesions that were greater than 1.4 mm^3 in size. Using spectral CT (dual-energy) images, a deep learning-based DC-U-Net model [89] created to identify and segregate spinal metastases in lung cancer attained the same level of performance as an expert. For the treatment of spinal bone metastasis in lung cancer patients on MRI images, researchers from 117 different institutions proposed a deep approach that uses the AdaBoost algorithm for image classification and the Chan-Vese (CV) algorithm to segment the lesion; this method achieved a high classification accuracy of 96.55%. The researchers used MRI scans to make their findings. A deep learning network [90] that was trained on 2,880 annotated CT images from 114 patients with prostate cancer was able to effectively detect bone lesions and classify them as benign or malignant. Clinical decision making relies heavily on accurate volume estimates of metastatic lesions. With the help of 100 CT scans, 84 researchers have trained a CNN method to automatically classify metastatic lesions and determine their volume. The outcomes were like those obtained by a knowledgeable radiologist.

Bone metastasis can be detected using a deep learning model, and the primary tumor where metastatic lesions originated from can also be determined. Researchers have developed a deep learning-based DCE-MRI analysis approach [91] for detecting bone metastases in the spine and determining whether the tumor originated in the lung. When it came to predicting the main cancer location when comprehensive PET/CT was not available, the deep learning model had a higher accuracy than both hotspot-based and radiomics-based techniques, achieving a score of 0.81.

9.5.3 Use of Deep Learning on Pathology Images for Diagnosing Bone Cancer

Images obtained using tissues that have been formalin-fixed and paraffin-embedded (FFPE) are the ones that are typically relied on for making a routine diagnosis of bone cancer. When it comes to determining a tumor's clinical prognosis and how it will react to treatment, the histopathology that is revealed by tissue pictures that have been stained with H&E and immunohistochemistry (IHC) for certain biomarkers may give vital information. Digital histologically evaluated (H&E) tissue images have recently surpassed pathology slides for use in tumor diagnosis and localization utilizing deep learning methods.

A CNN model was recommended as a classifier for classifying osteosarcoma WSIs into necrotic tumor, viable tumor, and nontumor in H&E-stained pictures with accuracy of 91.2%. The training data consisted of 263 necrotic tumor tiles, 536 nontumor tiles, and 345 viable tumor tiles. These tiles were annotated by two pathologists [92]. The CNN model's subtype classification and the tumor's spatial extent over the WSIs were visualized using tumor prediction maps. In contrast, the researchers demonstrated a CNN model with similar accuracy (92.4%), precision (97%), and F1-score (95%) results. When implemented to osteosarcoma, a DS-Net classifier that was made up of ASN and CN neurons and trained utilizing paired data and a unique residual block dubbed DRB was able to accurately identify between the viable and necrotic parts of the tumor with an average accuracy of 95.1%. The use of a CNN classifier [93] which is additionally capable of classifying subtypes of soft tissue sarcoma from histological slides resulted in a significant improvement in the accuracy of pathologists, increasing it from 46.3% to 87.1%.

The deep learning model not only helped with tumor detection but also assisted with the use of a statistical method for analyzing survival and predicting the outcome of sarcoma cases [93]. With an AUC value of 0.91 and accuracy of 88.9%, CNN classifiers trained on H&E-stained tissue pictures proved beneficial for the survival analysis of leiomyosarcoma patients. Class activation maps were also employed to visualize the image areas and characteristics that the model detected. They indicated that the predicted regions of "dead" were connected to parameters such as a lack of lymphoid infiltrates, a significant intercellular matrix, the existence of intratumoral bleeding, and an abundance of tumor-associated arteries, all of which are recognized as good prognostic criteria for tumors [93].

9.6 Conclusion

The application of machine learning and deep learning techniques to the evaluation of risk, illness prediction, and the detection of bone cancer has shown promising results. In this chapter, we concluded that a correct diagnosis of bone cancer is difficult and that AI-based machine learning and deep learning techniques play a key role in overcoming obstacles such as noise reduction, accuracy, and stages of bone cancer detection. In a country like India, where the death rate is high and the doctor-to-patient ratio is relatively low, a computer-based method in a healthcare setting for early diagnosis of bone cancer has proven to be quite effective. This situation explains why cancer diagnosis relies so much on medical imaging.

References

1. Ottaviani, G., Jaffe, N., Eftekhari, F., Raymond, A.K., Yasko, A.W., *Pediatric and adolescent osteosarcoma*. Springer Science & Business Media, New York City, 2010.
2. Ritter, J. and Bielack, S.S., Osteosarcoma. *Ann. Oncol.*, 21, vii320–5, 2010 Oct 1.
3. Tu, C., Yang, K., Wan, L., He, J., Qi, L., Wang, W., Lu, Q., Li, Z., The crosstalk between lncRNAs and the Hippo signalling pathway in cancer progression. *Cell Prolif.*, 53, 9, e12887, 2020 Sep.
4. He, J., Ling, L., Liu, Z., Ren, X., Wan, L., Tu, C., Li, Z., Functional interplay between long non-coding RNAs and the Wnt signaling cascade in osteosarcoma. *Cancer Cell Int.*, 21, 1, 1–7, 2021 Dec.
5. Ferguson, J.L. and Turner, S.P., Bone cancer: Diagnosis and treatment principles. *Am. Fam. Physician*, 98, 4, 205–213, 2018 Aug 15.

6. Leite, T.C., Watters, R.J., Weiss, K.R., Intini, G., Avenues of research in dietary interventions to target tumor metabolism in osteosarcoma. *J. Transl. Med.*, 19, 1–3, 2021 Dec.
7. Ogrinc, N., Caux, P.D., Robin, Y.M., Bouchaert, E., Fatou, B., Ziskind, M., Focsa, C., Bertin, D., Tierny, D., Takats, Z., Salzet, M., Direct water-assisted laser desorption/ionization mass spectrometry lipidomic analysis and classification of formalin-fixed paraffin-embedded sarcoma tissues without dewaxing. *Clin. Chem.*, 67, 11, 1513–1523, 2021 Nov.
8. Wu, T.T., Zheng, R.F., Lin, Z.Z., Gong, H.R., Li, H., A machine learning model to predict critical care outcomes in patient with chest pain visiting the emergency department. *BMC Emerg. Med.*, 21, 1, 1–3, 2021 Dec.
9. Binhssan, A., Enchondroma tumor detection. *Int. J. Adv. Res. Comput. Commun. Eng.*, 4, 6, 1–4, 2015 Jun.
10. Savage, R.S. and Yuan, Y., Predicting chemoinsensitivity in breast cancer with' omics/digital pathology data fusion. *R. Soc. Open Sci.*, 3, 2, 140501, 2016 Feb 10.
11. Madabhushi, A. and Lee, G., Image analysis and machine learning in digital pathology: Challenges and opportunities. *Med. Image Anal.*, 33, 170–175, 2016 Oct 1.
12. Xiang, L., Qiao, Y., Nie, D., An, L., Lin, W., Wang, Q., Shen, D., Deep auto-context convolutional neural networks for standard-dose PET image estimation from low-dose PET/MRI. *Neurocomputing*, 267, 406–16, 2017 Dec 6.
13. Bylund, N.E., Andersson, M., Knutsson, H., Interactive 3D filter design for ultrasound artifact reduction, in: *IEEE International Conference on Image Processing 2005*, vol. 3, IEEE, pp. III–728, 2005 Sep 14.
14. Hameed, S.A., Radi, M.A., Gaata, M.T., Medical image classification approach based on texture information. *Iraqi J. Inf. Technol.*, 8, 3, 1–14, 2018.
15. Singh, S., Singh, Y., Vijay, R., An evaluation of features extraction from lung CT images for the classification stage of malignancy. *IOSR J. Comput. Eng. (IOSR-JCE)*, 01, 2278–8727, 2015.
16. Aishwariya, R., Geetha, M.K., Archana, M., Computer-aided fracture detection of x-ray images. *IOSR J. Comput. Eng.*, 8, 2278–2661, 2013.
17. Chu, G., Lo, P., Ramakrishna, B., Kim, H., Morris, D., Goldin, J., Brown, M., Bone tumor segmentation on bone scans using context information and random forests, in: *Medical Image Computing and Computer-Assisted Intervention–MICCAI 2014: 17th International Conference, Boston, MA, USA, September 14-18, 2014, Proceedings, Part I 17*, Springer International Publishing, pp. 601–608, 2014.
18. Deniz, C.M., Xiang, S., Hallyburton, R.S., Welbeck, A., Babb, J.S., Honig, S., Cho, K., Chang, G., Segmentation of the proximal femur from MR images using deep convolutional neural networks. *Sci. Rep.*, 8, 1, 16485, 2018 Nov 7.
19. Kermany, D.S., Goldbaum, M., Cai, W., Valentim, C.C., Liang, H., Baxter, S.L., Identifying medical diagnoses and treatable diseases by image-based deep learning. *Cell*, 172, 5, 1122–1131, e9, 2018.

20. AlDubayan, S.H., Conway, J.R., Camp, S.Y., Witkowski, L., Kofman, E., Reardon, B., Han, S., Moore, N., Elmarakeby, H., Salari, K., Choudhry, H., Detection of pathogenic variants with germline genetic testing using deep learning vs standard methods in patients with prostate cancer and melanoma. *JAMA*, 324, 19, 1957–1969, 2020 Nov 17.
21. Chung, S.W., Han, S.S., Lee, J.W., Oh, K.S., Kim, N.R., Yoon, J.P., Kim, J.Y., Moon, S.H., Kwon, J., Lee, H.J., Noh, Y.M., Automated detection and classification of the proximal humerus fracture by using deep learning algorithm. *Acta Orthop.*, 89, 4, 468–473, 2018 Jul 4.
22. Štajduhar, I., Mamula, M., Miletić, D., Uenal, G., Semi-automated detection of anterior cruciate ligament injury from MRI. *Comput. Methods Programs Biomed.*, 140, 151–64, 2017 Mar 1.
23. Xue, Y., Zhang, R., Deng, Y., Chen, K., Jiang, T., A preliminary examination of the diagnostic value of deep learning in hip osteoarthritis. *PLoS One*, 12, 6, e0178992, 2017 Jun 2.
24. Jamaludin, A., Lootus, M., Kadir, T., Zisserman, A., Urban, J., Battié, M.C., Fairbank, J., McCall, I., Genodisc Consortium, ISSLS PRIZE IN BIOENGINEERING SCIENCE 2017: Automation of reading of radiological features from magnetic resonance images (MRIs) of the lumbar spine without human intervention is comparable with an expert radiologist. *Eur. Spine J.*, 26, 1374–1383, 2017 May.
25. Yune, S., Lee, H., Kim, M., Tajmir, S.H., Gee, M.S., Do, S., Beyond human perception: Sexual dimorphism in hand and wrist radiographs is discernible by a deep learning model. *J. Digit. Imaging*, 32, 665–671, 2019 Aug 15.
26. Koitka, S., Demircioglu, A., Kim, M.S., Friedrich, C.M., Nensa, F., Ossification area localization in pediatric hand radiographs using deep neural networks for object detection. *PLoS One*, 13, 11, e0207496, 2018 Nov 16.
27. Abdel Razek, A.A., Alksas, A., Shehata, M., AbdelKhalek, A., Abdel Baky, K., El-Baz, A., Helmy, E., Clinical applications of artificial intelligence and radiomics in neuro-oncology imaging. *Insights Imaging*, 12, 1–7, 2021 Dec.
28. Heindel, W., Gübitz, R., Vieth, V., Weckesser, M., Schober, O., Schäfers, M., The diagnostic imaging of bone metastases. *Dtsch. Ärztebl. Int.*, 111, 44, 741, 2014 Oct.
29. Reddy, C.K., Anisha, P.R., Raju, G.V., A novel approach for detecting the tumor size and bone cancer stage using region growing algorithm, in: *2015 International Conference on Computational Intelligence and Communication Networks (CICN)*, IEEE, pp. 228–233, 2015 Dec 12.
30. Ananda, R.S. and Thomas, T., Automatic segmentation framework for primary tumors from brain MRIs using morphological filtering techniques, in: *2012 5th International Conference on Biomedical Engineering and Informatics*, IEEE, pp. 238–242, 2012 Oct 16.
31. Chaudhary, A. and Singh, S.S., Lung cancer detection on CT images by using image processing, in: *2012 International Conference on Computing Sciences*, IEEE, pp. 142–146, 2012 Sep 14.

32. Podgorelec, V., Kokol, P., Stiglic, B., Rozman, I., Decision trees: An overview and their use in medicine. *J. Med. Syst.*, 26, 445–463, 2002 Oct.
33. Dalwadi, M.N., Khandhar, D.N., Wandra, K.H., Automatic boundary detection and generation of region of interest for focal liver lesion ultrasound image using texture analysis. *IJARCET*, 2, 2369–2373, 2013 Jul.
34. Lahsasna, A., Ainon, R.N., Zainuddin, R., Bulgiba, A., Design of a fuzzy-based decision support system for coronary heart disease diagnosis. *J. Med. Syst.*, 36, 3293–3306, 2012 Oct.
35. Polat, K. and Güneş, S., Breast cancer diagnosis using least square support vector machine. *Digital Signal Process.*, 17, 4, 694–701, 2007 Jul 1.
36. Liu, H.X., Zhang, R.S., Luan, F., Yao, X.J., Liu, M.C., Hu, Z.D., Fan, B.T., Diagnosing breast cancer based on support vector machines. *J. Chem. Inf. Comput. Sci.*, 43, 3, 900–907, 2003 May 27.
37. Akay, M.F., Support vector machines combined with feature selection for breast cancer diagnosis. *Expert Syst. Appl.*, 36, 2, 3240–3247, 2009 Mar 1.
38. Nguyen, C., Wang, Y., Nguyen, H.N., Random forest classifier combined with feature selection for breast cancer diagnosis and prognostic. *J. Biomed. Sci. Eng.*, 6, 1–10, 2013.
39. Cherry, K.M., Wang, S., Turkbey, E.B., Summers, R.M., Abdominal lymphadenopathy detection using random forest, in: *Medical Imaging 2014: Computer-Aided Diagnosis*, vol. 9035, pp. 381–386, SPIE, San Diego, California, United States, 2014 Mar 18.
40. Das, A. and Bhattacharya, M., A study on prognosis of brain tumors using fuzzy logic and genetic algorithm based techniques, in: *2009 International Joint Conference on Bioinformatics, Systems Biology and Intelligent Computing*, IEEE, pp. 348–351, 2009 Aug 3.
41. Schaefer, G. and Nakashima, T., Data mining of gene expression data by fuzzy and hybrid fuzzy methods. *IEEE Trans. Inf. Technol. Biomed.*, 14, 1, 23–29, 2009 Oct 20.
42. Zhao, W. and Davis, C.E., Swarm intelligence based wavelet coefficient feature selection for mass spectral classification: An application to proteomics data. *Anal. Chim. Acta*, 651, 1, 15–23, 2009 Sep 28.
43. Chang, P.C., Lin, J.J., Liu, C.H., An attribute weight assignment and particle swarm optimization algorithm for medical database classifications. *Comput. Methods Programs Biomed.*, 107, 3, 382–392, 2012 Sep 1.
44. Chen, H.L., Yang, B., Wang, G., Wang, S.J., Liu, J., Liu, D.Y., Support vector machine based diagnostic system for breast cancer using swarm intelligence. *J. Med. Syst.*, 36, 2505–2519, 2012 Aug.
45. Mishra, A. and Suhas, M.V., Classification of benign and malignant bone lesions on CT images using random forest, in: *2016 IEEE International Conference on Recent Trends in Electronics, Information & Communication Technology (RTEICT)*, IEEE, pp. 1807–1810, 2016 May 20.
46. Sinthia, P. and Sujatha, K., A novel approach to detect bone cancer using K-means clustering algorithm and edge detection method. *ARPN J. Eng. Appl. Sci.*, 11, 13, 8002–8007, 2016 Jul.

47. Kumar, R. and Suhas, M.V., Classification of benign and malignant bone lesions on CT imagesusing support vector machine: A comparison of kernel functions, in: *2016 IEEE International Conference on Recent Trends in Electronics, Information & Communication Technology (RTEICT)*, IEEE, pp. 821–824, 2016 May 20.
48. Asuntha, A. and Srinivasan, A., Bone cancer detection using artificial neural network. *Indian J. Sci. Res.*, 17, 2, 56–63, 2018.
49. Kurdi, S.Z., Ali, M.H., Jaber, M.M., Saba, T., Rehman, A., Damaševičius, R., Brain tumor classification using meta-heuristic optimized convolutional neural networks. *J. Pers. Med.*, 13, 2, 181, 2023 Jan 20.
50. Reddy, C.K., Anisha, P.R., Prasad, L.N., A novel approach for detecting the bone cancer and its stage based on mean intensity and tumor size. *Recent Researches Appl. Comput. Sci.*, 20, 1, 162–171, 2016.
51. Ambalkar, S.S. and Thorat, S.S., Bone tumor detection from MRI Image using machine learning. *Int. Res. J. Eng. Technol. (IRJET)*, 5, 5, 6667–6670, 2018.
52. Mutasa, S., Varada, S., Goel, A., Wong, T.T., Rasiej, M.J., Advanced deep learning techniques applied to automated femoral neck fracture detection and classification. *J. Digital Imaging*, 33, 1209–1217, 2020 Oct.
53. Almeida, D.F., Astudillo, P., Vandermeulen, D., Three-dimensional image volumes from two-dimensional digitally reconstructed radiographs: A deep learning approach in lower limb CT scans. *Med. Phys.*, 48, 5, 2448–2457, 2021 May.
54. Barbosa Jr., E.J., Gefter, W.B., Ghesu, F.C., Liu, S., Mailhe, B., Mansoor, A., Grbic, S., Vogt, S., Automated detection and quantification of COVID-19 airspace disease on chest radiographs: A novel approach achieving expert radiologist-level performance using a deep convolutional neural network trained on digital reconstructed radiographs from computed tomography-derived ground truth. *Invest. Radiol.*, 56, 8, 471–479, 2021 Aug 1.
55. Tembine, H., Deep learning meets game theory: Bregman-based algorithms for interactive deep generative adversarial networks. *IEEE Trans. Cybern.*, 50, 3, 1132–1145, 2019 Jan 1.
56. He, Y., Pan, I., Bao, B., Halsey, K., Chang, M., Liu, H., Peng, S., Sebro, R.A., Guan, J., Yi, T., Delworth, A.T., Deep learning-based classification of primary bone tumors on radiographs: A preliminary study. *EBioMedicine*, 62, 1–8, 2020 Dec 1.
57. Papandrianos, N., Papageorgiou, E.I., Anagnostis, A., Development of convolutional neural networks to identify bone metastasis for prostate cancer patients in bone scintigraphy. *Ann. Nucl. Med.*, 34, 824–832, 2020 Nov.
58. Pi, Y., Zhao, Z., Xiang, Y., Li, Y., Cai, H., Yi, Z., Automated diagnosis of bone metastasis based on multi-view bone scans using attention-augmented deep neural networks. *Med. Image Anal.*, 65, 101784, 2020 Oct 1.
59. Shao, X., Zhang, H., Wang, Y., Qian, H., Zhu, Y., Dong, B., Xu, F., Chen, N., Liu, S., Pan, J., Xue, W., Deep convolutional neural networks combine Raman

spectral signature of serum for prostate cancer bone metastases screening. *Nanomed.: Nanotechnol. Biol. Med.*, 29, 102245, 2020 Oct 1.

60. Fu, Y., Xue, P., Ji, H., Cui, W., Dong, E., Deep model with Siamese network for viable and necrotic tumor regions assessment in osteosarcoma. *Med. Phys.*, 47, 10, 4895–4905, 2020 Oct.
61. Nabid, R.A., Rahman, M.L., Hossain, M.F., Classification of osteosarcoma tumor from histological image using sequential RCNN, in: *2020 11th International Conference on Electrical and Computer Engineering (ICECE)*, IEEE, pp. 363–366, 2020 Dec 17.
62. Do, N.T., Jung, S.T., Yang, H.J., Kim, S.H., Multi-level seg-unet model with global and patch-based x-ray images for knee bone tumor detection. *Diagnostics*, 11, 4, 691, 2021 Apr 13.
63. Yin, P., Mao, N., Chen, H., Sun, C., Wang, S., Liu, X., Hong, N., Machine and deep learning based radiomics models for preoperative prediction of benign and malignant sacral tumors. *Front. Oncol.*, 10, 564725, 2020 Oct 16.
64. Vanel, D., Bittoun, J., Tardivon, A., MRI of bone metastases. *Eur. Radiol.*, 8, 1345–1351, 1998 Sep.
65. Lecouvet, F.E., Larbi, A., Pasoglou, V., Omoumi, P., Tombal, B., Michoux, N., Malghem, J., Lhommel, R., Vande Berg, B.C., MRI for response assessment in metastatic bone disease. *Eur. Radiol.*, 22538/2353, 1986–1997, 2013 Jul.
66. Eweje, F.R., Bao, B., Wu, J., Dalal, D., Liao, W.H., He, Y., Luo, Y., Lu, S., Zhang, P., Peng, X., Sebro, R., Deep learning for classification of bone lesions on routine MRI. *EBioMedicine*, 68, 1–9, 2021 Jun 1.
67. Huang, L., Xia, W., Zhang, B., Qiu, B., Gao, X., MSFCN-multiple supervised fully convolutional networks for the osteosarcoma segmentation of CT images. *Comput. Methods Programs Biomed.*, 143, 67–74, 2017 May 1.
68. Zhang, R., Huang, L., Xia, W., Zhang, B., Qiu, B., Gao, X., Multiple supervised residual network for osteosarcoma segmentation in CT images. *Comput. Med. Imaging Graph.*, 63, 1–8, 2018 Jan 1.
69. Qu, Y., Li, X., Yan, Z., Zhao, L., Zhang, L., Liu, C., Xie, S., Li, K., Metaxas, D., Wu, W., Hao, Y., Surgical planning of pelvic tumor using multi-view CNN with relation-context representation learning. *Med. Image Anal.*, 69, 101954, 2021 Apr 1.
70. Chen, B., Zeng, Y., Liu, B., Lu, G., Xiang, Z., Chen, J., Yu, Y., Zuo, Z., Lin, Y., Ma, J., Risk factors, prognostic factors, and nomograms for distant metastasis in patients with newly diagnosed osteosarcoma: A population-based study. *Front. Endocrinol.*, 12, 672024, 2021 Jul 30.
71. Navarro, F., Dapper, H., Asadpour, R., Knebel, C., Spraker, M.B., Schwarze, V., Schaub, S.K., Mayr, N.A., Specht, K., Woodruff, H.C., Lambin, P., Development and external validation of deep-learning-based tumor grading models in soft-tissue sarcoma patients using MR imaging. *Cancers*, 13, 12, 2866, 2021 Jun 8.
72. El-Hennawy, G., Moustafa, H., Omar, W., Elkinaai, N., Kamel, A., Zaki, I., Farid, N., El-Kholy, E., Different 18F-FDG PET parameters for the prediction

of histological response to neoadjuvant chemotherapy in pediatric Ewing sarcoma family of tumors. *Pediatr. Blood Cancer*, 67, 11, e28605, 2020 Nov.
73. Saleh, M.M., Abdelrahman, T.M., Madney, Y., Mohamed, G., Shokry, A.M., Moustafa, A.F., Multiparametric MRI with diffusion-weighted imaging in predicting response to chemotherapy in cases of osteosarcoma and Ewing's sarcoma. *Brit. J. Radiol.*, 93, 1115, 20200257, 2020 Nov 1.
74. Huang, B., Wang, J., Sun, M., Chen, X., Xu, D., Li, Z.P., Ma, J., Feng, S.T., Gao, Z., Feasibility of multi-parametric magnetic resonance imaging combined with machine learning in the assessment of necrosis of osteosarcoma after neoadjuvant chemotherapy: A preliminary study. *BMC Cancer*, 20, 1, 1–9, 2020 Dec.
75. Kim, J., Jeong, S.Y., Kim, B.C., Byun, B.H., Lim, I., Kong, C.B., Song, W.S., Lim, S.M., Woo, S.K., Prediction of neoadjuvant chemotherapy response in osteosarcoma using convolutional neural network of tumor center 18F-FDG PET images. *Diagnostics*, 11, 11, 1976, 2021 Nov.
76. Smrke, A., Tam, Y.B., Anderson, P.M., Jones, R.L., Huang, P.H., The perplexing role of immuno-oncology drugs in osteosarcoma. *J. Bone Oncol.*, 31, 100400, 2021 Dec 1.
77. Raskin, K.A., Schwab, J.H., Mankin, H.J., Springfield, D.S., Hornicek, F.J., Giant cell tumor of bone. *JAAOS-J. Am. Acad. Orthop. Surg.*, 21, 2, 118–26, 2013 Feb 1.
78. He, Y., Guo, J., Ding, X., van Ooijen, P.M., Zhang, Y., Chen, A., Oudkerk, M., Xie, X., Convolutional neural network to predict the local recurrence of giant cell tumor of bone after curettage based on pre-surgery magnetic resonance images. *Eur. Radiol.*, 29, 5441–5451, 2019 Oct 1.
79. Liu, Y., Yang, P., Pi, Y., Jiang, L., Zhong, X., Cheng, J., Xiang, Y., Wei, J., Li, L., Yi, Z., Cai, H., Automatic identification of suspicious bone metastatic lesions in bone scintigraphy using convolutional neural network. *BMC Med. Imaging*, 21, 1, 1–9, 2021 Dec.
80. Mercolini, F., Zucchetta, P., Jehanno, N., Corradini, N., Van Rijn, R.R., Rogers, T., Cameron, A., Scarzello, G., Coppadoro, B., Minard-Colin, V., Gallego, S., Role of 18F-FDG-PET/CT in the staging of metastatic rhabdomyosarcoma: A report from the European paediatric Soft tissue sarcoma Study Group. *Eur. J. Cancer*, 155, 155–162, 2021 Sep 1.
81. Davila, D., Antoniou, A., Chaudhry, M.A., Evaluation of osseous metastasis in bone scintigraphy. *Semin. Nucl. Med.*, 45, 1, 3–15, 2015 Jan 1. WB Saunders.
82. Elfarra, F.G., Calin, M.A., Parasca, S.V., Computer-aided detection of bone metastasis in bone scintigraphy images using parallelepiped classification method. *Ann. Nucl. Med.*, 33, 866–874, 2019 Nov.
83. Kadomoto, S., Yaegashi, H., Nakashima, K., Iijima, M., Kawaguchi, S., Nohara, T., Shigehara, K., Izumi, K., Kadono, Y., Nakajima, K., Mizokami, A., Quantification of bone metastasis of castration-resistant prostate cancer

after enzalutamide and abiraterone acetate using bone scan index on bone scintigraphy. *Anticancer Res.*, 39, 5, 2553–2559, 2019 May 1.

84. Cheng, D.C., Liu, C.C., Hsieh, T.C., Yen, K.Y., Kao, C.H., Bone metastasis detection in the chest and pelvis from a whole-body bone scan using deep learning and a small dataset. *Electronics*, 10, 10, 1201, 2021 May 18.
85. Cheng, D.C., Hsieh, T.C., Yen, K.Y., Kao, C.H., Lesion-based bone metastasis detection in chest bone scintigraphy images of prostate cancer patients using pre-train, negative mining, and deep learning. *Diagnostics*, 11, 3, 518, 2021 Mar 15.
86. Zhao, Z., Pi, Y., Jiang, L., Xiang, Y., Wei, J., Yang, P., Zhang, W., Zhong, X., Zhou, K., Li, Y., Li, L., Deep neural network based artificial intelligence assisted diagnosis of bone scintigraphy for cancer bone metastasis. *Sci. Rep.*, 10, 1, 17046, 2020 Oct 12.
87. Han, S., Oh, J.S., Lee, J.J., Diagnostic performance of deep learning models for detecting bone metastasis on whole-body bone scan in prostate cancer. *Eur. J. Nucl. Med. Mol. Imaging*, 1, 1–1, 2021 Aug 7.
88. Minarik, D., Enqvist, O., Trägårdh, E., Denoising of scintillation camera images using a deep convolutional neural network: A Monte Carlo simulation approach. *J. Nucl. Med.*, 61, 2, 298–303, 2020 Feb 1.
89. Fan, X., Zhang, X., Zhang, Z., Jiang, Y., Deep learning-based identification of spinal metastasis in lung cancer using spectral CT images. *Sci. Program.*, 2021, 1–7, 2021 Jun 28.
90. Masoudi, S., Mehralivand, S., Harmon, S.A., Lay, N., Lindenberg, L., Mena, E., Pinto, P.A., Citrin, D.E., Gulley, J.L., Wood, B.J., Dahut, W.L., Deep learning based staging of bone lesions from computed tomography scans. *IEEE Access*, 9, 87531–87542, 2021 Apr 20.
91. Lang, N., Zhang, Y., Zhang, E., Zhang, J., Chow, D., Chang, P., Hon, J.Y., Yuan, H., Su, M.Y., Differentiation of spinal metastases originated from lung and other cancers using radiomics and deep learning based on DCE-MRI. *Magn. Reson. Imaging*, 64, 4–12, 2019 Dec 1.
92. Arunachalam, H.B., Mishra, R., Daescu, O., Cederberg, K., Rakheja, D., Sengupta, A., Leonard, D., Hallac, R., Leavey, P., Viable and necrotic tumor assessment from whole slide images of osteosarcoma using machine-learning and deep-learning models. *PLoS One*, 14, 4, e0210706, 2019 Apr 17.
93. Foersch, S., Eckstein, M., Wagner, D.C., Gach, F., Woerl, A.C., Geiger, J., Glasner, C., Schelbert, S., Schulz, S., Porubsky, S., Kreft, A., Deep learning for diagnosis and survival prediction in soft tissue sarcoma. *Ann. Oncol.*, 32, 9, 1178–1187, 2021 Sep 1.

Index

Printed in the USA/Agawam, MA
September 16, 2026

910661.067